Manual of
Skin Diseases of the Dog and Cat

Manual of Skin Diseases of the Dog and Cat

Second Edition

Sue Paterson MA VetMB DVD DipECVD MRCVS
RCVS and European Specialist in Veterinary Dermatology
Head of Dermatology and Director Rutland House Referral Hospital
St Helens, Merseyside

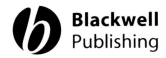

Blackwell Publishing

This edition first published 2008
© 1998, 2000, 2008 Blackwell Publishing

Blackwell Publishing was acquired by John Wiley & Sons in February 2007. Blackwell's publishing programme has been merged with Wiley's global Scientific, Technical, and Medical business to form Wiley-Blackwell.

Registered office
John Wiley & Sons Ltd, The Atrium, Southern Gate, Chichester, West Sussex, PO19 8SQ, United Kingdom

Editorial office
9600 Garsington Road, Oxford, OX4 2DQ, United Kingdom

For details of our global editorial offices, for customer services and for information about how to apply for permission to reuse the copyright material in this book please see our website at www.wiley.com/wiley-blackwell.

The right of the author to be identified as the author of this work has been asserted in accordance with the Copyright, Designs and Patents Act 1988.

All rights reserved. No part of this publication may be reproduced, stored in a retrieval system, or transmitted, in any form or by any means, electronic, mechanical, photocopying, recording or otherwise, except as permitted by the UK Copyright, Designs and Patents Act 1988, without the prior permission of the publisher.

Wiley also publishes its books in a variety of electronic formats. Some content that appears in print may not be available in electronic books.

Designations used by companies to distinguish their products are often claimed as trademarks. All brand names and product names used in this book are trade names, service marks, trademarks or registered trademarks of their respective owners. The publisher is not associated with any product or vendor mentioned in this book. This publication is designed to provide accurate and authoritative information in regard to the subject matter covered. It is sold on the understanding that the publisher is not engaged in rendering professional services. If professional advice or other expert assistance is required, the services of a competent professional should be sought.

First published 1998 and 2000 as *Skin Diseases of the Dog* and *Skin Diseases of the Cat* by Blackwell Science Ltd
Second edition published by Blackwell Publishing 2008

Library of Congress Cataloging-in-Publication Data

Paterson, Sue.
 Manual of skin diseases of the dog and cat / Sue Paterson. – 2nd ed.
     p. ; cm.
 Originally published as two separate works: Skin diseases of the dog / Sue Paterson. 1998, and Skin diseases of the cat / Sue Paterson. 2000.
 Includes bibliographical references and index.
 ISBN-13: 978-1-4051-6753-6 (pbk. : alk. paper)
 ISBN-10: 1-4051-6753-X (pbk. : alk. paper) 1. Dogs–Diseases–Handbooks, manuals, etc. 2. Cats–Diseases–Handbooks, manuals, etc. 3. Veterinary dermatology–Handbooks, manuals, etc. I. Paterson, Sue. Skin Diseases of the Dog. II. Paterson, Sue. Skin Diseases of the Cat. III. Title.
 [DNLM: 1. Dog Diseases–Handbooks. 2. Cat Diseases–Handbooks. 3. Skin Diseases–veterinary–Handbooks. SF 992.S55 P297m 2008]

SF992.S55P37 2008
636.7′08965–dc22
                              2007039707

A catalogue record for this book is available from the British Library.

Set in 10/12pt Sabon by Aptara Inc., New Delhi, India
Printed in Singapore by C.O.S. Printers Pte Ltd

1 2008

Contents

Dedication vi
Acknowledgements vi
Abbreviations vii

1. Introduction – structure and function 1
2. Approach to the case 9
3. Diagnostic tests 13
4. Bacterial skin disease 26
5. Fungal skin disease 57
6. Viral, rickettsial and protozoal diseases 82
7. Parasitic skin disease 100
8. Endocrine and metabolic skin disease 136
9. Otitis externa 162
10. Allergic skin disease 173
11. Immune mediated skin disease 188
12. Alopecia 214
13. Nutritional skin disease 231
14. Congenital and hereditary skin diseases 238
15. Pigment abnormalities 259
16. Psychogenic skin disease 268
17. Keratinisation defects 277
18. Miscellaneous skin diseases in the dog 292
19. Miscellaneous skin diseases in the cat 304
20. Environmental skin diseases 317
21. Neoplastic and non-neoplastic tumours 326

Index 350

Dedication

To Richard, Sam and Matt

Acknowledgements

To all the staff especially the dermatology crew (Steve, Laura, Bernie, Emma and Lydia) at Rutland House as well as "the boys" for putting up with my madness, my friend and co-conspirator Janie and of course to all our loyal referring veterinarians without whom I would not have a day job.

Thanks,
Sue

Abbreviations

Dose schedule and measurement units:

sid	once daily
bid	twice daily
tid	three times daily
qid	four times daily
eod	every other day
po	by mouth
sq	by subcutaneous injection
sc	subcutaneously
iv	by intravenous injection
im	by intramuscular injection
mm	millimetres
cm	centimetres
kg	kilograms
mg	milligrams
ml	millilitres

General:

BMZ	basement membrane zone
IRS	inner root sheath
ORS	outer root sheath
DTM	dermatophyte test medium
SDA	Sabouraud's dextrose agar
MRSA	methicillin resistant *Staphylococcus aureus*
EMG	electromyogram
MRI	magnetic resonance imaging
HA	hospital acquired
CA	community acquired
BCG	bacille Calmette–Guerin
DTM	dermatophyte test medium
ELISA	enzyme-linked immunosorbent assay
CDV	canine distemper
FeLV	feline leukaemia virus
FIV	feline immunodeficiency virus
FIP	feline infectious peritonitis
FRV	feline rhinotracheitis virus
FCV	feline calici virus
FSV	feline sarcoma virus
ADV	Aujeszky's disease virus
FHV1	feline herpes virus 1
TSH	thyroid-stimulating hormone
ALT	alanine transaminase/ alanine aminotransferase/ alanine transferase
SAP	serum alkaline phosphatase
ALP	alkaline phosphatase
SAT	serum aspartate transaminase
AST	aspartate transaminase
TT4	total thyroxine
FT4	free thyroxine
TT3	total triiodothyronine
FT3	free triiodothyronine

SAP	serum alkaline phosphatase	TEN	toxic epidermal necrolysis
LDH	lactate dehydrogenase	EM	erythema multiforme
ACTH	adrenocorticotrophic hormone	CM	Chiari-like malformation
CRF	corticotropin-releasing factor	SM	syringomyelia
IGF-1	insulin-like growth factor – 1	EB	epidermolysis bullosa
NME	necrolytic migratory erythema	WKS	Waardenburg–Klein syndrome
SLE	systemic lupus erythematosus	VKH	Vogt–Koyanagi–Harada-like syndrome
ANA	antinuclear antibody test	FOPS	feline orofacial pain syndrome
LE	lupus erythematosus	TVT	transmissible venereal tumour
CAD	cold agglutinin disease	SCC	squamous cell carcinoma

Please note that some of the drugs mentioned in this book are not licensed specifically for use in animals. It is the veterinary surgeons responsibility to ensure that where possible a licensed drug should be used and the veterinary cascade should be followed.

Introduction – structure and function

Dermatological diseases remain some of the most common and frustrating problems presented to veterinary surgeons in practice. All veterinary practitioners can expect up to 20% of their caseload to include skin cases, and as such they should have a thorough grounding in dermatology. The pet owning client now has the opportunity to seek specialist advice through a referral from their veterinary surgeon. Therefore, the generalist should not only exhibit competence in the management of common diseases, but should also have the ability to identify those requiring specialised care, whether they are unusual manifestations of everyday problems or rare dermatoses.

The skin is one of the most important organs in the canine and feline body. It is crucial for the provision of a wide range of functions. These include the following:

- Effective barrier to prevent loss of water, electrolytes and macromolecules
- Mechanical protection from chemical, physical and microbial damage
- Elasticity to allow movement
- Production of adnexa, e.g. hair and claws
- Nerve sensors to allow the perception of heat, cold, pressure, pain and itch
- Temperature regulation
- Storage of vitamins, electrolytes, water, fat, carbohydrates and protein
- Immune regulation to prevent development of infection and neoplasia
- Antibacterial and antifungal activity
- Vitamin D production
- Pigment production to protect against solar damage
- Communication as to the health of the individual and sexual identity
- Secretion via epitrichial, atrichial and sebaceous glands
- Excretion

Structure of the skin

Epidermis

This is the most superficial layer of the skin and is composed of multiple layers of cells. There are four distinct cell types:

- Keratinocytes ~ 85%
- Langerhans cells ~ 3–8%
- Melanocytes ~ 5%
- Merkel cells ~ 2%

Keratinocytes

These cells form the bulk of the epidermis. They are constantly reproducing and pushing upwards from the stratum basale to replace those cells above them. As they move into the outermost layers of the epidermis they are shed as dead horny cells. They have a variety of functions in both providing structural support for the skin and playing a role in epidermal immunity as

- they produce structural keratins,
- are phagocytic and capable of processing antigens,
- produce cytokines (IL-1, IL-3, prostaglandins, leukotrienes, interferon) to stimulate or inhibit the immune response.

Langerhans cells

These are mononuclear dendritic cells that form an important part of the immune surveillance of the skin. They can be found basally or suprabasilar. Their principal functions are

- antigen processing and presentation to helper T lymphocytes,
- induction of cytotoxic T lymphocytes directed to modified alloantigens,
- production of cytokines including IL-1, and
- phagocytic activity.

Melanocytes

These are dendritic cells found within the basal layer of the epidermis, outer root sheath, hair matrix of the hair follicle and ducts of sebaceous and sweat glands. In the epidermis, each melanocyte communicates via its dendritic projections with 10–20 keratinocytes to form the 'epidermal melanin unit'. Each melanocyte produces eumelanin or pheomelanin within melanosomes through series of steps from tyrosine. Melanosomes containing pigment migrate to the end of dendrites and transfer melanin to adjacent epidermal cells. They have a variety of important functions:

- production of protective colouration and for sexual attraction,
- barrier against ionising radiation,
- scavengers for cytotoxic radicals,
- contribution to inflammatory response via production of cytokines.

Merkel cells

These are dendritic epidermal cells confined to the basal cell layer of the epidermis or just below.

They are predominantly found in tylotrich pads and hair follicle epithelium. Their principal functions are

- specialised slow-adapting mechanoreceptors,
- influencing cutaneous blood flow and sweat production,
- coordinating keratinocytes proliferation,
- controlling of hair cycle by maintaining and stimulating hair follicle stem cell population.

Epidermal structure

The epidermis in the dog and cat is a very thin structure; it is only 2–3 nucleated cells thick not including the horny cell layer. In haired skin it is 0.1–0.5 mm thick and in the footpads and planum nasale up to 1.5 mm. It can be divided into different layers working from the inner to the outer layers; these are as follows:

- Stratum basale – basal cell layer
- Stratum spinosum – spinous/prickle cell layer
- Stratum granulosum – granular cell layer
- Stratum lucidum – clear cell layer
- Stratum corneum – horny cell layer

Stratum basale

This is made up of a single layer of columnar cells, tightly adherent to the basement membrane. It is mostly made up of keratinocytes. Hemidesmosomes are located along the inner aspect of the basal keratinocytes. These structures act to anchor the epidermis to the basement membrane zone. The basal cell layer is the initial site of keratin production.

Stratum spinosum

This layer is generally 1–2 cells thick except in footpads, nasal planum and at mucocutaneous junctions where there may be up to 20 cell layers. Cells within it are polyhedral to flattened cuboidal in shape. The 'prickles' or desmosomes are intercellular bridges that mediate adhesion between keratinocytes. Keratinocytes within this layer synthesise lamellar granules, which are important in the barrier function of the skin. Keratin production also accelerates in the stratum spinosum and is formed into bundles.

Stratum granulosum

The granular cell layer is not always present in haired skin, where it occurs it is made up of a layer of 1–2 flattened cells. In non-haired skin it may be up to 4–8 cells thick. The cells contain keratohyaline granules, which are rich in profilaggrin. Within this layer profilaggrin is converted to filaggrin, which acts to bind keratin filaments as the cornified envelope starts to form. Lamellar granules migrate to the periphery of the cells and discharge their contents, rich in phospholipids and ceramides, into intercellular space to form lipid-rich lamellae between cells. Degeneration of cell organelles and the nucleus starts in this level.

Stratum lucidum

This is a compact layer of dead keratinocytes only found in footpads and nasal planum.

Stratum corneum

This is the outermost layer of the epidermis and consists of multiple layers of flattened cornified cells. These are constantly shed to balance the proliferation of basal cells. On the canine trunk it is about 47 cells thick. The transit time from the stratum basale to stratum corneum is approximately 22 days. The cells have an internal scaffold of keratin/filaggrin and an external lipid-rich cornified cell envelope.

Basement membrane zone (BMZ)

This is the area that separates the epidermis from the dermis. The functions of this area are as follows:

- Acting to anchor the epidermis to the dermis.
- Maintaining a functional and proliferative epidermis.
- Maintaining tissue architecture and acting as a physical barrier.
- Aiding wound healing.
- Regulating nutrition between the epithelium and the underlying connective tissue.

The BMZ can be divided into four components; moving from the epidermis to the dermis it can be divided into

- basal cell plasma membrane – contains the anchoring hemidesmosomes of basal cells,
- lamina lucida,
- lamina densa,
- sublamina dense – contains anchoring fibrils and dermal microfibril bundles.

Dermis

The dermis is part of the body's connective tissue system; it accounts for most of the tensile strength and elasticity of the skin. It is made from a combination of insoluble fibres (collagen and elastin) and soluble polymers (proteoglycans and hyaluronan).

Fibrous components resist tensile forces. The soluble polymers help dissipate compressive forces. The dermis is composed of four main components:

- fibres
- ground substance
- cells
- epidermal appendages, arrector pili muscles, blood and lymph vessels

Fibres

The dermal fibres are produced by fibroblasts and are collagenous, reticular or elastic.

Collagenous fibres (collagen)

These account for about 90% of all dermal fibres and 80% of the extracellular matrix. They form thick bands of multiple protein fibrils. They provide tensile strength and some elasticity.

Collagen types are as follows:

- Predominant collagen types in the dermis are fibrillar and collagen I (87%), III (10%), V (3%).
- Collagen VI present as microfibrils.
- Collagen IV (lamina densa) and collagen V (lamina lucida) found in BMZ.
- Collagen VII found in anchoring fibrils of BMZ.

Reticular fibres (reticulin)
These fibres form a network of fine branching structures.

Elastin fibres
These fibres account for about 4% of the extracellular matrix. They are single fine branching structures bordering collagen bundles. They give the skin much of its elasticity.

Ground substance
The ground substance is produced by fibroblasts. It is composed of glycosaminoglycans linked to proteoglycans. It fills the space around all the other structures to provide dermal support. It contributes to water storage, lubrication, growth and development.

Cells
The normal dermis is sparsely populated with cells. Fibroblasts and dermal dendrocytes are found throughout the dermis. Melanocytes are found around superficial blood vessels and around hair bulbs. Mast cells can also be found around superficial dermal blood vessels and appendages. Other cells that can be seen in very small numbers in normal skin are neutrophils, eosinophils, lymphocytes, histiocytes and plasma cells.

Epidermal appendages

Arrector pili muscles
These are smooth muscles that originate in superficial dermis and insert at the bulge region of primary hair follicle. They are present in all haired skin especially prominent in neck and rump. Contraction of muscle raises the hair (piloerection).

They are under cholinergic nerve control. Piloerection is associated with 'flight or fight'. It is also important as a mechanism for thermoregulation and emptying sebaceous glands.

Blood vessels
Three intercommunicating plexuses of arteries and veins are found within the dermis:

- deep plexus, which supplies the subcutis, lower portions of hair follicle and epitrichial sweat gland;
- middle plexus, which supplies the arrector pili muscle, middle portion of hair follicle and sebaceous gland;
- superficial plexus, which supplies upper portion of hair follicles and sends capillary loops up to the epidermis.

Arteriovenous anastomoses are the connections between arteries and veins found especially in the deep dermis that allows blood to bypass the capillary bed; they are most commonly seen in the extremities.

Lymph vessels
These arise from capillary networks in superficial dermis and surround adnexal structures. The vessels that arise from these networks drain into a subcutaneous lymphatic plexus. Lymphatics control the microcirculation of the skin. Their main functions are as follows:

- draining away debris and excess matter that results from daily wear and tear in the skin;
- serving as channels for the return of proteins and cells from tissues to blood stream;
- linking the skin and regional lymph nodes;
- carrying material that has penetrated the skin, e.g. solvents, topical drugs, vaccines inflammatory products.

Nerves
The nerve supply to the skin can be divided into a dermal network, hair follicle network and specialised end organs within the dermis. Sensory nerves can be either thermoreceptors (cold

or warm units) thought to be in the epidermis or mechanoreceptors (Pacinian corpuscle, Ruffini corpuscles), which are spread throughout the skin. Mechanoreceptors are also associated with hairs; either large guard hairs or tylotrich hairs (G and T hair units) or all hair, especially down hairs (D hair units). Motor nerves supply the arrector pili muscle and the epitrichial sweat gland.

Hair follicle

The hair follicle can be divided into three sections:

- Infundibulum, which extends from the entrance of sebaceous gland to epithelial surface.
- Isthmus, extending from the entrance of sebaceous gland to the attachment of arrector pili muscle.
- Inferior segment, extending from the attachment of arrector pili muscle to the dermal papilla.

The dog and cat both have compound hair follicle. A cluster consists of 2–5 large primary hairs surrounded by groups of smaller secondary (down) hairs. One of the primary hairs is the largest (central primary hair) and the others are smaller (lateral primary hairs). Each primary hair can have 5–20 secondary hairs accompanying it.

Each primary hair has an arrector pili muscle, sebaceous gland and sweat (epitrichial) gland. Each secondary hair usually has only a sebaceous gland. Primary hairs emerge independently through individual holes; the secondary hairs emerge through a common hole. Two specialised forms of tactile hairs are found in mammalian skin; these are the sinus hairs and tylotrich hairs:

- Sinus hairs (vibrissae, whiskers) are found on the muzzle, lips, eyelid, face and throat, also on the palmar aspect of the carpus of cats. Hairs are thick, stiff and tapered distally. They are thought to act as slow-adapting mechanoreceptors.
- Tylotrich hairs are scattered amongst normal body hairs. Follicles are larger than the surrounding ones and contain a single stout hair and an annular complex of neurovascular tissue at the level of the sebaceous gland. These hairs are thought to act as rapid acting mechanoreceptors.

Structure of the hair follicle

The hair follicle has five major components:

- dermal hair papilla
- hair matrix
- hair
- inner root sheath
- outer root sheath

Dermal hair papilla
Extension of dermal connective tissue covered by basement membrane.

Hair matrix
The hair matrix is made up of nucleated epithelial cells covering the dermal papilla that give rise to the hair and inner root sheath.

Hair
The hair is made up of three parts – medulla, cortex and cuticle:

- Medulla, which is the innermost region composed of longitudinal rows of cuboidal cells.
- Cortex, composed of cornified spindle-shaped cells, containing pigment to colour the hair.
- Cuticle, the outermost layer of flattened cornified anuclear cells, these form 'tiles' that interlock with the cuticle of the inner root sheath.

Secondary (down) hairs have a narrower medulla and more prominent cuticle than primary hairs. Lanugo hairs have no medulla.

Inner root sheath (IRS)
The function of the IRS is to mould the hair within it, which is accomplished by hardening in advance

of the hair. It is composed of three concentric layers all of which contain eosinophilic granules (trichohyalin granules). Working from the innermost layer outwards, these layers are as follows:

- IRS cuticle single layer of overlapping cells that point towards the hair bulb and interlock with cells of hair cuticle.
- Huxley's layer consisting of 1–3 nucleated cell layers.
- Henle's layer – a single layer of anuclear cells.

Outer root sheath (ORS)

The ORS is a downward extension of the epidermis. It is thickest towards the epidermis and thinnest towards the hair bulb. In the infundibulum normal keratinisation occurs in the same way as the epidermis with the formation of keratohyaline granules. In the isthmus trichilemmal keratinisation occurs. Below the level of the isthmus no keratinisation occurs as ORS is covered by IRS. The ORS is surrounded by two other structures, which are the basement membrane (glassy membrane), a downward extension of the epidermal basement membrane, and the fibrous root sheath, which is a layer of thick connective tissue.

Arrector pili muscle

See Section 'Epidermal appendages'.

Sebaceous gland

The sebaceous glands are distributed throughout haired skin. They are not found in the footpads or nasal planum. They open through a duct into hair follicle canal in the infundibular region. They tend to be large and numerous in sparsely haired areas especially mucocutaneous junctions and interdigital spaces, dorsal neck, rump and chin (submental organ) and dorsal tail (tail gland, supracaudal organ, preen gland). Sebaceous glands have an abundant blood supply and are innervated: their oily sebum secretion thought to be under hormonal control; androgens causing hypertrophy and hyperplasia; oestrogens and glucocorticoids causing involution. Sebaceous gland secretion is thought to be predominantly triglycerides and wax esters this mixes with fatty acids derived from follicular bacteria to make the sebum excreted onto the skin surface. Functions of sebum include

- physical barrier by lubrication and hydration of skin and hairs,
- chemical barrier (sebum/sweat emulsion has antimicrobial activities),
- pheromonal properties.

Sweat gland

Two types are recognised: the epitrichial (apocrine) or atrichial (eccrine) sweat glands.

Epitrichial (apocrine)

These are distributed throughout haired skin but not found in footpad or nasal planum. These structures are located below sebaceous glands and open through duct into hair follicle canal in the infundibular region above sebaceous gland opening. They are large and numerous in sparsely haired areas as sebaceous glands. They have a rich blood supply but are not innervated. Their control is thought to be by diffusion of neurotransmitters from the circulation. The secretions from these glands are thought to help act as a chemical barrier as the secretion is especially rich in IgA. Epitrichial sweat is also thought to have pheromonal properties.

Atrichial (eccrine)

Atrichial sweat glands are only found in footpads and are not associated with hairs. They have a rich nerve supply; direct nerve control thought to occur.

The hair cycle

The hair cycle is made up of three main parts: anagen, catagen and telogen.

Anagen (growing phase)

A new hair bulb forms and germ cells at the base of follicle extend down to surround the dermal papilla deep in the dermis. A well-developed spindle-shaped dermal papilla covered by hair matrix ('ball and claw' appearance) can be identified to form the hair bulb. Hair matrix cells are often heavily melanised and show mitotic activity. A hair plucked in anagen shows a large expanded root that is moist and glistening, often pigmented and square at the end.

Catagen (intermediate phase)

During this phase hair growth stops and the dermal papilla moves away from matrix cells as hair moves up in dermis.

Telogen (resting phase)

During this phase the dermal papilla separates from the bulb of matrix cells ('club' hair appearance). The pigment is lost from bulb and there is no visible mitotic activity. Hairs plucked in telogen show a tapered club root with little or no pigment.

Subcutis (hypodermis)

This is the deepest and thickest layer of the skin; it is 90% triglyceride by weight. There is no subcutis in the lips, cheek, eyelid, external ear and anus. Fibrous bands that are continuous with the fibrous structures of the dermis penetrate and lobulate the subcutaneous fat into lobules of lipocytes. These form attachments of the skin to underlying fibrous skeletal components. Superficial portions of the subcutis project into the deeper layers of dermis to provide additional protection to some of the deeper structures. Functions of the subcutis include

- an energy reserve,
- important in thermogenesis and insulation,
- protective padding and support,
- maintaining surface contours,
- steroid reservoir, site of steroid metabolism and oestrogen production.

Table 1.1 Resident and transient bacteria of the canine skin.

Resident organisms – dog skin	Transient organisms – dog skin
Skin • *Micrococcus* spp. • Coagulase negative staphylococcus esp. *S. epidermidis, S. xylosus* • Alpha haemolytic streptococci • *Clostridium* spp. • *Propionibacterium acnes* • *Acinetobacter* spp. • Gram negative aerobes **Hairs** • *Micrococcus* spp. • Gram negative aerobes • *Bacillus* spp. • *Staphylococcus intermedius* (seeded from mucosa) **Hair follicles** • *Micrococcus* spp. • *Propionibacterium acne* • *Streptococci* • *Bacillus* spp. • *Staphylococcus intermedius* (seeded from mucosa) **Mucosal sites** • *Staphylococcus intermedius* (nares, oropharynx and anal ring)	**Skin** • *Escherichia coli* • *Proteus mirabilis* • *Corynebacterium* spp. • *Bacillus* spp. • *Pseudomonas* spp.

Cutaneous ecology

Both canine and feline skins have a normal microflora. Bacteria are located in the superficial epidermis and infundibulum of the hair follicles. The normal flora is a mixture of micro-organisms that live in symbiosis. These so-called 'normal inhabitants' can be classified as resident or transient (see Tables 1.1 and 1.2):

- Resident organisms can successfully multiply on normal skin.

Table 1.2 Resident and transient bacteria of the feline skin.

Resident organisms – cat skin	Transient organisms – cat skin
Micrococcus spp.	Beta haemolytic streptococci
Coagulase negative staphylococcus esp. *S. simulans*	*E. Coli* *P. mirabilis*
Alpha haemolytic streptococci *Acinetobacter* spp.	*Pseudomonas* spp. *Alcaligenes* spp.
Coagulase positive staphylococcus esp. *S. intermedius, S. aureus*	Bacillus spp. *Staphylococcus* spp. (coagulase positive)
	Staphylococcus spp. (coagulase negative except *S. simulans*)

- Transient organisms do not multiply on the normal skin of most animals. They can be cultured from normal skin but are of no significance unless they become involved in the pathological process as secondary invaders.

In some situations, bacteria from other body sites can be important as pathogens. In bite wounds in cats the pathogenic organisms are usually those derived from the mouth flora (Table 1.3).

Faecal contamination of skin and soft tissue, especially where wounds are licked, can lead to faecal anaerobes becoming pathogens (Table 1.4).

Table 1.3 Normal flora of the feline mouth.

Normal mouth flora of the cat
Pasteurella multocida Beta haemolytic streptococci *Corynebacterium* spp. *Actinomyces* spp. *Bacteroides* spp. *Fusobacterium* spp.

Table 1.4 Faecal contaminants of the canine and feline skin.

Faecal contaminants of skin – dog and cat (anaerobes)
Actinomyces spp. *Clostridium* spp. *Peptostreptococcus* spp. *Bacteroides* spp. *Fusobacterium* spp. *Prevotella* spp.

Selected references and further reading

Campbell, K.L. (ed) and Lichtensteiger, C.A. (2004) Structure and function of the skin. In: *Small Animal Dermatology Secrets*. pp. 1–9. Hanley and Belfus, Philadelphia

Haake, A.R. and Holbrook, K. (1999) The structure and development of the skin. In: Freedberg, I.M. et al. (eds). *Fitzpatrick's Dermatology in General Medicine*. 5th edn. pp. 70–113. McGraw-Hill, New York

Jenkinson, D.M. (1990) Sweat and sebaceous glands and their function in domestic animals. In: von Tscharner, C. and Halliwell, R.E.W. (eds). *Advances in Veterinary Dermatology I*. p. 229. Bailliere Tindall, Philadelphia

Kwochka, K.W. (1993) The structure and function of epidermal lipids. *Vet Dermatol*, **4**, 151

Mason, I.S. and Lloyd, D.H. (1993) Scanning electron microscopical studies of the living epidermis and stratum corneum in dogs. In: Ihrke, P.J. et al. (eds). *Advances in Veterinary Dermatology II*. p. 131. Pergamon, Oxford

Scott, D.W. (1990) The biology of hair growth and its disturbance. In: von Tscharner, C. and Halliwell, R.E.W. (eds). *Advances in Veterinary Dermatology I*. pp. 3–33. Bailliere Tindall, Philadelphia

Scott, D.W. et al. (2001) Structure and function of the skin. In: *Muller and Kirk's Small Animal Dermatology*. 6th edn. pp. 1–70. WB Saunders, Philadelphia

Suter, M.M. et al. (1997) Keratinocyte biology and pathology. *Vet Dermatol*, **8**, 67

Approach to the case

History taking

Time is always the most important limiting factor when taking a history from a client. Often, it is impossible to assess a patient during a normal consultation and it is tempting to prescribe a symptomatic treatment during a busy clinic. This is a justifiable practice providing the therapy that is supplied does not compromise the ability to investigate the problem more thoroughly at a later date. Antibiotics, antihistamines and topical therapy in the form of shampoos will rarely complicate a diagnosis. The response of a patient to such treatments can often help in directing further tests. Symptomatic steroid therapy is rarely indicated and often makes further investigations impossible in the short term.

History taking needs to be logical and different clinicians approach their questioning in a different manner. Often, the emphasis will be changed depending on the initial owner complaint.

History forms are used extensively by some clinicians, but the author does not use a pre-printed sheet as she feels that this tends not to encourage relevant questioning that can be varied for each case. The history itself can be divided into six sections.

Owner complaint

It is important to assess how reliable your owner is. Owners can mislead a clinician by failing to give an accurate history. Other members of the family present in a consultation can often provide useful information, especially children. At this stage, decide whether you are dealing with a pruritic disease, seborrhoeic problem, pustular disease, etc. This can help with the emphasis of your questioning.

General details

The age, sex, breed, colour and weight of the animal can give important clues to the nature of the disease. For example, demodex is more usually found in young dogs; certain breeds are predisposed to particular diseases.

General health

- Level of activity, e.g. lethargy, poor exercise tolerance in canine hypothyroidism or hyperactivity in feline hyperthyroidism.

- Sexual behaviour, e.g. abnormal attention to other dogs in cases of Sertoli cell tumours.
- Appetite/thirst is often increased in hyperadrenocorticism and in steroid administration.
- Feeding, especially the types of food, changes of diet, titbits, supplements; are cats being fed elsewhere?
- Gastrointestinal signs; e.g., signs of colitis can be associated with dietary intolerances.
- Urogenital signs, e.g. cystitis associated with hyperadrenocorticism.
- Cardio-thoracic signs of a bradycardia are often seen in canine hypothyroidism; previous history of respiratory disease in a kitten may be an indicator of a naso-pharyngeal polyp.
- Central nervous system signs, e.g. fits may occur in hyperadrenocorticism, or otitis interna may be associated with long-standing allergic otitis.
- Locomotor system signs, e.g. polyarthritis associated with systemic lupus erythematosus; lameness can also be seen with onychodystrophy in dogs and nail bed problems, e.g. pemphigus foliaceus, in cats.
- Eye disease, e.g. conjunctivitis, may be seen with allergy in both dogs and cats; keratoconjunctivitis sicca may accompany canine hypothyroidism.
- Ear disease may be seen as an extension of an allergic or endocrine disorder.
- Weight loss – associated with neoplasia, diabetes, chronic systemic disorders.

Environmental history

- Other in contact animals, either pets or wild animals, e.g. foxes and hedgehogs in cases of dogs or small rodents for hunting cats, which can be a source of cat pox (Figure 2.1).
- Human contacts – owner contagion especially ringworm, scabies, cheyletiella (Figure 2.2), flea bites.
- Animal's environment, e.g., does the dog live indoors or outdoors? What types of bedding are used? Does the pet sleep on the owner's bed?
- Holidays/kennelling; especially if the pet improved in a kennelled environment.

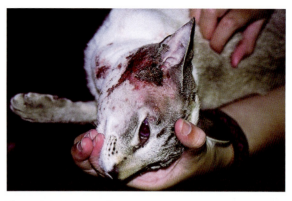

Figure 2.1 Lesions of cat pox in a Siamese cat.

Dermatological history

- When did the symptoms first appear?
- What part of the body was first affected?
- Progression of the disease; has there been evidence of any seasonality?
- Is pruritus present?

Previous therapy

- What previous therapy has been given?
- How has the pet responded to previous treatment?

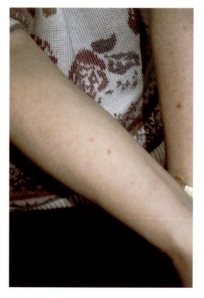

Figure 2.2 Papular lesions of *Cheyletiella* on the arms of an owner.

- Flea treatment; especially which products are used, how often and when it was last used?
- Topical treatment; when was the dog last shampooed, have any cream or lotions been applied?

Examination of the animal

Once a history has been taken the animal can be examined. A general physical inspection should be undertaken in every case. A more detailed examination of some organ systems can be undertaken where indicated. Ophthalmological, neuromuscular examination including cranial nerve reflexes may be indicated in some systemic diseases.

Physical examination

It is important to have adequate space, good owner and pet cooperation (sedation of the pet may be necessary) and good lighting.

Before even touching the dog or cat it is important to assess the animal's general appearance (Figure 2.3), demeanour, body condition. After that the examination should be logical to include the following:

- Temperature, pulse and respiratory rate.
- Mouth – especially the gums and palate (Figure 2.4) looking for abnormalities of colour, petechiation (Figure 2.5), lesions such as ulcers and erosions.
- Ears/eyes – are often affected as an extension of the skin disease.
- Palpation of peripheral lymph nodes – lymphadenopathy can be seen with neoplastic disease or infections.
- Auscultation of the chest – bradycardia (hypothyroidism), tachycardia (hyperthyroidism).
- Abdominal palpation – abdominal masses, hepatomegaly in endocrine disease.
- Musculature – masticatory muscles can be atrophic with dermatomyositis, facial asymmetry with cranial nerve damage in otitis media, pot bellied appearance in hyperadrenocorticism.

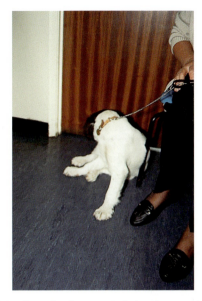

Figure 2.3 Does the dog scratch during the consultation?

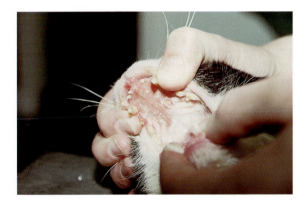

Figure 2.4 Eosinophilic granuloma on the soft palate.

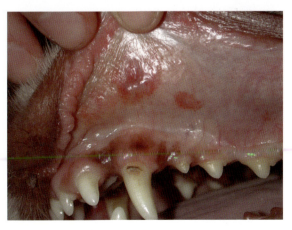

Figure 2.5 Petechiation on the gums of a dog.

- Genitalia: male – scrotal masses, gynaecomastia with sex hormone imbalances; female – vulval enlargement seen with sex hormone imbalances.

Dermatological examination

This should include the whole of the skin and all of the mucous membranes:

- Has the animal given you any dermatological clues whilst it has been in the room? Is dog scratching during the consultation? Is the cat over grooming?

General assessment of the coat

- Presence of scales suggestive of increased epidermal turn over or crust often associated with superficial infection with bacteria or dermatophytes.
- Hair colour/texture – is the coat faded, have primary hairs been lost?

Skin

It is important to check the inaccessible areas of the skin, always turn the animal over to check the ventral abdominal skin (Figure 2.6) as well as inside the mouth and ears; the perianal skin; interdigital spaces and footpads. Assessment of the skin should include the following.

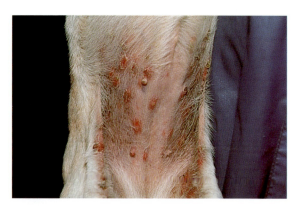

Figure 2.6 Ventral abdominal skin showing primary pustular and papular lesions.

Glabrous (non-haired) skin

- Skin quality – atrophic/inelastic with hyperadrenocorticism, skin fragility syndrome.
- Skin temperature – often cool in hypothyroidism.
- Colour – pallor, erythema, hyperpigmentation, jaundice.
- Primary and secondary lesions – pustules, papules, comedones, etc.

Haired skin

- Will the hair epilate easily?
- Are there areas of stubble suggesting the hair has been chewed out?
- Do the hairs look unusual – are there follicular casts?
- Is there evidence of pigment abnormalities on the hairs?

After taking a careful history and completing a physical and dermatological examination, the clinician should be in a position to compile a list of differential diagnoses. This helps in deciding which further diagnostic tests are required. It is often not necessary to perform every test on each animal. This can also act as a guide to the owners at an early stage as to the possible causes of the disease, the prognosis, and what diagnostic investigations are to be undertaken. It is important at this stage to discuss a treatment plan with the owner including the potential costs.

Selected references and further reading

Bloom, P. (2004) Diagnostic techniques in dermatology. In: Campbell, K.L. (ed) *Small Animal Dermatology Secrets*. pp. 21–33. Hanley and Belfus, Philadelphia

Medleau, L. and Hnilica, K. (2006) Diagnostic techniques. In: *Small Animal Dermatology A Color Atlas and Therapeutic Guide*. 2nd edn. pp. 12–24. WB Saunders, Philadelphia

Scott, D.W. et al. (2001) Diagnostic methods. In: *Muller and Kirk's Small Animal Dermatology*. 6th edn. WB Saunders, Philadelphia

Diagnostic tests 3

Initial diagnostic tests

There can be no excuse not to perform a basic diagnostic panel on all cases. Many laboratories now offer a skin panel as part of their service. However, despite careful packaging of samples prior to posting they rarely arrive at the laboratory in the state they left the practice. A good quality microscope is essential, but other than this expense initial diagnostic tests require a minimal amount of outlay for equipment.

Minimum database for skin disease for both the cat and dog:

- Wet paper test
- Coat brushings
- Diascopy
- Acetate tape impression smears of coat and skin
- Skin scrapings – superficial and deep
- Hair plucking/trichography
- Cutaneous cytology – impression smears, fine needle aspirate

In addition, in the cat (all cases) and inflammatory skin disease dog:

- Fungal culture

Minimum database for otitis in cat or dog:

Ear flap

- Acetate tape impression smears skin
- Skin scrapings – superficial and deep
- Hair plucking/trichography
- Impression smears/exudate from lesions

External ear canal

- Ear discharge – unstained and stained

Wet paper test

The coat is brushed onto a piece of wet paper. Flea faeces will show up as red streaks (Figure 3.1). This should be undertaken in all cases of pruritic skin disease, especially where there is dorsal involvement. It is important to check if the pet has been shampooed recently. False positive tests are common in cats due to the fact that faeces are groomed out of the coat.

Coat brushings

The coat is brushed onto dry paper (Figure 3.2) and can be examined with a hand lens to look for

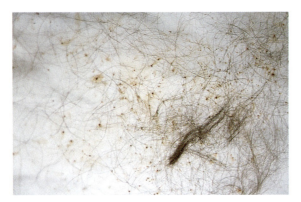

Figure 3.1 Wet paper test; flea faeces appear as red streaks on wet paper.

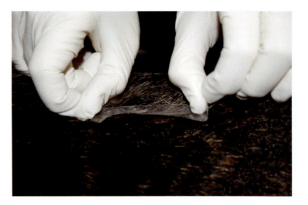

Figure 3.3 Tape stripping hair from the dorsum.

surface parasites, e.g. cheyletiella, lice. Alternatively, the material on the paper can be mounted in either potassium hydroxide of liquid paraffin and examined under the microscope.

Diascopy

This is a useful and simple technique to assess the difference between vasodilation and haemorrhage. A glass slide is placed over an erythematous lesion and gentle pressure is applied:

- Erythematous lesions blanche when pressure is applied as they are caused by dilated blood vessels.
- Haemorrhagic lesions do not blanche when pressure is applied as they are caused by red blood cell leakage out of vessels.

Acetate tape impression smears

This technique can be performed on the skin or hair.

Hair

The tape is pressed repeatedly onto the coat to pick up eggs from the hairs (Figure 3.3), e.g. cheyletiella, lice as well as parasites on the surface of the skin, e.g. lice, trombicula. This is a useful technique to trap some of the fast moving parasites, which can often be seen with the naked eye. It can also be used to identify flea faeces. Selection of site is important in the cat where samples should be taken from areas where the cat is unable to lick, e.g. the back of the neck.

Skin

The tape is pressed firmly onto an alopecic area of skin, which may be clipped if necessary. Site selection is important. Thickened lichenified skin is most likely to reveal evidence of yeast infection. The author will usually rub the tape gently with a thumbnail to ensure good contact of the tape with the skin. A modified Wright's stain such as Diff-Quik can then be applied to the tape, which is then carefully inverted with the adhesive slide downwards onto a microscope slide for examination. As the tape acts as a cover slip, the sample can be examined under high power (100× oil immersion) if necessary. This method can be used to identify surface bacteria; yeast, especially

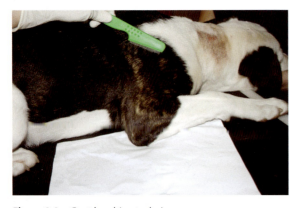

Figure 3.2 Coat brushing technique.

Table 3.1 Mounting material for skin scrapes – advantages and disadvantages.

Liquid paraffin	Potassium hydroxide
Non-irritant to skin	Potential skin irritant
Will not clear the sample	Will clear the sample by digesting keratin
Does not kill the mites, which can thus be identified by movement across the slide	Mites killed
Mites will curl up if the sample is not examined soon after it is taken, making mite identification difficult	Mites well preserved and observation of body parts easier, esp. cheyletiella

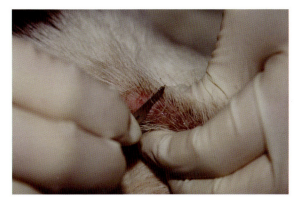

Figure 3.4 Skin scraping technique.

Malassezia; parasites, especially surface living demodex *Demodex corniei* (dog) *Demodex gatoi* (cat).

Skin scrapings

Skin scrapes are essential as part of any basic dermatological investigation. Scrapes may be taken into either liquid paraffin or 10% potassium hydroxide. When liquid paraffin is used a few drops can be gently added to the sample before a cover slip is added. When potassium hydroxide is used the sample is best left to stand for 10–15 minutes and may be gently warmed before examining as this allows the potassium hydroxide to digest keratin to clear the field. There are advantages and disadvantages of both mounting materials (see Table 3.1).

Superficial skin scraping

A scalpel blade should be blunted by gently rubbing on the microscope slide prior to use. It is moistened with either 10% potassium hydroxide or liquid paraffin to provide better collection of material and scraped through the coat and superficial layers of the skin. There are advantages and disadvantages of using each mounting material; these are listed in Table 3.1. Hair may be gently clipped away if the coat is very thick. The scalpel blade is normally held perpendicular to the skin and the scraping should be in the direction of the hair coat. Material should be spread thinly onto the slides. Multiple samples should be taken from non-excoriated areas. When potassium hydroxide is used, the slides may be gently warmed to break up keratin and/or left to stand for 10–15 minutes prior to examination.

Deep skin scraping

The technique is identical to that for superficial scrapings except that scrapings should be taken to a depth where the skin is erythematous and mild capillary ooze is seen (Figures 3.4 and

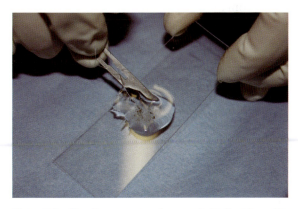

Figure 3.5 The skin scrape may be mounted in liquid paraffin or potassium hydroxide.

Table 3.2 Ectoparasites and most appropriate tests to identify them.

Parasite	Methods that are most useful to identify	Comments
Cheyletiella spp.	Superficial skin scrapes, tape strips, coat brushing	False negative in animals grooming excessively
Demodex canis	Deep skin scrapes, hair plucks, skin biopsy	Skin scrapes false negatives on thickened lesions and from shar-peis; biopsy and hair pluck better; choose areas of comedones for scraping
Demodex corniei	Superficial skin scrapes, tape strips	
Demodex cati	Deep skin scrapes, hair plucks, skin biopsy	Choose areas of comedones for scraping
Demodex gatoi	Superficial skin scrapes, tape strips	Lateral shoulder may be predilection site
Felicola subrostratus	Superficial skin scrapes, tape strips, coat brushing	
Fleas	Wet paper test, tape strips, coat brushing	False negative in animals grooming excessively
Linognathus setosus	Superficial skin scrapes, tape strips	
Lynxacarus radosky	Superficial skin scrape, tape strip, coat brushing	
Neotrombicula autumnalis	Superficial skin scrape, tape strip	
Notoedres cati	Superficial skin scrape, tape strip	
Otodectes cynotis	Superficial skin scrape, tape strip (skin) wax examination	
Sarcoptes scabiei	Deep skin scrape	False negatives common, predilection sites ear tips and lateral elbows; serology and empirical therapy also useful
Trichodectes canis	Superficial skin scrape, tape strip, coat brushing	

3.5). The skin may be pinched to express the mites from the follicles. Different depths of scraping are needed to identify different ectoparasites (Table 3.2).

Hair plucking/trichography

Hair plucks are a useful way to assess a variety of different factors including the presence of fungal infection, trauma, shaft defects and hair growth phase (Figure 3.6).

Hair tip

Examination of the tip is particularly useful in cats where damage to the hair tips suggests

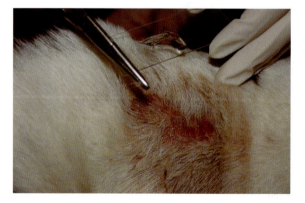

Figure 3.6 Hair plucking for trichography.

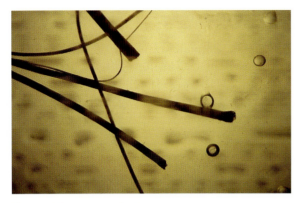

Figure 3.7 Traumatised hair suggesting excessive grooming.

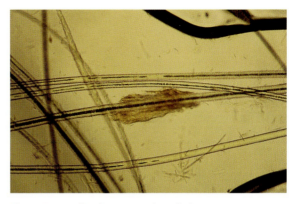

Figure 3.9 Follicular casts on hair shafts.

self-inflicted trauma (Figure 3.7). In hair loss through endocrine disease, the tip remains finely tapered (Figure 3.8).

Hair shaft

Dermatophyte ectothrix spores can be identified on the shafts of the hairs. Spores appear as small spherical structures in rows along the shaft. Pigment changes such as clumping of pigment along the shaft are typical of colour mutant alopecia follicular dysplasia. Follicular casts can be seen in sebaceous adenitis, follicular dystrophy, demodicosis and hyperadrenocorticism (Figure 3.9). Ectoparasite eggs such as cheyletiella and lice can be seen attached to hair shafts (Figure 3.10). Other shaft abnormalities such as trichorrhexis nodosa have been recorded but are rare (Figure 3.11).

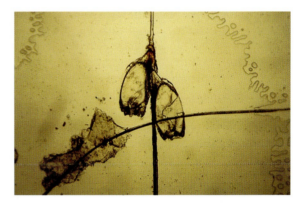

Figure 3.10 Lice eggs cemented to hair shafts.

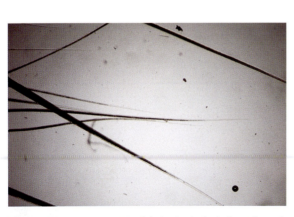

Figure 3.8 Non-traumatised hair tip in hair loss through endocrine disease.

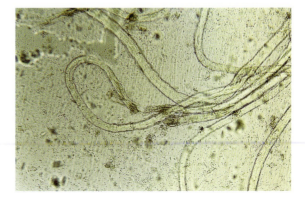

Figure 3.11 Trichorrhexis nodosa showing 'paint brush-like' splitting of hair shafts.

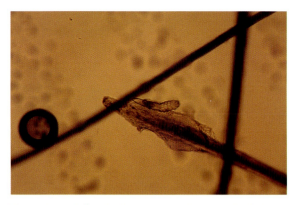

Figure 3.12 Follicular demodex on bulb of hair plucked from an area of comedone formation.

Hair bulbs

Examination of the bulbs allows assessment of the stage of the growth cycle of each hair. Parasites such as demodex can also be seen at the level of the hair bulb (Figure 3.12):

- Telogen hairs have elongated unpigmented spear-shaped roots (Figure 3.13). These are hairs in the resting phase and are most commonly seen in endocrine disease. Most hairs in normal dogs will be in this stage.
- Anagen hairs have bent club shaped roots that are heavily pigmented (Figure 3.13). These are growing hairs and should be identified in samples from normal dogs. In dogs with prolonged growth phase, e.g. poodles, most hairs will be in this stage.

Cutaneous cytology

Cytological examination is a useful technique that allows the clinician to look for the presence of infection (bacteria, yeast, fungi) and also assess infiltrating cell types (neoplastic, inflammatory cells, acanthocytes).

Three techniques may be employed:

- Direct impression smears
- Examination of pustule contents
- Fine needle aspirates

Direct impression smears

This technique is suitable for any exudative lesion, e.g. erosions, ulcers, papules and furuncles, or for obtaining samples from the undersides of crusts.

- None exudative lesions can be picked with a sterile 25 gauge needle to express fluid.
- The microscope slide is gently pressed onto the lesion to collect exudates (Figure 3.14).
- The sample may be air dried or carefully warmed to dry (the author uses a small handheld hair dryer).
- The slide is stained using a modified Wright's stain (Diff-Quik) and gently rinsed and dried again.
- The sample should always be examined on low power ($10\times$ objective) initially to select areas for close inspection, subsequently on high power ($40\times$) or under oil immersion ($100\times$).

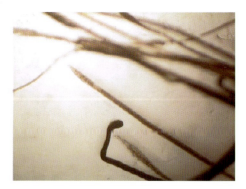

Figure 3.13 Anagen hair bulb in lower half of picture is dark and curled. Telogen hair bulb is long, thin and unpigmented.

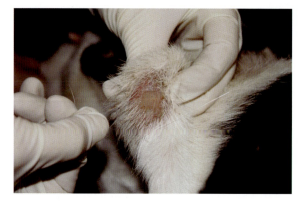

Figure 3.14 Impression smear of exudative lesion.

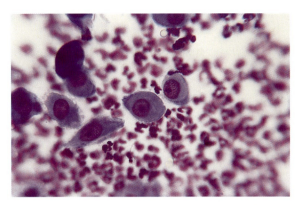

Figure 3.15 Acanthocytes from a sterile pustule in the case of pemphigus foliaceus.

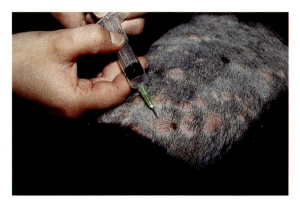

Figure 3.16 Fine needle aspirates from plaques on a dog's dorsum.

Examination of pustule contents

This method is useful for pustular lesions to identify if they have an infectious or sterile aetiology. The pustule should be picked with a sterile 25 gauge needle and the contents gently pressed onto the slide. It should be stained as above. Findings include the following:

- Bacteria plus degenerate neutrophils identified in bacterial infection.
- Acanthocytes (rounded nucleated keratinocytes), non-degenerate white blood cells (usually neutrophils and eosinophils) seen in immunological diseases such as pemphigus (Figure 3.15).
- Demodex mites, bacteria and degenerate neutrophils can be seen in follicular demodex.

Fine needle aspirates

Aspirates are most suitable for nodular lesions especially neoplastic and pyogranulomatous disease:

- A 21–23 gauge needle attached to a 2 or 5 ml syringe should be used (Figure 3.16).
- The lesion should be sterilised with spirit and immobilised between finger and thumb.
- The needle is inserted into the lesion whilst pressure is applied to the plunger to create negative pressure. The needle can be constantly repositioned within the lesion without removing it, to draw up as much material as possible.
- The pressure on the needle should be released before the needle is withdrawn. The sampling should be stopped if there is evidence of blood in the hub of the needle.
- The needle is then removed and the plunger withdrawn to fill the syringe with air.
- The needle is then replaced and the contents of the needle expressed onto a clean microscope slide.
- The material may be gently smeared if necessary and stained as above. The slide should be scanned initially on a low power ($4\times$ or $10\times$) to identify areas of interest before using high power ($40\times$) or oil immersion ($100\times$).

Fungal culture

Dermatophyte culture should be undertaken in any inflammatory canine skin disease and any feline skin problem. A sterile toothbrush, hairbrush or carpet square coat brushing can be used (Figure 3.17).

Sampling lesions

- Samples of hair and scale can be collected by brushing the lesion and an area of at least 3 cm^2 around its periphery. Alternatively, sterile forceps can be used to pick off scale, crust and hair.
- Wood's lamp examination of hairs may help select suitable hairs for sampling.

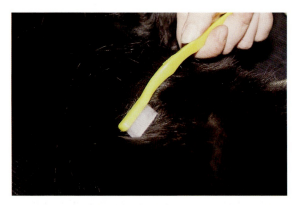

Figure 3.17 Tooth brushing from coat for dermatophyte culture.

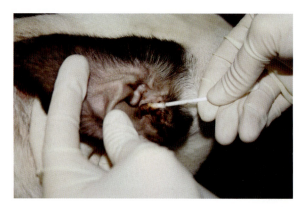

Figure 3.18 Collection of ear wax using a cotton swab.

- Nail clippings can also be cultured in cases of onychomycosis by clipping the nail and then grinding it up or shaving it and sprinkling onto the culture medium.

Sampling non-lesional skin/asymptomatic carriers

- A toothbrush is best employed to comb through the whole coat.

Choice of culture medium

- Samples can be bedded on dermatophyte test medium (DTM) or else Sabouraud's dextrose agar (SDA). Care should be taken to rest the samples on the surface and not embed them in the medium.
- DTM has the advantage of producing a colour change as dermatophytes grow, but macroconidia production is generally better on SDA.
- The plates should be checked daily for growth. Dermatophyte colonies appear as white fluffy or buff-coloured colonies. Pigmented colonies are almost always contaminants.
- Dermatophytes lead to a colour change on the medium from yellow to red. Colonies sporulate poorly on DTM but colonies can be collected in many cases by the use of acetate tape touched onto the surface to collect macroconidia, which can subsequently be stained and mounted.

Examination of ear wax

Both plain unstained samples and stained samples should be examined from the external ear canal (Figure 3.18). This procedure can be used to make initial decisions for treatment, possibly pending cultures, and can also be used to monitor the progress of the disease.

Initial sampling

- Plain sample is prepared by rolling wax collected on a cotton wool swab from the external ear canal onto a microscope slide (Figure 3.19). The sample should then be examined unstained. Initially, this should be done on low power (4×, 10×) rarely is a higher power needed. *Demodex* spp. and *Otodectes cynotis* can be identified by this technique.

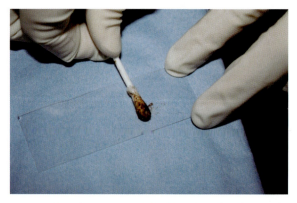

Figure 3.19 The cotton swab is rolled along the slide and air dried.

Diagnostic tests

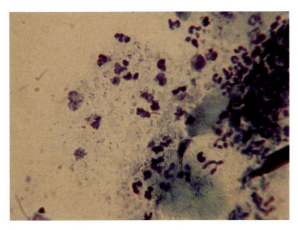

Figure 3.20 Degenerate neutrophils and bacteria on a stained sample of ear wax.

- Wax may also be collected and prepared in the same way but air dried or gently warmed and then stained with Diff-Quik. Examination should be performed with both low and high power objectives. This technique will identify different cell types and micro-organisms such as bacteria (rods and cocci, Figure 3.20) or yeast (Figure 3.21).

Follow-up samples

- These samples should be taken at different points during therapy.
- Assessment of the inflammatory infiltrate and micro-organisms helps to make judgements on the progression of the disease and response to therapy.

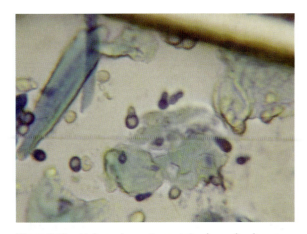

Figure 3.21 Malassezia yeast on a stained sample of ear wax.

Further diagnostic tests

Initial investigations will give information as to which further tests are deemed necessary. It is important to discuss these again with the owner at this stage.

Culture

Culture has become a more important tool in investigation, especially since methicillin resistant *Staphylococcus aureus* (MRSA) isolates have been identified in small animals. Bacterial culture is probably not indicated in all cases of bacterial pyoderma; however, it should be undertaken in certain circumstances (see Table 3.3).

The main groups of pathogens that can be cultured are as follows:

- Bacteria: sterile swabs or tissue culture can be submitted for aerobic or anaerobic culture.
- Fungi: hair, scale and crust can be submitted for growth on DTM or SDA.
- Yeast: contact plates are usually employed to look for Malassezia.

Superficial bacterial culture

Sterile swabs can be used to collect moist exudates from the skin or for absorbing pustule contents from pricked pustules. In ears, samples should be taken before any cleaning takes place. The more chronic the lesion the more important it is to look for anaerobic bacteria as well as aerobic pathogens. It is important to inform the laboratory if you are suspicious of an unusual or zoonotic organism, e.g. nocardia, mycobacterium or MRSA.

Deep bacterial culture

Samples from deep lesions are best taken as sterile biopsy samples. Samples once harvested should be placed in a transport swab container or else sterile saline and delivered to the laboratory as quickly as possible.

Table 3.3 Indications for bacteriology culture.

Indications for bacteriology culture	Comment
Cytology reveals cocci and there has been no response to (1) appropriate antibiotic at (2) correct dose for (3) appropriate length of time	High clinical suspicion of resistant staphylococcus possible MRSA
Cytology reveals evidence of cocci and rods or just rods	Difficult to predict antibiotic therapy; multiple antibiotics may be needed
Deep pyoderma	A long course of antibiotics is required so early appropriate antibiotic therapy is needed
Chronic disease – where glucocorticoids and multiple antibiotic treatments have been used	May be overgrowth of commensals or anaerobes with unpredictable sensitivity
German shepherd dog pyoderma	Often unpredictable sensitivity and multiple pathogens

Biopsy

Biopsy can provide an enormous amount of information if appropriate samples are taken. Ideally, samples should be from early lesions and where possible primary lesions should be biopsied. The major indications for biopsy include the following:

- Suspected neoplastic lesions (Figure 3.22).
- Ulcerative or vesicular lesions.
- Skin disease unresponsive to rational therapy.
- Unusual or serious skin disease, especially when the dog is systemically unwell.
- To make a diagnosis where expensive or potentially dangerous drugs are to be used.

Often a biopsy will not give a definitive diagnosis but will allow the clinician to place a disease within a general group. The main categories are as follows:

- Neoplasia
- Infection and deep parasites (folliculitis, cellulites, furunculosis, demodicosis)
- Immune mediated disease, e.g. autoimmune disease, vasculitis
- Endocrine disease, e.g. hyperadrenocorticism, follicular dysplasia
- Keratinisation disorders, e.g. sebaceous adenitis, primary seborrhoea
- Allergy and superficial parasites (fleas, sarcoptes, etc.)

Types of biopsy

- Punch biopsy: 6 mm or 8 mm biopsy sample.
- Excisional biopsy.
- Nail biopsy/amputation (see section on nail disease).

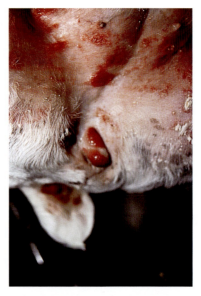

Figure 3.22 Erythroderma with scale, nodules and plaques in a dog with epitheliotrophic lymphoma. Such presenting signs warrant biopsy.

Table 3.4 Biopsy techniques.

Procedure	Comments
Select an appropriate area for biopsy	Choose primary lesions, e.g. pustules, vesicles Chronically damaged skin and secondary lesions, e.g. ulcers, lichenification and alopecia, rarely provide good diagnostic information
Select multiple areas to biopsy	Sample at least three areas and different representative lesions; footpad and nasal lesions are difficult to biopsy but provide useful information
Clip the area gently but do not prep the skin	Overpreparation of the skin can remove crust and scale, which is useful diagnostically; cleaning can affect tissue culture results
Inject a small bleb of local anaesthetic into the subcutaneous skin	Suitable agents include lidocaine, novocaine and articaine
Punch biopsy: use a disposable punch (6–8 mm); place over the lesion; apply gentle pressure and twist the punch	If a blunt punch is used it can distort the tissue by producing shearing forces and give unreliable results
Once the full thickness of skin has been penetrated the punch can be withdrawn	Care should be taken over delicate structures to ensure they are not damaged
Excisional biopsy: an elliptical excision is made around a lesion with a scalpel blade	This technique is useful for larger lesions also nose, footpads and ear flaps
Fine forceps should be used to grab the subcutaneous fat on the sample and any adherent fat can be snipped with fine forceps to release it	If the epidermis is grasped or heavy forceps are used, the sample can be damaged
Mount the sample on a piece of card	Allows the pathologist to orientate the sample for processing
Place in 10% formalin solution	Ensure that the sample is in at least 10× its own volume of formalin to ensure that it is adequately preserved
Ensure that the submission form contains a detailed clinical history and a list of differential diagnoses	Providing the pathologist with information allows them to provide you with more useful information
Submit to a pathologist with a level of expertise in dermatohistopathology	Subtle or rare diseases may not be recognised by a general pathologist
Once the sample has been removed the wound may be closed using sutures or staples	

For biopsy techniques, see Table 3.4.

Allergy testing

Allergy testing can be performed to identify offending allergens in both cases of food allergy and atopic dermatitis. In vitro tests (serology) are available for food allergy, and both in vitro (serology) and in vivo (intradermal skin testing) are available for atopic dermatitis.

Serology testing

These tests rely on the identification of antigen-specific antibody levels and are available for both environmental allergens and food allergens. The use of serology to identify food allergic individuals remains controversial with questions asked about the sensitivity and specificity of these tests. The author prefers to use a carefully selected food trial followed by dietary challenge to investigate food-allergic individuals. Serology testing for

Table 3.5 Advantages and disadvantages of serological versus intradermal allergy tests.

Serological tests	Intradermal tests
Can be performed by veterinary surgeon in practice	Needs to be performed by experienced operator
No outlay for diagnostic kit so individual animals can be tested, but test is relatively expensive	Expensive intradermal allergens need to be purchased; a kit should contain at least 40 allergens; it is a cost-effective procedure provided multiple tests are performed within the shelf life of the kit
Allergens tested are those offered by central laboratory	Allergens tested can be individualised for specific area
Animal does not require sedation or clipping Glucocorticoid withdrawal is probably indicated; antihistamines may not interfere with testing	Animal needs sedation and clipping Glucocorticoid and antihistamine withdrawal is needed prior to testing
No check to see if the animals' test has been affected by inadequate drug withdrawal	Use of histamine (positive control) and sterile diluent (negative control) allows investigator to decrease the risk of false negative and positive results
False negative results can be seen in allergic animals that subsequently have positive intradermal allergy tests and successfully respond to vaccines	A higher percentage of dogs produce meaningful positive reactions to intradermal allergy testing than serology
Animal stress during the procedure should not interfere with test results	Animal stress during the procedure may lead to false negative results
Good results are seen with allergen-specific immunotherapy based on serological testing	Response to allergen-specific immunotherapy is recognised as being superior when based on intradermal tests compared to serology

environmental allergens does produce good results and does have significant advantages over intradermal allergy testing (see Table 3.5).

Intradermal allergy testing

Intradermal allergy testing is considered to be the gold standard test for the identification of environmental allergens in atopic dermatitis. It is the author's and indeed most veterinary dermatologists' preferred test. Intradermal allergy testing involves measuring the allergic response in the skin, which is the target reaction for the allergy reaction (Figure 3.23). These tests also have advantages and disadvantages (see Table 3.5).

Trial therapy

A therapeutic trial can be employed in a variety of situations and can be used as a justifiable shortcut when owner's funds are inadequate to allow a more detailed investigation. The use of anti-inflammatories is rarely indicated as a therapeutic trial, and in the author's opinion immunosuppressive therapy in any form should *never* be

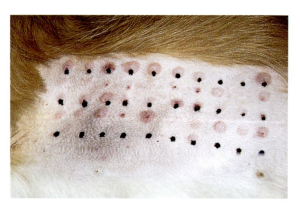

Figure 3.23 Intradermal allergy tests to a variety of environmental allergens. Positive reactions are represented as erythematous weals.

used without stringent efforts to make a diagnosis. Situations where trial therapy may be used include the following:

- Anti-parasitic therapy – in cases of suspected scabies, flea allergic dermatitis.
- Antibiotics – in pustular disease to assess if the aetiology is an infectious or sterile disease.
- Food trial – where a diet is suspected as a cause of the disease – food allergy, zinc responsive disease.
- Drug withdrawal – in cases where the lesions may have been caused by a reaction to a drug.

The reader is referred to the specific sections for more detailed descriptions of further diagnostic tests that may be employed.

In endocrine disease or where the dog or cat is thought to have cutaneous lesions as a manifestation of systemic disease, blood tests may be needed. These may include

- routine haematology and biochemistry,
- viral screens in cats,
- endocrine screen including thyroid function tests,
- dynamic function tests, ACTH stimulation test, low/high dose dexamethasone suppression test.

There will be situations where the dermatologist or veterinary surgeon needs to redirect a skin case to another discipline for further investigation:

- Ultrasonography, e.g. for visualisation of adrenal glands in hyperadrenocorticism or liver architecture in necrolytic migratory erythema.
- Radiography to diagnose calcinosis cutis or underlying bone pathology in acral lick granuloma.
- Electrocardiogram (ECG) may identify cardiac abnormalities seen with hypothyroidism.
- Electromyogram (EMG) to identify abnormal traces seen with dermatomyositis or in endocrine disease.
- Advanced diagnostic imaging, e.g. magnetic resonance imaging (MRI) in cases of chronic ear disease or in pruritus associated with neurological disease.

Once a diagnosis has been made it is important to again discuss with the owner the long-term prognosis for the animal, the success rate for the therapy, and the length of course of the treatment. Is a short course of drugs required or can the owner expect the dog to be on therapy for life? What are the side effects of therapy? What happens if the disease is not treated? What will it all cost? This procedure can often take as long as the initial consultation, but is as important. If the owner appreciates which diagnostic tests have been undertaken and the seriousness of the disease, then long-term client compliance is much better.

Selected references and further reading

Bloom, P. (2004) Diagnostic techniques in dermatology. In: Campbell, K.L. (ed) *Small Animal Dermatology Secrets*. pp. 21–33. Hanley and Belfus, Philadelphia

Dunstan, R.W. et al. (2004) A guide to taking skin biopsies: a pathologist's perspective. In: Campbell, K.L. (ed) *Small Animal Dermatology Secrets*. pp. 34–42. Hanley and Belfus, Philadelphia

Medleau, L. and Hnilica, K. (2006) Diagnostic techniques. In: *Small Animal Dermatology: A Color Atlas and Therapeutic Guide*. 2nd edn. pp. 12–24. WB Saunders, Philadelphia

Scott, D.W. et al. (2001) Diagnostic methods. In: *Muller and Kirk's Small Animal Dermatology*. 6th edn. WB Saunders, Philadelphia

Bacterial skin disease 4

General

The primary pathogen in the dog is *Staphylococcus intermedius*. Staphylococcus is thought to be a resident of the mucosae, especially the nasal, anal, genital tract areas, and is seeded to the skin through grooming or other activities. It is rare for it to cause an infection without an underlying factor. Almost any skin condition may lead to infection but the most common triggers are allergy, keratinisation disorders and follicular diseases. In deep pyodermas non-resident organisms such as *Pseudomonas* spp., *Actinomyces* spp., *Nocardia* spp. *and Mycobacteria* spp. can be isolated.

Bacterial skin infection in the cat is rare. Subcutaneous abscesses are the most common forms of infection usually due to bite wounds. Feline superficial and deep infections are almost always associated with other underlying disease processes such as metabolic or immunological abnormalities. The primary pathogen in superficial infections is *S. intermedius*. In deep pyoderma many different aerobic and anaerobic bacteria including *Pasteurella multocida*, beta-haemolytic streptococcus, *Actinomyces* spp. *Bacteroides* spp. and *Fusobacterium* spp. can be identified.

Pyoderma can be classified according to depth as follows:

- Surface
- Superficial
- Deep

Surface pyoderma

Outermost layers of the epidermis are involved. It can be seen as

(a) acute moist dermatitis (hot spot, wet eczema),
(b) intertrigo complex.

Acute moist dermatitis

Cause and pathogenesis
Acute moist dermatitis as its name suggests is a rapidly developing surface bacterial infection that is created by the animal as a result of self-inflicted trauma, which may be licking, rubbing or chewing. It is common in dogs and rare in cats. No breed predilection is recognised. Most cases occur in the summer and autumn. Fleas are the most common inciting trigger.

The site of the lesions can give a clue to the underlying cause. Most lesions are found on the trunk (fleas), tail base (fleas, impacted anal glands), lateral thigh (fleas), neck (allergy) face (otitis) (Figure 4.1). Other causes include the following:

Bacterial skin disease

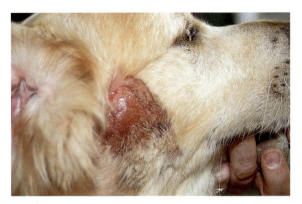

Figure 4.1 Acute moist dermatitis secondary to otitis externa. Typical appearance of erythema with exudation and self-inflicted trauma.

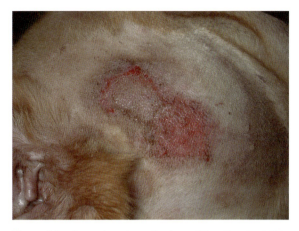

Figure 4.3 Area of acute moist dermatitis without satellite lesions.

- Allergy – atopy (Figure 4.2), food, flea allergy.
- Ectoparasites – cheyletiella, lice.
- Localised pain – arthritis, soft tissue pain especially anal glands, dental problems.
- Otitis externa.
- Trauma – bites, injection reaction.
- Hygiene – poor coat condition, inadequate grooming (especially long coated dogs).
- Hyperthermia secondary to hyperthyroidism.
- Psychogenic – flanks or tail (especially in oriental cat breeds).

Clinical signs
Localised area of moist erythematous exudation (Figure 4.3). Margins are clearly defined. Typically, the lesion is surrounded by halo of erythematous skin. If the central lesion is surrounded by papules or pustules, so-called satellite lesions, the dermatitis is not confined to the surface and is a superficial or deep pyoderma.

Differential diagnosis
- Superficial or deep localised pyoderma
- Demodicosis
- Dermatophytosis
- Neoplasia especially mast cell tumour, sebaceous gland adenocarcinoma (dog), squamous cell carcinoma (cat)
- Eosinophilic granuloma (cat)
- Ulcerative dermatitis with linear subepidermal fibrosis (cat)

Diagnosis
- History, e.g. presence of otitis, poor flea control.
- Clinical signs – the presence of satellite lesions suggest a deeper infected process, which requires more aggressive antibiotic treatment.
- Skin scrape.
- Cytology – reveals degenerate neutrophils and often mixed bacteria.
- Fungal culture.

Treatment
- Check for underlying causes, especially if a recurrent problem. Flea control is important in all cases.
- Clip area (if necessary under sedation).

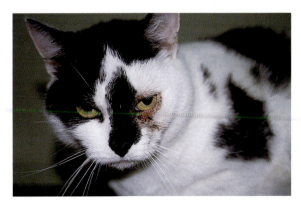

Figure 4.2 Acute moist dermatitis caused through face rubbing in an allergic cat.

- Use a collar or equivalent to break self-perpetuating itch/scratch cycle.
- Topical therapy should be used to
  - dry the skin, e.g. 5% aluminium acetate or calamine lotion applied 2–3 times daily for 2–7 days;
  - cleanse the skin, e.g. antibacterial shampoo containing acetic acid, benzoyl peroxide, chlorhexidine, ethyl lactate used prior to drying agents;
  - decrease pruritus, e.g. topical antibiotic and steroid combinations for short-term use only (up to 7 days), e.g. fusidic acid/betamethasone.
- Systemic glucocorticoid therapy may be used if there is no evidence of bacterial colonisation beyond the surface, e.g. prednisolone 1 mg/kg po sid (dogs) or 2 mg/kg po sid (cats) for 5–10 days.

Intertrigo complex (skin fold pyoderma)

Cause and pathogenesis

Intertrigo complex occurs where skin folds become colonised with pathogenic organisms. Other factors that contribute are the maceration of the skin through overgrooming, tear staining or urine scalding. Bacterial involvement is common but intertrigo can occur where bacteria are seen in conjunction with or with only yeast and/or surface demodex. Different anatomical locations provide different micro-environments to allow commensal organisms to multiply and cause disease. These include most commonly the following:

- Bacteria – *S. intermedius, Pseudomonas* spp. (Figure 4.4)
- Yeast – *Malassezia pachydermatis* (dog), *Malassezia sympodialis* (cat)
- Ectoparasites – *Demodex canis* (dog), *Demodex gatoi* (cat)

Types of intertrigo (see Table 4.1)

- Lip fold
- Facial fold
- Vulval fold
- Tail fold

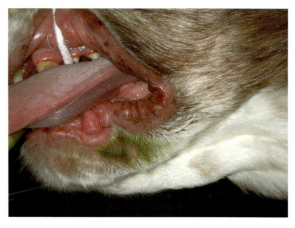

Figure 4.4 Pseudomonas colonisation of lip fold in a spaniel.

- Body fold
- Interdigital folds
- Scrotal folds

Diagnosis

- Cytology of lesions with direct impression smear or acetate tape stained with Diff-Quik to look for bacteria and yeast.
- Skin scrapings to check for parasite involvement (See section on diagnosis for techniques).
- Culture and sensitivity is rarely needed.

Treatment

Medical therapy:

- Medical therapy is preferable where possible but is often life long.
- Cleansing of the infected area can be undertaken with medicated wipes, shampoos or sprays.
- Topical cleansing dependent on pathogen:
  - Bacteria – acetic acid, benzoyl peroxide, chlorhexidine or ethyl lactate.
  - Yeast – boric acid, clotrimazole, ketoconazole or miconazole.
- Topical protectants/creams depend on pathogen:
  - Gram positive bacteria – fusidic acid, neomycin.
  - Gram negative bacteria – silver sulphadiazine, polymyxin.
  - Yeast – clotrimazole, miconazole.

Table 4.1 Intertrigo – different presentations.

Site of fold dermatitis	Breed incidence	Concurrent disease	Organism involved commonly	Specific therapy
General comments	*Not an exclusive list*	*Must be identified and treated if possible*	*Not an exclusive list*	*General medical therapy; see specific agents under treatment below*
Lip fold dogs	Spaniels	Dental disease, e.g. calculi, gingivitis any disease causing excessive salivation	*Malassezia* spp. *Staphylococcus* spp. *Pseudomonas* spp.	Topical cleansing and emollient protection Surgical cheiloplasty
Facial fold dogs	Brachiocephalic breeds, e.g. bulldog (Figure 4.5), Boxer	Primary eye disease causing epiphora, e.g. distichiasis Secondary corneal disease can occur due to rubbing	*Malassezia* spp. *Staphylococcus* spp. *Demodex* spp.	Topical cleansing and emollient protection Surgical removal of facial folds
Facial fold cats	Persians other short faced breeds (Figure 4.6)	Primary eye disease causing ocular discharge, e.g. infectious or allergic conjunctivitis	*Malassezia* spp. *Staphylococcus* spp. *Demodex* spp.	Topical cleansing and emollient protection Facial fold resection
Vulval fold dogs		Often due to immature vulva due to early spaying or urinary tract disease (Figure 4.7), e.g. cystitis, urolithiasis	*Staphylococcus* spp. *Pseudomonas* spp.	Topical cleansing and emollient protection Vulvaplasty
Tail fold dogs	Bulldogs	Corkscrew tail often due to poor docking (Figure 4.8)	*Malassezia* spp. *Staphylococcus* spp. *Pseudomonas* spp.	Topical cleansing and emollient protection Surgical 'filleting' of end of tail to remove bone
Body fold dogs	Spaniels, bassets, bloodhounds, shar-pies esp. on neck	More common in obese animals	*Malassezia* spp. *Staphylococcus* spp.	Topical cleansing and emollient protection
Body fold cats	Mammary folds most commonly	Most common in obese cats and those with mammary hyperplasia due to hormonal therapy or lactation	*Staphylococcus* spp.	Topical cleansing and emollient protection
Interdigital folds dogs	Gun dogs, Boxers (Figure 4.9)	Underlying atopy leading to foot licking	*Malassezia* spp. *Staphylococcus* spp.	Topical cleansing
Interdigital folds cats	Devon Rex (Figure 4.10) possible associated with keratinisation disorder or allergy	Possible associated with keratinisation disorder or allergy	*Malassezia* spp. *Staphylococcus* spp.	Topical cleansing ± systemic anti-yeast drugs
Scrotal folds dogs	Entire males	Often associated with allergy	*Malassezia* spp.	Topical cleansing and emollient protection

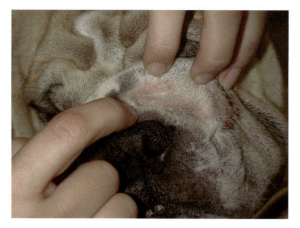

Figure 4.5 Surface infection in a bulldog's facial fold.

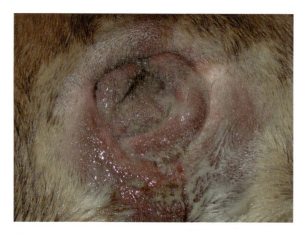

Figure 4.8 Surface infection is a corkscrew tail fold of a bulldog.

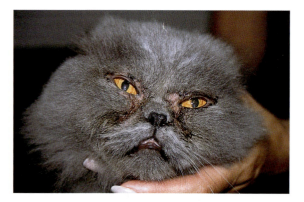

Figure 4.6 Facial fold pyoderma in a Persian cat.

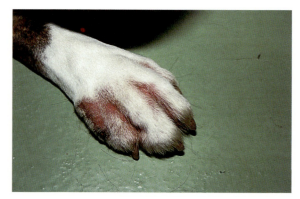

Figure 4.9 Interdigital intertrigo with malassezia infection in an atopic Boxer.

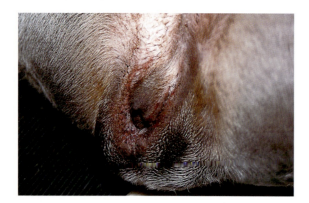

Figure 4.7 Surface infection due to incontinence in an old bitch.

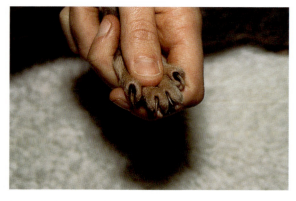

Figure 4.10 Nail fold *Malassezia* in a Devon Rex.

Adjunct therapy:

- Where necessary underlying disease needs to be addressed, e.g. weight reduction programme for obese animals, castration for scrotal folds, dental therapy for gingivitis. Investigation and therapy of allergy, demodicosis, bladder, eye disease.

Surgical therapy:

- Surgical therapy should only be undertaken when medical therapy has been unsuccessful and underlying disease has been controlled. It should not be a substitute for medical therapy.
- Surgical intervention involves removal of the excessive folds. Most commonly applied to the face, vulva and lips.

Superficial bacterial infection (superficial pyoderma)

Superficial bacterial infection involves the epidermis and the intact follicle and does not extend deeper into the dermis or involve damage to the hair follicle.

Types

(a) Impetigo
(b) Folliculitis
(c) Mucocutaneous pyoderma
(d) Methicillin resistant *Staphylococcus aureus*
(e) Dermatophilosis

Impetigo

Subcorneal pustules especially found in sparsely haired areas usually on the ventral abdominal skin.

Cause and pathogenesis
Canine juvenile impetigo (Figure 4.11) – usually staphylococcus seen in young dogs secondary to the following:

- Parasitism (fleas, cheyletiella, endoparasites)
- Poor hygiene

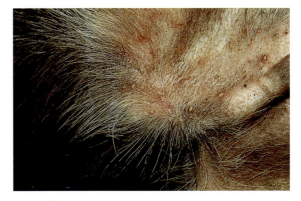

Figure 4.11 Juvenile impetigo in a young dog.

- Inadequate nutrition
- Systemic disease, e.g. distemper

Feline juvenile impetigo – bacteria involved usually staphylococcus, *P. multocida* or beta-haemolytic streptococcus. Most common causes are

- overgrooming of kittens by queen,
- systemic disease, e.g. cat flu.

Canine adult onset bullous impetigo (Figure 4.12) – caused by staphylococcus but may also be caused by Gram negative bacteria. Older dogs secondary to the following:

- Endocrine disease
- Debilitating disease, e.g. internal neoplasia

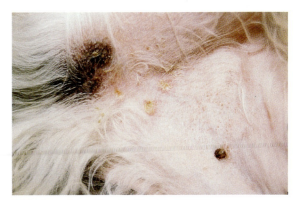

Figure 4.12 Bullous impetigo caused by staphylococcus in a dog with hypothyroidism.

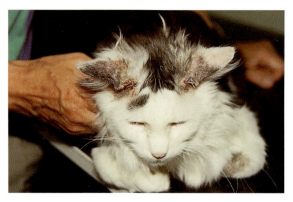

Figure 4.13 Adult onset impetigo on the ear secondary to atopy.

Feline adult onset impetigo – causal organisms as feline juvenile disease. Secondary to the following:

- Viral immunosuppression, e.g. FeLV, FIV, pox virus
- Debilitating disease, e.g. neoplasia
- Endocrine disease, e.g. hyperadrenocorticism
- Allergy especially atopy (Figure 4.13)

Clinical signs
- Non-follicular pustules, rupture to form papules and crusts. Pruritus variable.
- Distribution can be generalised but often seen on hairless ventral abdominal areas.
- Small non-follicular pustules on glabrous skin ruptured to form epidermal collarettes, papules and crust.
- Adult onset bullous impetigo clinical signs as feline disease and juvenile canine disease except the pustules are large and flaccid. These rupture causing loss of large areas of epidermis.

Differential diagnosis
Canine disease:

- Sterile pustular disease, e.g. pemphigus foliaceus, sterile eosinophilic pustulosis
- Demodicosis
- Dermatophytosis

Feline disease:

- Miliary dermatitis
- Dermatophytosis
- Sterile pustular disease

Diagnosis
- History and clinical signs
- Skin scrapings
- Cytology of lesions – degenerate neutrophils with bacteria
- Culture and sensitivity
- Fungal culture (especially cats)
- Identification of underlying disease where appropriate

Treatment
- Juvenile impetigo/feline adult onset impetigo:
  - Where possible identify and treat underlying causes; however, the condition can regress spontaneously in kittens and puppies as general health and immune status improves.
  - Antibacterial shampoos, spray or wipes containing acetic acid, benzoyl peroxide, chlorhexidine, ethyl lactate can be used 2–3 times weekly until cure, approximately 10 days.
  - Topical antibiotic creams (without steroid) can be used on localised lesions; suitable products contain fusidic acid or neomycin.
  - Antibiotics are rarely necessary. In severe cases 3 weeks of antibiotics required and for 7 days beyond clinical resolution (see Table 4.2, oral antibiotics for superficial bacterial skin disease).
- Canine adult onset bullous impetigo:
  - Identification of underlying disease is important to prevent recurrence.
  - Antibacterial shampoos as juvenile impetigo above.
  - Antibiotics used for 10 days beyond clinical cure based on culture and sensitivity if necessary.

Mucocutaneous pyoderma

Bacterial infection of the mucocutaneous junction usually affects the lips and perioral skin. Uncommon condition only recorded in dogs.

Table 4.2 Antibacterial therapy for superficial and deep bacterial infection – see also under specific diseases.

Antibiotic	Dose rate	Indications
Amikacin[1]	5–10 mg/kg sq bid	Gram negative rods, atypical mycobacteria; *M. avium*
Amoxicillin	11–22 mg/kg po bid/tid	Cat bite abscesses
Ampicillin	20 mg/kg po bid/qid	*Actinomyces, Nocardia, Dermatophilus*
Cephalexin	25 mg/kg po bid	*Nocardia, Dermatophilus*
Clavamox (amoxicillin/clavulanate)	12.5–25 mg/kg po bid – tid	Cat bite abscesses, staphylococcal infections
Clindamycin	5.5 mg/kg po bid	*Nocardia*, cat bite abscesses, staphylococcal infections
Clofazimine	2–12 mg/kg po bid long courses up to 6 months required	Feline leprosy
Enrofloxacin	5.0 mg/kg po bid	Gram negative rods, atypical mycobacteria; *M. avium*; staphylococcal infections
Lincomycin	22 mg/kg po bid	Staphylococcal infections, *Dermatophilus*
Penicillin G procaine	10–15 mg/kg im or sq bid	*Actinomyces*
Potentiated sulphonamides (trimethoprim/sulphonamide)	Dose is mg of total product 30 mg/kg po bid	*Actinobacillus, Nocardia*
Rifampin[2]	5 mg/kg po bid	Feline leprosy
Streptomycin	10 mg/kg im or sc sid	*Actinobacillus*, plaque
Tetracycline	10–22 mg/kg po bid – tid	*Actinomyces*, L-form bacteria plaque

Note: For full list of abbreviations see front of book.
[1] Nephrotoxic drug – monitor renal function.
[2] Hepatotoxic drug – monitor hepatic function.

Cause and pathogenesis
Unknown cause. Bacteria involved usually coagulase positive staphylococcus.

Clinical signs
- Any age or sex. German shepherd dogs and German shepherd dog crosses appear to be predisposed.
- Mucocutaneous erythema, swelling followed by crusting and erosion (Figure 4.14).
- Lesions often bilaterally symmetrical usually painful leading to self-inflicted trauma.

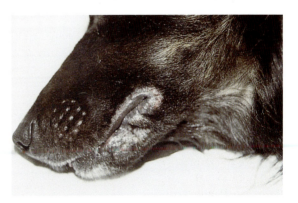

Figure 4.14 Mucocutaneous pyoderma in a German shepherd dog.

- Most common sites: commissures of the mouth but also nares, eyelids, vulva, prepuce and anus.

Differential diagnosis
- Intertrigo complex
- Demodicosis
- Dermatophytosis
- Malassezia dermatitis
- Autoimmune skin disease
- Epitheliotropic lymphoma

Diagnosis
- History and clinical signs.
- Skin scrapings.
- Cytology of lesions – degenerate neutrophils with bacteria usually cocci.
- Culture and sensitivity – rarely needed.
- Fungal culture.
- Histopathology reveals signs of epidermal hyperplasia, superficial epidermal pustules with crusting. Lichenoid infiltrate dermatitis with mixed dermal infiltrate.

Treatment
- Clipping and cleansing of area; may need sedation to achieve this.
- Antibacterial shampoos or wipes containing acetic acid, benzoyl peroxide, chlorhexidine or ethyl lactate.
- Topical ointments, e.g. fusidic acid (cocci on cytology) flamazine (rods on cytology) twice daily for 14 days then twice weekly.
- Systemic antibiotics indicated in severe cases, based on culture and sensitivity a minimum of 3–4 weeks (see Table 4.2).
- Relapses require long-term maintenance therapy with topical and/or systemic treatment.

Bacterial folliculitis

A superficial infection leading to the formation of follicular pustules caused by bacterial infection of the intact hair follicle. Common disease in the dog and rare in the cat.

Cause and pathogenesis
In dogs major pathogen is *S. intermedius*. *Staphylococcus schleiferi* is also isolated especially in dogs with chronic disease and multiple antibiotic therapies. Methicillin resistant *S. aureus* (MRSA) (see notes below on this pathogen) is also recognised as a significant pathogen in dogs and cat. In cats commonly the bacteria involved include staphylococcus (both coagulase positive and negative), *P. multocida* and beta-haemolytic streptococcus.

Bacterial infection is introduced into the skin by grooming and self-inflicted trauma.

Some of the most common predisposing factors include the following:

- Ectoparasites – demodex, scabies, fleas.
- Endocrinopathy – hypothyroidism (dog) hyperthyroidism (cat), hyperadrenocorticism.
- Allergy – food, atopy (Figure 4.15), fleas.
- Immunosuppression – iatrogenic, e.g. glucocorticoids, cyclosporines, progestagens, cytotoxic drugs; disease neoplasia (lymphoma), viral disease (cats, FeLV, FIV, FIP).

Clinical signs
- Short coated breeds – small tufts of hair leading to alopecia usually seen on the dorsum and producing a moth-eaten appearance (Figure 4.16).

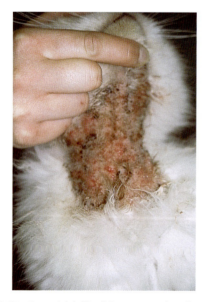

Figure 4.15 Bacterial folliculitis on ventral neck secondary to atopy.

Bacterial skin disease 35

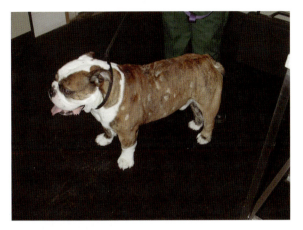

Figure 4.16 Short coat folliculitis in a bulldog.

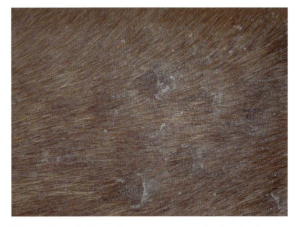

Figure 4.18 Epidermal collarettes on the flanks of a dog.

- Long coated breeds – increased hair loss leading to thinning of the coat before progressing, eventually leading to alopecia (Figure 4.17). Coat often dull and lacks lustre with excessive scaling.
- Primary lesions include follicular pustules (pustule hair protruding), papules as well as epidermal collarettes (Figure 4.18), crusts, target lesions (Figure 4.19), excoriation and alopecia with variable pruritus.
- Distribution depends on predisposing factors. Primary lesions are most obvious on glabrous skin; alopecia is noticeable on the dorsum and flanks.

Differential diagnosis
Other follicular diseases in dog and cat:

- Dermatophytosis
- Demodicosis
- Scabies
- Pemphigus foliaceus/erythematosus
- Miliary dermatitis (cat)

Diagnosis
- Skin scraping.
- Fungal examination – microscopy and culture.
- Cytology – degenerate neutrophils with evidence of bacteria with phagocytosis.
- Culture and sensitivity – sample should be taken from an intact pustule where possible.
- Histopathology from an intact pustule reveals non-specific interfollicular superficial dermatitis, with perifolliculitis and folliculitis.

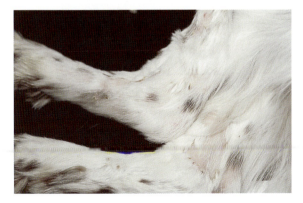

Figure 4.17 Erythema alopecia and hair loss due to staphylococcal folliculitis.

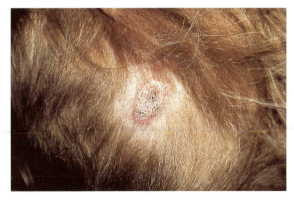

Figure 4.19 Target lesion typical of staphylococcal infection.

Treatment

- Topical therapy may be useful but is not a substitute for systemic antibiotics. Suitable topical agents include those listed under therapy of impetigo.
- Systemic antibiotics based on culture and sensitivity. Antibiotics suitable for empirical therapy include clindamycin, potentiated sulphonamides and cephalexin (see Table 4.2). Minimum courses of treatment 21–28 days (10 days beyond clinical cure).
- If pyoderma occurs within 3 months of cessation of treatment, then appropriate tests to identify predisposing factors are essential, e.g. endocrine/allergy test.
- Where a poor response to antibiotic therapy is seen, i.e. primary pustular lesions are still present whilst the animal is on therapy, consider antibiotic resistance (MRSA) or a sterile pustular disease.

Methicillin resistant *S. aureus*

A long discussion on MRSA is beyond the scope of this book. The following is intended as a brief outline only.

Cause and pathogenesis

Many different MRSA isolates have been identified. These can be categorised into 11 clonal groups: 5 are hospital acquired (HA) and 6 are community acquired (CA). Most of the cases identified in the UK in humans are HA isolates and belong to the epidemic (E) clones E15 and E16.

The carriage rate of MRSA in companion animals is unknown. However, isolates in the UK from small animal cases have identified HA-MRSA clones E15 and E16 suggesting that infection came from a human source. It would appear that there is a common link between MRSA infection in small animals and a hospital or health care worker contact. Situations where MRSA infection should be suspected are detailed in Table 4.3.

Clinical signs

- Skin lesions.
- Clinical lesions can be indistinguishable from those of non-MRSA infections in cats and dogs.

Table 4.3 Situations where MRSA should be suspected.

- Patients with non-healing wounds
- Patients with non-antibiotic responsive infections where previous cytology and/or culture indicates that staphylococci are involved
- Patients from known MRSA positive households or those belong to health care workers
- Patients with a history of chronic antibiotic therapy
- Patients that have been hospitalised after orthopaedic surgery
- Patients from a veterinary environment where there has been previous cases of MRSA

- Infection can produce signs similar to those of autoimmune disease with severe erosions and ulceration (Figure 4.20) often involving the mucocutaneous junctions in addition to the skin (Figure 4.21).
- Infection may also affect surgical wounds, especially following orthopaedic surgery or indwelling catheters.

Diagnosis

- Clinical signs, history especially failure to respond to antibiotic therapy.
- Culture – swabs should be submitted in transport medium to a laboratory capable of isolating MRSA and accurately reporting antibiotic

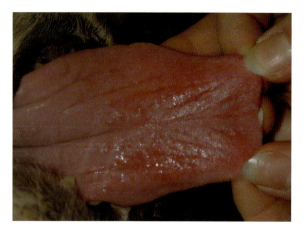

Figure 4.20 Oral ulceration seen as a result of MRSA infection.

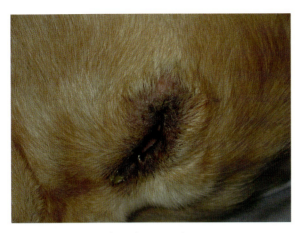

Figure 4.21 Periocular infection with MRSA.

sensitivity. MRSA control measures should be implemented whilst awaiting the bacteriology results. These include institution of strict hygiene measures and barrier nursing within the veterinary environment.
- Owners should be warned of the potential zoonotic risk, especially if immunocompromised individuals are in contact with the pet.

Treatment of MRSA
- Antibiotic selection should be based on culture and sensitivity. MRSA infection is often sensitive to potentiated sulphonamides and clindamycin, which are good empirical selections if there is a high level of suspicion of MRSA pending sensitivity results.
- Antibiotic therapy should be continued for at least 10 days beyond clinical cure and may be needed for up to 6 weeks.
- Most animals with MRSA will survive providing appropriate antibiotic therapy is instituted. Death is attributable to the underlying condition or inappropriate use of glucocorticoids and not the MRSA in most cases.
- It is suggested that most animals with MRSA infections have mucosal colonisation, although it is unclear whether this is a cause or consequence of infection. If the animal remains colonised, potential risks and precautions must be discussed with the owner.

Dermatophilosis

Rare superficial crusting dermatosis caused by *Dermatophilus congolensis* seen in both cats and dogs.

Cause and pathogenesis
Farm animals are usually source of infection. Predisposing factors:

- Moisture required for zoospore release.
- Skin trauma required to allow cutaneous penetration, e.g. ectoparasites, trauma.

Clinical signs
- Rare disease.
- Lesions usually occur on the dorsum, also face, ears and feet.
- Early lesions, papules and pustules developing into crusts.
- 'Paint brush' lesions – crusts containing embedded hair with ulcerated purulent areas.

Differential diagnosis
- Other pustular diseases, e.g. impetigo, pemphigus foliaceus, staphylococcal folliculitis.
- Seborrhoeic disease.
- Dermatophytosis.
- Zinc responsive dermatosis.

Diagnosis
- History and clinical signs.
- Direct smear of underside of crust stained with Diff-Quik – parallel rows of cocci 'rail road track'. In chronic cases this is often negative.
- Culture and sensitivity of crusts and exudate.
- Skin biopsy reveals a hyperplastic superficial perivascular dermatitis with a palisading crust of orthokeratotic parakeratosis and leukocytes.

Treatment
- Removal of predisposing factors.
- Systemic antibiotics based on culture and sensitivity. Ampicillin, cephalosporins, lincomycin useful for empirical therapy 10–14 day course (for doses, see Table 4.2).

- Crust removal using antiseborrhoeic shampoo, e.g. benzoyl peroxide is useful.

Deep bacterial infections (deep pyoderma)

Infection of deeper tissues of the dermis and often the subcutis. Infection starts as a surface or follicular insult that spreads to deeper structures and breaks out of the follicles. There are always underlying causes for the infection, which must be identified. Deep pyoderma is common in dogs and rare in cats.

Localised deep pyoderma – predisposing factors include the following:

- Self-inflicted trauma
- Wounds
- Foreign body (Figure 4.22)
- Subcutaneous abscesses (especially in cats)

Generalised deep pyoderma – predisposing factors include the following:

- Ectoparasites especially demodicosis
- Allergy
- Systemic disease causing immuno-incompetence
- Inappropriate treatment with an ineffective antibiotic or with corticosteroids

Types:

(a) Subcutaneous abscesses
(b) Furunculosis
(c) Pyotraumatic dermatitis
(d) Nasal furunculosis
(e) Chin pyoderma (canine acne)
(f) Pododermatitis
(g) German shepherd dog pyoderma
(h) Acral lick dermatitis
(i) Anaerobic cellulitis

Subcutaneous abscesses

Bite wounds are the most common reason for subcutaneous abscesses. They are the most common form of localised deep pyoderma in the cat.

Cause and pathogenesis

- Most commonly seen in all male cats prone to fighting (Figure 4.23).
- Small puncture wound from cat's canine teeth injects bacteria into the skin.
- Bacteria involved usually those of feline oral cavity, i.e. *P. multocida*, beta-haemolytic streptococcus, *Bacteroides* spp. and fusiform bacilli.
- The wound heals rapidly and a local infection develops over 48–72 hours.

Clinical signs

- Swollen area covered only by a small crust
- Common sites – tail base, shoulder, neck, leg and neck

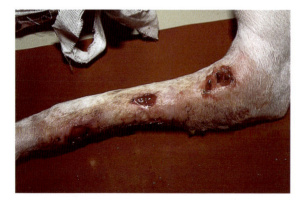

Figure 4.22 Localised deep pyoderma due to penetrating foreign body in the forelimb.

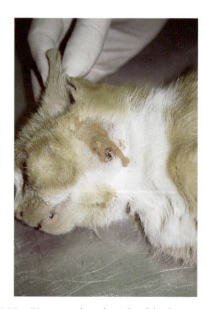

Figure 4.23 Bite wound on the side of the face.

- Area warm and painful to touch
- Animal often febrile
- Localised lymphadenopathy

Differential diagnosis
- Other less common bacteria infections
  - *Mycobacteria* spp.
  - *Yersinia pestis*
  - *Nocardia* spp.
  - *Actinomyces* spp.
- Fungal mycetoma
- Neoplasia
- Foreign body

Diagnosis
- History and clinical signs
- Aspiration of exudates – typical purulent material
- Cytology of exudates – mixed inflammatory cells with mixed bacterial population
- Response to therapy

Treatment
- Surgical drainage (sedation is often required).
- Flushing of the abscess with saline or chlorhexidine (0.025%) or EDTA tris/chlorhexidine solution.
- Antibiotics 7–10 days. Amoxicillin, clindamycin can be used for empirical therapy (see Table 4.2).
- Uncomplicated localised abscesses should heal uneventfully with appropriate therapy.
- Intact male cats should be castrated.
- If there is failure to heal, an immunosuppressive factor should be sought or other differentials explored.

Furunculosis

Furunculosis occurs when rupture of deeply infected follicles occurs within the dermis, infection spreads to involve deep levels of the dermis. Most commonly seen in dogs; rare in cats.

Cause and pathogenesis
Initial insult to follicle can be caused by bacteria, especially *S. intermedius*, but also by Gram negative bacteria such as *Pseudomonas* spp. (Figures 4.24 and 4.25). Mixed populations are common.
Underlying diseases include the following:

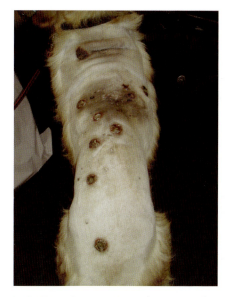

Figure 4.24 Deep Gram negative infection in a dog.

- Endocrinopathy – hypothyroidism (Figure 4.26) (dog), hyperadrenocorticism.
- Ectoparasites especially demodex, scabies.
- Primary keratinisation disorders.
- Immunosuppression through systemic disease (Figure 4.27) or through inappropriate use of anti-inflammatory drugs, e.g. glucocorticoids, cyclosporines, progestagens.
- Autoimmune skin and immune mediated disease.
- Allergy.

Clinical signs
- Depends on severity and extent of disease. Most commonly seen on pressure points and

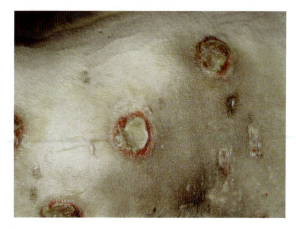

Figure 4.25 Close-up of dog in Figure 4.24.

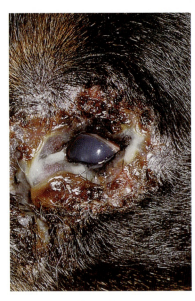

Figure 4.26 Periocular furunculosis secondary to hypothyroidism.

on the trunk, but can occur anywhere on the body.
- Early mild lesions – discrete papules progressing to ulcerated pustules and haemorrhagic bullae with crusting.
- Severe lesions – red/purple papules/bullae with fistulation discharging exudate, marked crusting.
- Lymphadenopathy is common.
- Animal usually depressed, anorexic and pyrexic.

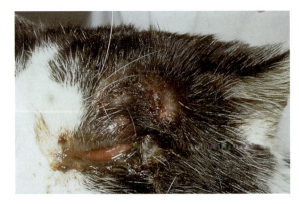

Figure 4.27 Periocular cellulitis in an immunosuppressed cat. (Source: Picture courtesy of P. Boydell.)

Differential diagnosis
- Autoimmune disease especially sterile pustular diseases
- Drug eruption
- Erythema multiforme
- Neoplasia
- Deep fungal infection

Diagnosis
- History and clinical signs.
- Cytology of exudates, stained with Diff-Quik. Mixed inflammatory infiltrate with bacteria often cocci also rods.
- Skin scrapings.
- Fungal culture.
- Bacteriology – culture and sensitivity (aerobic and anaerobic):
  - Surface swabs may give unrepresentative results due to contamination with oral flora, tissue culture usually better taken from biopsy.
- Biopsy – deep suppurative to pyogranulomatous folliculitis with furunculosis.
- Investigation of underlying cause.

Treatment
- Any underlying cause should be identified and treated.
- Antibiotics based on culture and sensitivity 6–8 weeks minimum at least 2 weeks beyond clinical cure.
- Clipping and cleansing lesions – under sedation/GA if necessary. Often large areas of the dog need to be clipped out.
- Deep cleansing bath soaks and whirlpool treatment may be useful.
- Antibacterial washes/soaks, e.g. acetic acid, chlorhexidine, ethyl lactate (see topical therapy for impetigo). Benzoyl peroxide may be too harsh on open sores.
- Calamine lotion to dry lesions.
- Treatment of underlying conditions essential.
- If there is concurrent pruritus then an Elizabethan collar should be used to prevent self-traumatisation, or sedating antihistamines, e.g. promethazine 12.5–50 mg po bid; glucocorticoids are contraindicated.

Pyotraumatic folliculitis

Clinical appearance similar to acute moist dermatitis/hot spot, but is a deep infective process and therefore different management. Common in dogs and uncommon in cats.

Cause and pathogenesis
- As for acute moist dermatitis – may be a progression from the surface infection; often other immunosuppressive factors are present, e.g. concurrent immunosuppressive disease. In cats may be secondary to viral disease, e.g. FeLV, FIV.
- Predisposed dog breeds: golden retriever, Labrador retriever.

Clinical signs
- Thickened, plaque-like skin – usually neck, cheek, rump.
- Satellite papules and pustules indicate deep infective process compared to localised surface lesions in a true 'hot spot' (Figure 4.28).

Differential diagnosis
- Acute moist dermatitis (surface infection)
- Neoplasia
- Eosinophilic granuloma (cat)

Diagnosis
As for furunculosis.

Treatment
- As for furunculosis.
- Elizabethan collar may help reduce traumatisation.

Nasal folliculitis/furunculosis

Cause and pathogenesis
- Deep infection of bridge of nose extending around nostrils, uncommon in dogs and rare in cats.
- May be created by trauma to the area, especially due to rooting or associated with insect bites.
- Predisposed breeds: German shepherd dog, English bull terrier, Border collie.

Clinical signs
- Acute papules and pustules (Figure 4.29) rapidly progressing to furunculosis with associated erythema, alopecia and swelling.
- Lesion usually painful.
- Lesions only affect the haired area of the skin and there is sparing of the planum nasale unlike autoimmune skin disease.
- Scarring usually occurs.

Differential diagnosis
- Autoimmune skin disease
- Drug eruption
- Dermatomyositis
- Demodicosis
- Dermatophytosis especially *Trichophyton mentagrophytes*

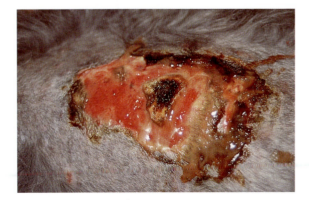

Figure 4.28 Pyotraumatic dermatitis due to atopy in a hypothyroid dog; note the presence of satellite lesions to denote deep infective process.

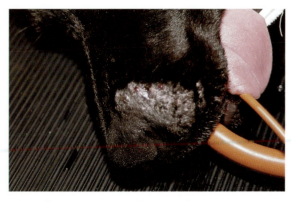

Figure 4.29 Nasal furunculosis in a Labrador secondary to allergy.

- Sterile nasal eosinophilic folliculitis/furunculosis
- Mosquito bite hypersensitivity (cat)

Diagnosis
- As for furunculosis.
- Cytology reveals signs of mixed inflammatory infiltrate with bacteria usually *Staphylococcus* spp. Polymorphs are mostly neutrophils compared to eosinophilic folliculitis, which is exclusively eosinophilic with few bacteria.

Treatment
- As for furunculosis.
- Topical treatment is difficult to use because of the pain of the lesions; however, if possible gently applied warm water soaks may be used daily to decrease scarring and remove crust.
- Prognosis good but scarring can occur.

Chin pyoderma (canine acne)

Deep folliculitis/furunculosis of the chin and lips of young dogs; very rare in cats.

Cause and pathogenesis
- Follicular damage initially sterile caused by trauma to the chin from
  - lying on hard floors,
  - friction from chew toys,
  - pruritus due to allergy.
- Bacterial infection occurs secondarily to trauma.
- Androgens limited role as condition can be seen in neutered dogs and females.
- Genetic predisposition may exist. Predisposed dog breeds: large short coated especially English bulldog, Great Dane, mastiffs and Boxer (Figure 4.30).

Clinical signs
- Initial signs non-painful, non-pruritic comedones.
- Alopecia, follicular papules develop into localised furunculosis.
- Serosanguinous discharge can be severe.

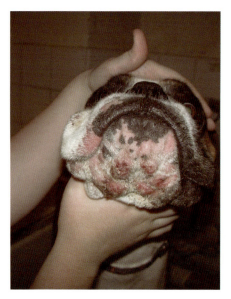

Figure 4.30 Chin furunculosis.

Differential diagnosis
- Demodicosis
- Dermatophytosis
- Contact dermatitis
- Juvenile cellulitis

Diagnosis
- History and clinical signs especially in predisposed breeds.
- Cytology – mixed inflammatory infiltrate with bacteria usually *Staphylococcus* spp.
- Skin scrapes to rule out demodex.
- Biopsy – folliculitis and furunculosis, often bacteria not seen on sections.

Treatment
- Remove and treat any underlying factors.
- Mild cases – benzoyl peroxide shampoo daily followed by fusidic acid cream. Should be applied daily until clinical remission, then every 3–5 days for maintenance.
- Severe cases – secondary bacterial infection with keratin and hair as foreign bodies in the skin.
- Antibiotics are needed for 4–6 weeks based on culture and sensitivity in combination with topical therapy.

- In many dogs response is complete and life long in others; long-term therapy is required.

Pododermatitis (interdigital pyoderma)

Cause and pathogenesis
Folliculitis and furunculosis of the feet often affect interdigital spaces. Initial lesions may be sterile and infection is secondary in many chronic cases. Common in dogs and rare in cats. Often referred to as interdigital cyst, these are not true cysts. There are numerous underlying causes; see Table 4.4.

Table 4.4 Causes of pododermatitis.

Lesion confined to a single foot	Lesions affect multiple feet
Foreign body, e.g. grass awn (Figure 4.31)	Contact irritant/allergy
Trauma – harsh flooring, rough ground	Allergy – food, atopy (Figure 4.32)
Conformation – due to orthopaedic disease or breed, e.g. Pekingese, bulldogs	Conformation – due to orthopaedic disease or breed, e.g. Pekingese, bulldogs
Fungal infection with dermatophytosis	Fungal infection with dermatophytosis
Neoplasia – squamous cell carcinoma, mast cell tumour, plasmacytoma	Neoplasia especially lymphoma
Abnormal weight bearing on that leg due to disease on another limb	Psychogenic lesions – nervous dogs, e.g. poodles
	Sterile pyogranulomas especially in English bulldog, dachshund, Great Dane, Boxer
	Ectoparasites, e.g. demodex, *Pelodera*, hookworms, ticks, Neotrombicula
	Bacterial infection due to immunodeficiency, endocrinopathy (Figure 4.33)

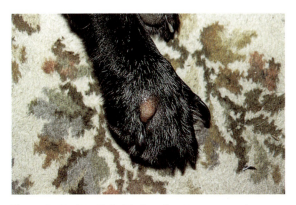

Figure 4.31 Interdigital lesion due to a penetrating grass seed.

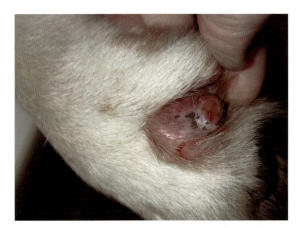

Figure 4.32 Interdigital lesions in an atopic Labrador.

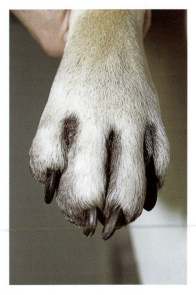

Figure 4.33 Multiple interdigital lesions secondary to hypothyroidism in a Great Dane.

Clinical signs
- Lesions found especially on the front feet.
- Interdigital erythema with pustules, nodules, fistulae, haemorrhagic bullae, fistulae, ulcers.
- Exudate variable, may be serosanguinous or haemorrhagic.
- Pruritus depends on cause, but usually painful, dog often lame.
- Predisposed breeds: English bulldog, Great Dane, English bull terrier, Boxer, German shepherd dog, Labrador retriever, golden retriever.

Diagnosis
As furunculosis, including the following:

- Cytology useful to assess degree of infection and make decision such as whether culture is needed:
    - Mixed inflammatory infiltrate usually cocci (*Staphylococcus* spp.) occasionally rods. If rods are present tissue culture indicated.
- Biopsy – suppurative to pyogranulomatous perifolliculitis, folliculitis, furunculosis. Nodular to diffuse pyogranulomatous dermatitis. Intralesional bacteria may be difficult to find.
- Investigation of underlying disease may include the following:
    - Radiography for bony changes underlying cutaneous lesions, radiopaque foreign bodies.
    - MRI may be necessary on occasions to identify foreign material.
    - Routine blood samples – endocrine tests.
    - Allergy investigation.

Treatment
Single lesions:

- Exploration of lesion under anaesthetic, flush dilute chlorhexidine/EDTA chlorhexidine.
- Antibiotics often not necessary.

Multiple lesions:

- Treatment of specific underlying disease is essential.
- Systemic antibiotics based on culture and sensitivity for 6–8 weeks and for at least 2 weeks beyond clinical cure. Secondary infection is common and thus should be eliminated in all cases before any anti-inflammatory therapy is prescribed.
- Cleansing antibacterial wipes may be useful for therapy and for maintenance after resolution.
- Foot soaks may be useful for 10–15 minute period in antibacterial washes, e.g. acetic acid, chlorhexidine, ethyl lactate or regular shampoos, if the dog will allow it.
- Topical antibiotics – fusidic acid (mupirocin 2% should be avoided in view of its use in cases of MRSA). Especially useful for treatment of early superficial lesions and for maintenance once deep infection has been treated.
- Sterile dermal granulomas – prednisolone 1 mg/kg po sid for 10 days, then alternate days.
- Protection of feet – boots, etc. Useful in chronic cases where there is pronounced secondary changes to the feet, such as abnormal healing of the pads that does not allow natural weight bearing.
- Fusion podoplasty can be undertaken as a salvage procedure in severe cases whereby all diseased interdigital tissue is removed and the digits are fused together.

German shepherd dog pyoderma

Deep folliculitis/furunculosis/cellulitis often idiopathic of middle-aged German shepherd dogs and German shepherd dog crosses of both sexes.

Cause and pathogenesis
It is thought that these dogs have an inherited immune incompetence triggered through an insult to the skin or immune system. Familial predisposition is often seen.

Bacterial infection is usually with coagulase positive *Staphylococcus* spp. However in chronic cases, especially those that have had multiple antibiotic treatments, overgrowth with commensal bacteria can cause infection.

Many contributory factors, no one cause in all cases:

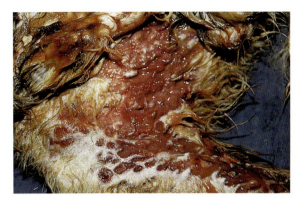

Figure 4.34 Severe furunculosis on the medical aspect of the hind leg in German shepherd dog pyoderma.

- Endocrine diseases especially hypothyroidism, also hyperadrenocorticism.
- Allergy especially flea allergic dermatitis, also atopy, food allergy.

Clinical signs
- Signs may be generalised but often start on dorsum, rump, ventral abdomen, uncommonly legs, head, neck.
- Lesions may start as typical signs of superficial pyoderma with papules, pustules but progress to deep-seated folliculitis/furunculosis, ulcers, haemorrhagic bullae, exudative lesions with serosanguineous exudate (Figure 4.34).
- Skin: painful and discoloured.
- Variable degrees of pruritus but can be severe self-inflicted trauma due to pruritus.
- Dogs debilitated, anorexic, pyrexic with weight loss seen in severe cases.

Diagnosis
As furunculosis.
- Cytology – mixed inflammatory infiltrate with bacteria often cocci (*Staphylococcus* spp.); however, rods can be seen.
- Antibiotic therapy is best based on culture and sensitivity taken from tissue culture.
- Strenuous efforts should be made to identify any underlying factors; supplementary tests should include the following:
  - ☐ Routine haematology and biochemistry
  - ☐ Thyroid function test
  - ☐ High levels of ectoparasite control especially fleas and scabies
  - ☐ Food trial
  - ☐ Allergy tests
  - ☐ Skin scrapes and biopsies for demodicosis

Treatment
- Important to identify and treat any contributory factors.
- Antibiotic and topical treatment as furunculosis.
- Dogs benefit from antibacterial soaks, gentle shampoo therapy and whirlpool baths.
- Clinical course variable; some cases resolve with treatment, especially if an underlying cause can be identified.
- In severe cases, relapses are common and these dogs require lifetime treatment.

Acral lick granuloma
- For investigation and underlying causes, see Chapter 16 – Psychogenic skin disease.
- There is almost always a deep infective process associated with this disease.
- Bacterial infection should be treated as localised furunculosis.

Anaerobic cellulitis

Deep bacterial infection dissecting through tissue planes. Uncommon in dogs and rare in cats.

Cause and pathogenesis
- Commonly seen after puncture wounds, especially bites and penetrating foreign bodies.
- Infection can also occur after surgery, trauma (Figure 4.35), burns and neoplasia.
- May also result as a progression from inadequately treated superficial pyoderma.

Clinical signs
- Poorly demarcated lesions, oedema, swelling and necrosis.
- Skin friable, dark, discoloured and will slough easily.
- Malodorous discharge from sinus tracts and furuncles often with crepitus.
- Bacteria involved include *Clostridium* spp. and *Bacteroides* spp. (Figure 4.36).
- Animal systemically ill, pyrexic, anorexic and lethargic.

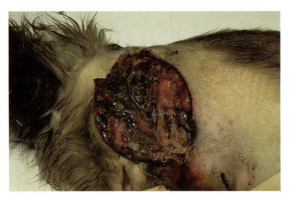

Figure 4.35 Anaerobic infection on the shoulder of a Pomeranian after a bite wound.

Diagnosis
- History and clinical signs.
- Exudative cytology – degenerate polymorphs with bacteria, rods and cocci.
- Skin scrapings.
- Culture and sensitivity should be for both aerobic and anaerobic infection from discharge or from tissue culture.

Treatment
- Surgical debridement may be necessary.
- Antibiotics based on culture and sensitivity may require 8–12 weeks of therapy and should be for 2 weeks beyond clinical cure. Useful drugs include clindamycin, cephalosporins and metronidazole.
- Topical therapy as furunculosis with antibacterial shampoos and soaks. Animals benefit from whirlpool baths.

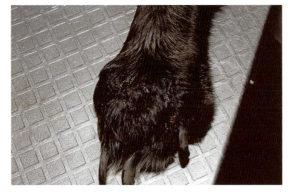

Figure 4.36 Anaerobic infection with *Bacteroides* spp. in a dog with chronic pododermatitis.

Uncommon pyogranulomatous bacterial infections

(a) Bacterial pseudomycetoma
(b) Mycobacterial infection
(c) Opportunistic mycobacteria
(d) Feline leprosy
(e) Actinomycosis
(f) Actinbacillosis
(g) Nocardiosis

Bacterial pseudomycetoma (botryomycosis)

Chronic pyogranulomatous infection caused by non-branching bacteria, which form tissue granules. Uncommon disease in dogs and cats.

Cause and pathogenesis
- Usually coagulase positive *Staphylococcus* spp., less commonly *Pseudomonas* spp., *Proteus* spp., *Streptococcus* spp. and *Actinobacillus* spp.
- Commonly seen after puncture wounds penetrating injury, bites, foreign body reaction.
- Pyogranuloma forms as host contains infection but cannot eliminate it.

Clinical signs
- Firm nodules usually non-painful and non-pruritic. May be single or multiple.
- Purulent discharge contains small white tissue grains (which are macroscopic colonies of bacteria).
- Site depends on initial insult; any area of body can be affected but extremities common.
- Lesions usually insidious onset.

Differential diagnosis
- Other infectious granulomas:
  - actinomycosis
  - nocardiosis
  - mycobacteria
  - *Yersinia pestis* (cat)
- Eumycotic mycetoma
- Dermatophytic pseudomycetoma

- Systemic mycosis
- Sterile pyogranulomatous disease
- Neoplasia

Diagnosis

- History and clinical signs especially presence of tissue grains.
- Cytology of exudates – typically neutrophils and macrophages with granules that are composed of dense bacterial colonies.
- Skin biopsy – examination should include special fungal and bacterial stains. Typical picture nodular to diffuse pyogranulomatous dermatitis and panniculitis with tissue grains containing bacteria.

Treatment

- Nodules need to be surgically excised.
- Post-operative antibiotics should be given for at least 4 weeks based on tissue culture.
- Without surgery antibiotics are rarely effective alone.
- Prognosis after appropriate therapy is good.

Mycobacterial infections

Cutaneous form of tuberculosis. Very rare mycobacterial infection in dogs and cats.

Cause and pathogenesis

- Most commonly, infection is passed from humans and contaminated meat or milk.
- Usually caused by *Mycobacterium tuberculosis*, *Mycobacterium bovis* and *Mycobacterium tuberculosis-bovis*.
- Rarely *M. avium* complex – environmental saprophyte of less public health concern.

Clinical signs

- Respiratory and gastrointestinal signs most common, leading to weight loss, cough, dyspnoea, vomiting or diarrhoea.
- Cutaneous lesions present as single/multiple ulcers, abscesses, plaques and nodules (Figure 4.37), especially on head, neck and limbs.

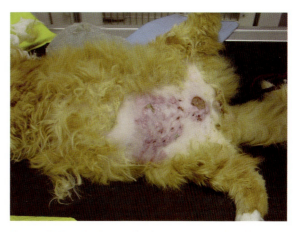

Figure 4.37 Mycobacterial infection on ventral abdomen of cat. (Source: Copyright 2008, Ellie Mardell.)

- Variable malodorous yellow/green discharge – no tissue grains present.
- Associated anorexia, pyrexia, and lymphadenopathy.

Differential diagnosis

As bacterial pseudomycetoma.

Diagnosis

- Radiography of chest to check for pulmonary lesions.
- Biopsy should include special stain for mycobacteria (Ziehl–Neelson) – nodular to diffuse pyogranulomatous dermatitis with variable numbers of intracellular acid fast, positive bacilli.
- Culture – laboratory needs to be alerted to use special media to harvest bacteria.
- Bacille Calmette–Guerin (BCG) or purified protein derivative intradermal test. Erythema with central necrosis is seen at the injection site 10–14 days if a positive result occurs.

Treatment

- Public health authority should be notified and asked for guidance.
- *M. tuberculosis* and *M. bovis* – euthanasia due to public health risk.
- If euthanasia is not an option then chemotherapy may be useful in some cases (see Table 4.5).

Table 4.5 Possible therapies for tuberculosis.

Mycobacterium	Drugs and dose rate
M. tuberculosis	Dogs and cats: isoniazid 10–20 mg/kg po sid plus ethambutol 15 mg/kg im sid Dogs only: pyrazinamide 15–40 mg/kg po sid plus rifampin 10–20 mg/kg bid/sid
M. bovis	Cats after surgical excision: rifampin 4 mg/kg po sid
M. tuberculosis/ M. bovis	Cats: rifampin 10–20 mg/kg po sid plus enrofloxacin 5–10 mg/kg po sid/bid plus clarithromycin 5–10 mg/kg po bid
M. avium	Dogs and cats: Doxycycline 10 mg/kg po bid or clofazimine 4 mg/kg po sid plus enrofloxacin 5–10 mg/kg po sid/bid plus clarithromycin 5 mg/kg po bid

- *M. avium* – antibiotic therapy may be used based on culture and sensitivity. Surgical removal of lesions or cryosurgery often produces only temporary success.

Opportunistic mycobacterial infections

Granulomatous disease caused by atypical mycobacterium, rare in dogs and uncommon in cats.

Cause and pathogenesis

- Free living saprophytic organisms usually harmless but can be facultative pathogens when inadvertently inoculated into the skin, usually through bites (Figure 4.38).
- Obese animals may be predisposed.
- Sources of infection include soil and artificial and natural water sources. Facultative pathogens include *M. fortuitum*, *M. chelonei*, *M. xenopi*, *M. smegmatis*, *M. phlei*, *M. thermoresistible* and *M. visibilis*. Cats most commonly *M. fortuitum* and *M. chelonei*.

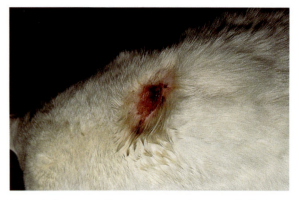

Figure 4.38 Atypical mycobacteria infection in flank.

- Not considered to be a zoonotic risk or contagious to other animals.

Clinical signs

- Lesions develop over several weeks at any site, usually localised at the site of inoculation.
- Present as chronic non-healing abscesses with fistulae, focal purple depressions intermingled with punctuate ulcers that drain serosanguinous or purulent discharge.
- Most commonly found caudal abdomen, lower back and pelvic areas, especially in cats adipose tissue of inguinal and caudal abdomen.
- Pain and lymphadenopathy variable.
- Lesions can expand to involve large areas of abdomen.
- Dissemination to internal organs is rare.
- Cats usually depressed, lethargic, anorexic, reluctant to move.

Differential diagnosis

As bacterial pseudomycetoma.

Diagnosis

- History and clinical signs.
- Cytology best undertaken by fine needle aspirates of closed lesions. Findings neutrophils, macrophages. Intracellular acid fast bacilli difficult to see with routine stains.
- Mycobacterial culture often successful in isolating organism compared to those of leprosy.

Table 4.6 Antibiotics useful for therapy of opportunistic mycobacteria.

Drug	Dose rate
Ciprofloxacin	62.5–125 mg/cat po bid
Clarithromycin	5–10 mg/kg po bid
Clofazimine	8 mg/kg po sid
Doxycycline or minocycline	5–12.5 mg/kg po bid or 25–50 mg/cat po tid or bid immediately after meals
Enrofloxacin	5–15 mg/kg po bid or 25–75 mg/cat po sid (use with care in cats due to potential retinal toxicity)
Marbofloxacin	2.75–5.5 mg/kg po bid

- Biopsy reveals nodular to diffuse pyogranulomatous dermatitis and panniculitis. Intralesional organisms may be difficult to find.

Treatment

- Spontaneous resolution uncommon.
- Wide surgical excision of infected tissue is necessary, taking care not to spread infection along tissue grains.
- Chemotherapy for relapses or if surgery not possible.
- Antibiotics based on sensitivity needed for long courses, 3–6 months, and should be continued for 6–8 weeks after clinical cure. Useful drugs are listed in Table 4.6.
- Doxycycline may be useful prophylactically after penetrating wounds in cats to prevent colonisation with atypical mycobacteria.
- Prognosis for cure is poor, although appropriate therapy and long-term therapy will allow the animal to live a good quality of life.

Feline leprosy syndrome

Granulomatous infection thought to be caused by two different acid fast organisms. Uncommon disease of cats.

Cause and Pathogenesis

- Infection caused by two poorly characterised mycobacterial species.
- Agents are difficult to culture and only identified on stained biopsy sections.
- Thought to be caused by *Mycobacterium lepraemurium* and an un-named mycobacterial species.

Clinical signs

M. lepraemurium: young cats <4 years of age:

- Rapidly progressive lesions in that widespread involvement may only take 2 months. Lesions are non-painful: single or multiple nodules often with non-healing fistulae. Lesions of variable size: a few mm up to 4 cm.
- Lesions can be found at any site but usually found on head or extremities as single or groups of nodules.
- Cat systemically well, no systemic spread to internal organs.

Unknown species: older cats >9 years with immunosuppressive disease, e.g. FeLV:

- Lesions start as localised, non-painful, non-ulcerated subcutaneous and cutaneous nodules on head or extremities.
- Lesions spread slowly over months to years and will occasionally affect internal organs.

Differential diagnosis

As bacterial pseudomycetoma.

Diagnosis

- History and clinical signs.
- Cytology from a fine needle aspirate or an impression smear – mixed inflammatory infiltrate with some intracellular acid fast bacilli that do not stain on routine smears.
- Biopsy reveals diffuse pyogranulomatous dermatitis and panniculitis with intracellular and extracellular acid fast bacilli. *M. lepraemurium* lesions tend to have caseous necrosis and moderate numbers of bacteria,

- Un-named bacilli have no caseous necrosis and large numbers of bacilli.
- Culture is almost always negative due to difficulty in growing the organisms.
- Polymerase chain reaction techniques can be used to identify the organisms DNA.

Treatment

M. lepraemurium:

- Complete surgical removal carries the highest success rate for single or well-circumscribed lesions. Risk with surgery of spreading infection along tissue lines.
- If surgical removal is not possible then medical therapy can be employed:
  - Clofazimine 8–10 mg/kg po sid or 50 mg/cat po every 48 hours. Long courses of therapy are needed and for at least 2–3 months after clinical cure.

Unknown mycobacterium:

- Surgical excision is rarely possible.
- Medical therapy may be useful using
  - clarithromycin 62.5 mg/cat po bid and rifampin 10–15 mg/kg po sid; therapy needs to be for several months and for at least 2 months beyond clinical cure.

Canine leproid granuloma syndrome

Cutaneous mycobacterial disease of dogs caused by an unknown mycobacterium.

Cause and pathogenesis

Thought to be caused by an environmental mycobacterium that is inoculated into the skin of dogs by biting flies. It has been reported on the African continent, America, New Zealand and Australia.

Clinical signs

- Lesions appear as single to multiple well-circumscribed subcutaneous nodules.
- Nodules range from a few mm to 5 cm in size and are non-painful and non-pruritic.
- Most commonly, lesions have been described on the head and dorsal ear folds.
- Dogs are systemically well, no spread to internal organs has been recognised.

Differential diagnoses

As bacterial pseudomycetoma.

Diagnosis

- History and clinical signs.
- Cytology from a fine needle aspirate: mixed inflammatory infiltrate mostly macrophages with a few to moderate numbers of medium length intracellular (within macrophages) and extracellular acid fast bacilli that do not stain on routine smears.
- Biopsy reveals diffuse pyogranulomatous dermatitis and panniculitis with intracellular and extracellular acid fast bacilli.
- Culture negative due to difficulty growing the organisms.
- Polymerase chain reaction techniques used to identify novel organisms DNA.

Treatment

- Self-limiting disease as lesions regress within 3–4 weeks.
- If lesions do not resolve then excisional surgery is best form of therapy.
- In severe refractory cases combination therapy with rifampin and clarithromycin or rifampin and doxycycline may be used.

Actinomycosis

Pyogranulomatous or suppurative disease caused by Gram positive anaerobic filamentous *Actinomyces* organisms, including *A. viscosus.*, *A. odontolyticus*. Rare in cats, uncommon in dogs.

Cause and pathogenesis

- Opportunistic commensals of gastrointestinal tract.

- Infection caused by contamination of penetrating wounds with *Actinomyces* spp., especially seen in outdoor and hunting dogs.

Clinical signs

Dogs:

- Insidious disease lesions can occur up to 2 years after injury.
- Firm to fluctuant painful abscesses seen at any site.
- Fistulae and exudate variable, discharge variable colour and consistency usually malodorous.
- Yellow-tan soft granules (macroscopic colonies of actinomycetes) seen in 50% of cases.
- Infection may spread to involve other organs: e.g. osteomyelitis, abdominal or thoracic cavity.

Cats:

- Most commonly seen as a pyothorax or as subcutaneous abscesses.
- Exudate from abscess malodorous, serosanguinous to purulent.

Differential diagnosis

As bacterial pseudomycetoma especially nocardiosis.

Diagnosis

- History and clinical signs.
- Direct smear of fine needle aspirates with Gram stain – suppurative to pyogranulomatous inflammation with mixed population of bacteria. Actinomycetes appear as Gram positive beaded filamentous organisms.
- Anaerobic culture is needed to identify organisms that can be difficult to culture.
- Biopsy reveals nodular to diffuse suppurative to pyogranulomatous dermatitis plus panniculitis. May contain tissue grains of Gram positive filamentous organisms.

Table 4.7 Drug therapies for Actinomycosis.

Drug	Dose rate
Penicillin G potassium po, sq, im, iv OR Penicillin V potassium po	60,000 U/kg tid
Clindamycin	5–10 mg/kg sq bid
Erythromycin	10 mg/kg po tid
Minocycline	5–25 mg/kg iv or po bid
Amoxicillin	20–40 mg/kg im, sq or po qid

Treatment

- Wide surgical excision preferable – risk of spread of infection along tissue planes.
- Debulk and chemotherapy if surgery not possible.
- Penicillin G potassium drug of choice. Other suitable drugs are listed with this in Table 4.7. Treatment is needed for 1 month after complete remission, minimum 3–4 months.
- Relapses common, prognosis for complete cure is guarded.

Actinobacillosis

Pyogranulomatous disease caused by Gram negative aerobic coccobacillus *Actinobacillus lignieresii*. Rare disease in dogs and cats.

Cause and pathogenesis

- Commensal of the oral cavity.
- Infection occurs by contamination of injury around face and mouth.

Clinical signs

- Lesions insidious onset, develop over weeks to months.
- Painful abscesses often neck and mouth.
- Exudate thick white/green – odourless.
- Yellow sulphur granules often present.

Differential diagnosis

As bacterial pseudomycetoma.

Diagnosis

- History and clinical signs.
- Direct smear of fine needle aspirate – Gram stain. Mixed inflammatory infiltrate Gram negative coccobacilli.
- Aerobic culture of pus.
- Biopsy – nodular to diffuse suppurative to pyogranulomatous dermatitis plus panniculitis. Tissue grains usually present

Treatment

- Wide surgical excision.
- Drainage, curettage and chemotherapy if surgery not possible.
- Useful drugs include sodium iodide (20 mg/kg or 0.2 mL/kg of 20% solution orally twice daily), streptomycin, sulphonamides, and tetracycline.
- Treatment for 1 month after remission therapy for a minimum 3–4 months.
- Relapses common and prognosis is guarded.

Nocardiosis

Pyogenic and suppurative infection caused by Gram positive, partially acid fast branching filamentous aerobe *Nocardia* sp. especially *N.asteroides, N.brasiliensis* Uncommon in dogs and rare in cats.

Cause and pathogenesis

- Soil saprophytes normally non-pathogenic.
- Infection by wound contamination, inhalation and ingestion.
- Common in immuno-compromised animals.

Clinical signs

- Localised nodules with cellulites and abscess formation. Secondary ulceration and fistulous tracts.
- Lesions tend to occur on areas of wounding, i.e. the limbs, feet (Figure 4.39) and abdomen (cats).

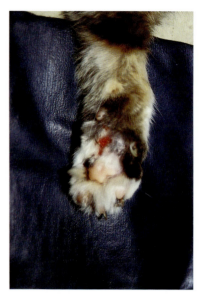

Figure 4.39 *Nocardia* infection on the footpad.

- Systemic signs include pyothorax, pyrexia, depression, inappetance and dyspnoea.
- Neurological signs may be present.

Differential diagnosis

As bacterial pseudomycetoma.

Diagnosis

- History and clinical signs.
- Direct smear of fine needle aspirate – Gram stain. Nocardia differ to *Actinomyces* spp. as partial acid fast and branch at right angles, can look like Chinese characters.
- Aerobic culture needed for isolation.
- Biopsy reveals a nodular to diffuse dermatitis with panniculitis often with tissue grains.

Treatment

- Surgical drainage in combination with antibiotic therapy.
- Antibiotic therapy based on culture and sensitivity where possible.
- Useful drugs include potentiated sulphonamides, ampicillin combined with erythromycin or cephalosporin.

- Treatment should be for at least 1 month after remission and a minimum 3–4 months.
- Prognosis guarded.

Plague

Rare zoonotic disease caused by facultative anaerobic Gram negative coccobacillus *Yersinia pestis*. Dogs resistant to infection. Uncommon disease in cats but they are susceptible.

Cause and pathogenesis

- Yersinia cannot penetrate broken skin but can invade mucous membranes.
- Cats are infected when eating infected rodent, which act as the reservoir for infection, and are bitten by rodent fleas, which act as the vector for Yersinia.
- 3 forms recognised – bubonic, pneumonic and septicaemic plague. Bubonic is most common
- Incubation period 1–2 days by ingestion or inhalation but 2–6 days by flea bite, penetrating wound or mucous membrane.
- Humans become infected by cats bringing home fleas or dead rodents or from feline body fluids, e.g. pus, saliva.

Clinical signs

- Usually occurs as an acute and fatal disease; 50% of cases bubonic plague present with skin signs.
- Localised abscesses occur near infection site, especially head and neck. Often lymph node abscessation occurs (bubo) with accompanying lymphadenopathy.
- Septicaemic and pneumonic form less common. Seen as pyrexia, anorexia, depression – up to 75% mortality, often not diagnosed until advanced and fatal.

Differential diagnosis

As bacterial pseudomycetoma as well as

- Wound infections
- Cat abscesses

Diagnosis

- History and clinical signs.
- Cytology of exudates or lymph node aspirate mixed inflammatory infiltrate with small Gram negative bipolar coccobacilli.
- Culture of exudate.
- Immunofluorescence of impression smears or polymerase chain reaction technique of exudates or lymph node aspirate to detect *Yersinia pestis* antigen.
- Serology – fourfold increase in antibody to *Yersinia pestis* in two samples taken 14 days apart.

Treatment

- Prompt therapy important due to rapid and fatal progression of the disease.
- Barrier nursing should be practiced and animals should be isolated as any fluids from infected animals are contagious.
- Antibiotics should be started at the earliest possible opportunity and given parenterally to avoid risk to veterinary staff or owner. A minimum of 3 weeks is required and should be extended well beyond clinical cure.
- Antibiotics based on culture and sensitivity where possible. Useful drugs are listed in Table 4.8.
- Flea treatment with a rapidly acting adulticide is essential.
- Abscesses should be lanced and flushed with 0.025% chlorhexidine.
- Asymptomatic in contacts may be treated with tetracycline 20 mg/kg po bid for 7 days.
- Prognosis is very poor unless cases are caught early.

Table 4.8 Drugs useful for therapy of plaque.

Drugs	Dosage
Gentamicin	2–4 mg/kg im or sq sid or bid
Chloramphenicol	15 mg/kg im or iv bid
Trimethoprim sulphadiazine	15 mg/kg im or iv bid

L-form infections

Skin infection caused by cell wall deficient bacteria similar to *Mycoplasma* spp. Disease is uncommon in cats and rare in dogs.

Cause and pathogenesis

Mode of infection is usually by contamination of bite wounds or surgical wounds.

Clinical signs

- Cutaneous signs include persistent and spreading cellulitis and synovitis, exudate non-odorous, often over joints.
- Systemic signs include commonly pyrexia, depressed and polyarthropathy.

Differential diagnosis

As bacterial pseudomycetoma.

Diagnosis

- History and clinical signs.
- Cytology of exudates – pyogranulomatous inflammation, bacteria cannot be seen.
- Culture unsuccessful unless special L-form medium is used.
- Biopsy – pyogranulomatous dermatitis with non-specific non-diagnostic pattern.
- Electron microscopy of fresh tissue reveals pleomorphic cell wall deficient organisms in macrophages.

Treatment

- Usually unresponsive to range of antibiotics usually used to treat pyoderma.
- Complete response seen to tetracycline at dose of 22 mg/kg po tid or doxycycline 5–10 mg/kg po bid. Treatment should be continued for 7–10 days beyond clinical cure.

Lyme borreliosis

Multisystemic disease caused by Gram negative spirochete *Borrelia burgdorferi*. Rare disease in both dogs and cats.

Cause and pathogenesis

Spread by hard-shelled ticks of the genus *Ixodes*.

Clinical signs

- Most common signs not cutaneous but polyarthropathy.
- Cutaneous lesions very rare and variable, tend to occur 1–2 weeks at site of tick bite.
- Urticaria, papules, acute moist dermatitis has all been recorded.

Diagnosis

- History and clinical signs.
- Serology – cross reactivity is seen with other species of spirochetes, so positive titre not diagnostic and a rising or falling titre is more useful.

Treatment

Antibiotics, especially tetracycline and ampicillin 10–14 days.

Bacterial skin infections associated with primary immunodeficiencies

Primary immunological defects lead to increased susceptibility to infection. These diseases should be considered when infection occurs in young animals where no cause can be identified.

Severe combined immunodeficiency

Both B and T cell lines non-functional.

Clinical signs

- Young puppies, basset hound predisposed.
- Severe bacterial pyoderma, otitis, diarrhoea and respiratory infections.
- Death before 4 months of age.

Treatment

Usually ineffective.

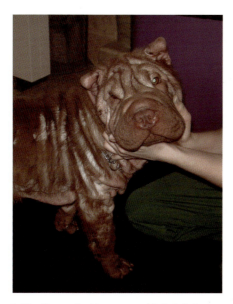

Figure 4.40 Shar-pei with suspected IgA deficiency.

Selective IgA deficiency

Deficiency of mucosal antibody IgA.

Clinical signs

- Young dogs especially shar-peis (Figure 4.40).
- Upper respiratory tract infections, otitis, staphylococcal pyoderma and atopic dermatitis.
- Not usually life threatening.

Treatment

Chronic antibiotic therapy.

Transient hypogammaglobulinaemia

Delayed onset of immunoglobulin synthesis seen in young puppies.

Clinical signs

Bacterial upper respiratory tract and skin infections start at 2–3 months of age.

Treatment

Spontaneous recovery occurs at 5–6 months of age.

Cyclic haematopoiesis

Cyclic fluctuation of all cellular blood elements.

Clinical signs

- Cyclic signs are seen during signs of neutropaenia approximately 8–12 days lasting 2–4 days.
- Grey collies predisposed.
- Recurrent gastrointestinal and skin infections occur.
- Haemorrhages associated with thrombocytopenia.
- Life expectancy approximately 3 years.

Treatment

Supportive antibiotic therapy – bactericidal drugs.

Granulocytopathy syndrome

Leukocyte adhesion molecule deficiency.

Clinical signs

- Young dogs, Irish setter predisposed.
- Recurrent bacterial dermatitis, gingivitis, osteomyelitis.

Treatment

Supportive antibiotic therapy – bactericidal drugs.

C3 deficiency

Lack of complement component important for a bacterial opsonisation.

Clinical signs

- Young dogs, Brittany spaniel predisposed.
- Recurrent Gram negative bacterial infections and *Clostridia* spp.

Treatment

Supportive antibiotic therapy – bactericidal drugs when possible.

Selected references and further reading

Davidson, E.B. (1998) Managing bite wounds in dogs and cats. Part I. *Compend Contin Educ*, **20**, 811

Davidson, E.B. (1998) Managing bite wounds in dogs and cats. Part II. *Compend Contin Educ*, **20**, 974

DeBoer, D.J. (1995) Management of chronic and recurrent pyoderma in the dog. In: Bonagura, J.D. (ed). *Kirk Current Veterinary Therapy XII*. p. 611. WB Saunders, Philadelphia

DeBoer, D.J. and Pukay, B.P. (1993) Recurrent pyoderma and immunostimulants. In: Ihrke, P.J. et al. (eds). *Advances in Veterinary Dermatology II*. p. 443. Pergamon, Oxford

Greene, C.E. et al. (1998) Antibacterial chemotherapy. In: Greene, C.E. and Kersey, R. (eds). *Infectious Diseases of the Dog and Cat*. pp. 185–205. WB Saunders, Philadelphia

Hall, J.A. (2004) Antimicrobial therapy. In: Campbell, K.L. (ed). *Small Animal Dermatology Secrets*. pp. 57–63. Hanley and Belfus, Philadelphia

Ihrke, P.J. and DeManuelle, T.C. (1999) German shepherd dog pyoderma: an overview and antimicrobial management. *Compend Contin Educ*, **21**, 44–49

Medleau, L. and Hnilica, K. (2006) Bacterial skin disease. In: *Small Animal Dermatology: A Color Atlas and Therapeutic Guide*. 2nd edn. pp. 26–61. WB Saunders, Philadelphia

Scott, D.W. et al. (2001) Bacterial Skin Disease *Muller and Kirk's Small Animal Dermatology*. 6th edn. pp. 274–335. WB Saunders, Philadelphia

Thomas, R.C. (2004) Principles of topical therapy. In: Campbell, K.L. (ed). *Small Animal Dermatology Secrets*. pp. 71–85. Hanley and Belfus, Philadelphia

Fungal skin disease 5

A mycosis (pl. mycoses) is a disease caused by a fungus.

Mycoses can be classified according to their depth of infection:

(1) Superficial
(2) Subcutaneous (intermediate)
(3) Systemic (deep)

Superficial mycoses

Fungal infections of the superficial layers of skin, hairs and claws:

(a) Dermatophytosis
(b) Candidiasis
(c) Malasseziasis

Dermatophytosis

Dermatophytosis is an infection of the hair shaft and stratum corneum caused by keratophilic fungi. Common in cats and dogs.

Cause and pathogenesis

- Usually caused by *Microsporum canis, Microsporum gypseum,* and *Trichophyton mentagrophytes.*
- Zoonotic infection (Figure 5.1).
- Transmission occurs from
  - infected animal (hair, scale),
  - environmental contamination,
  - fomites (grooming equipment, bedding).

Source of infection:

M. canis	zoophilic dermatophyte	reservoir usually cats
T. mentagrophytes	zoophilic dermatophyte	reservoir rodents
M. gypseum	geophilic dermatophyte	reservoir soil
T. erinacei	zoophilic dermatophyte	reservoir hedgehogs
M. persicolor	zoophilic dermatophyte	reservoir small rodents

Predisposing factors:

- Strong breed predilections exist in Persian cats (Figure 5.2), Jack Russell terriers (Figure 5.3), and Yorkshire terriers appear to be predisposed.
- Cell mediated immunity is important; factors affecting this predispose to infection:
  - young animals – delayed development of immunity and local skin mechanisms

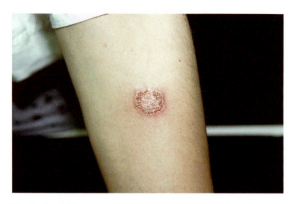

Figure 5.1 Ringworm lesion on owner caused by *M. canis*.

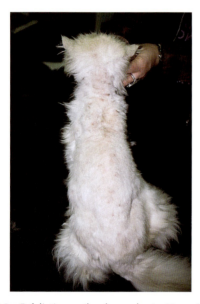

Figure 5.2 Exfoliative erythroderma due to *M. canis*.

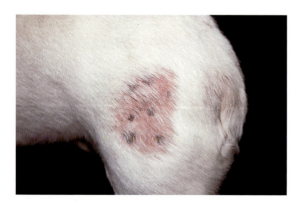

Figure 5.3 Folliculitis on the lateral aspect of a Jack Russell terrier due to *T. mentagrophytes*.

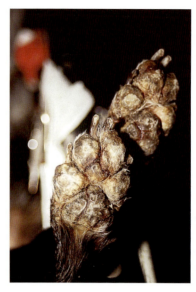

Figure 5.4 Superficial infection with *M. canis* of footpads in a dog with hepatocutaneous disease due to a pancreatic tumour.

- viral infection (FeLV, FIV, FIP)
- neoplasia (Figure 5.4)
- poor nutrition
- anti-inflammatory or immunosuppressive drug therapy
- pregnancy/lactation

Clinical signs

- Variable, dependent on type of fungus and post-immune status, lesions may be localised (Figures 5.5 and 5.6) or generalised (Figure 5.7). Pruritus is mild.

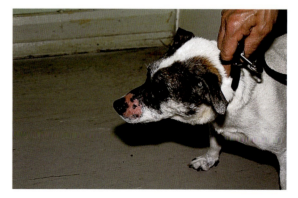

Figure 5.5 Scarring on the nose of a Jack Russell due to *T. mentagrophytes* infection.

Fungal skin disease 59

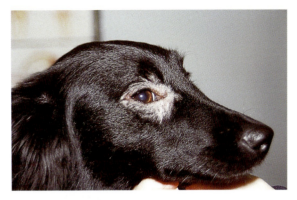

Figure 5.6 Typical crusting and scaling periocular lesions of *M. canis* in a collie.

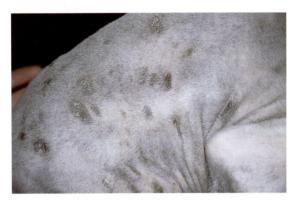

Figure 5.7 Diffuse alopecia with macular areas of hyperpigmentation caused by *M. canis*.

- 'Classical' lesion, circular patches of alopecia 'cigarette ash' scale usually seen on ears and extremities (Figure 5.8).
- Trichophyton infections also folliculitis and furunculosis confined to single leg (Figure 5.9).

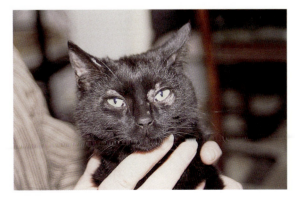

Figure 5.8 Typical periocular grey crusting seen with *M. canis* infection.

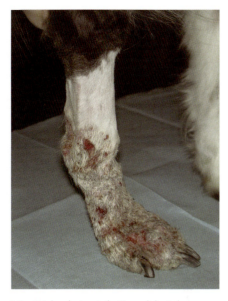

Figure 5.9 Trichophyton infection of dog's leg.

- Lesions heal leaving scarring alopecia.
- *M. persicolor* infections often generalised seborrhoea plus papulopustular crusts on face.
- Kerion localised, well-circumscribed exudative nodular lesion (Figure 5.10).
- Onychomycosis is a common presentation in dogs, very rare in cats. Usually *Trichophyton* spp. can affect one or more digits causing paronychia and onychodystrophy (Figure 5.11).
- In cats dermatophytosis can present as miliary dermatitis (Figure 5.12).
- Pseudomycetoma seen in Persian cats appears as ulcerated, discharging subcutaneous nodules, especially on the trunk and tail base (Figure 5.13).

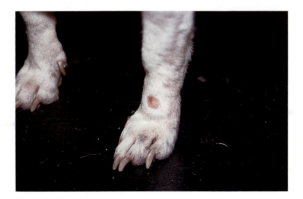

Figure 5.10 Kerion on carpus of dog.

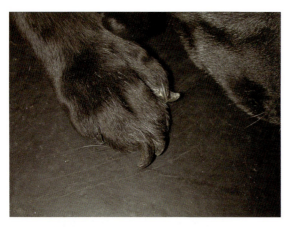

Figure 5.11 Onychomycosis in a Labrador.

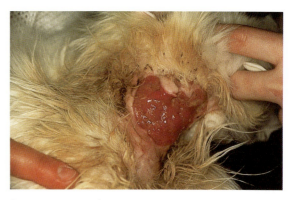

Figure 5.13 Pseudomycetoma in a Persian cat. (Source: Picture courtesy R. Bond.)

- Asymptomatic carrier state recognised in cats especially long-haired cats including Persians. Carrier state rare in dogs, except possibly the Yorkshire terrier.

Differential diagnosis

(a) Crusting follicular lesions:

- Staphylococcal folliculitis
- Demodicosis
- Pemphigus foliaceus
- Miliary dermatitis in cats (allergic causes)
- Ectoparasites (scabies, cheyletiella)

(b) Kerion:

- Acral lick granuloma
- Neoplasia especially squamous cell carcinoma, mast cell tumour

Diagnosis

- Ultraviolet (Wood's lamp, Figure 5.14) examination of hairs – apple green fluorescence on individually plucked hair shafts. Only 50% of *M. canis* infection fluoresces:
  - False negatives occur if Wood's lamp not warmed up, fluorescence destroyed by topical drugs, e.g. iodine.
  - False positives can occur if bacterial infection is present (not apple green fluorescence), topical medication on the hair may fluoresce.
- Microscopy of plucked hairs or scale in 10% potassium hydroxide or mineral oil. In positive cases arthrospores are often visible on hair shafts (Figure 5.15); these may be difficult to find.

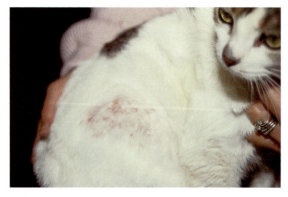

Figure 5.12 Widespread papulocrustous dermatitis due to *M. canis*.

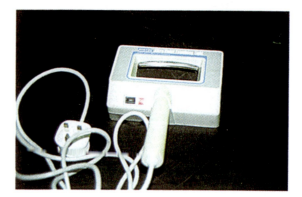

Figure 5.14 Wood's lamp should be turned on and allowed to warm up before being used.

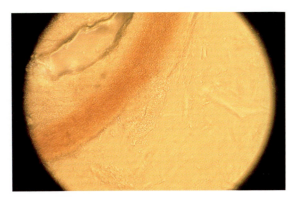

Figure 5.15 Arthrospores of *M. canis* on a plucked hair.

- Fungal culture using the MacKenzie method (Figures 5.16–5.19). Sterile toothbrush brushed through coat then implanted into culture medium. Dermatophyte test medium (DTM) or Sabouraud's dextrose agar:
  - False negatives on DTM – some isolates produce no colour change.
  - False positives on DTM – saprophytic fungi cause colour changes (Figure 5.20).
- Biopsy not always diagnostic. Histopathological findings variable include perifolliculitis, folliculitis, furunculosis, superficial perivascular dermatitis, follicular orthokeratosis or parakeratosis. Fungal hyphae can be seen on normal stains or special fungal stains may be necessary.

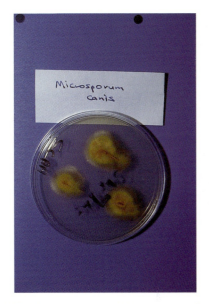

Figure 5.17 Reverse pigment *M. canis* on Sabouraud's dextrose agar.

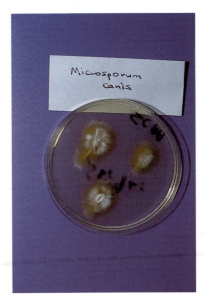

Figure 5.16 Colony morphology *M. canis* on Sabouraud's dextrose agar.

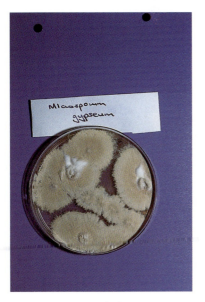

Figure 5.18 Colony morphology *M. gypseum* on Sabouraud's dextrose agar.

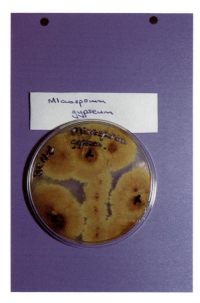

Figure 5.19 Reverse pigment *M. gypseum* on Sabouraud's dextrose agar.

Treatment

Animal
Topical treatment:

- Localised lesions gentle clipping.
- Lotion or cream applied twice daily up to 6 cm beyond active edge of the lesion until the lesions resolve (see Table 5.2).
- Generalised lesions whole body clip (probably not necessary if animal can be shampooed adequately).

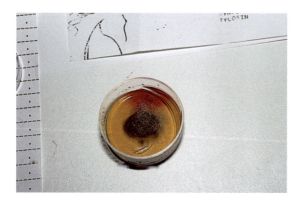

Figure 5.20 False-positive colour change caused by saprophytic fungi. Note colonies are black.

- Apply shampoo or rinse to whole body twice weekly (see Table 5.2).
- All treatment should be continued for 2 weeks after negative fungal cultures.

Systemic treatment:

- Indications – generalised dermatophytosis and any local lesions unresponsive after 3–4 weeks of topical treatment. It is often possible to resolve dermatophytosis in dogs with topical therapy alone; in cats systemic therapy is required in most cases.
- All of the systemic drugs for dermatophytosis are potentially teratogenic.
- Systemic therapy is usually needed for a minimum of 4–6 weeks and often doubles this in long-haired cats (see Tables 5.3 and 5.4).
- Onychomycosis may require 6–9 months of treatment.
- Treatment should continue until two negative cultures are obtained 3 weeks apart.

Environment including fomites
- Thorough cleaning is important. New types of vacuums that expel air may contaminate the environment so should be used with care.
- Liquid disinfection is useful, provided the chemicals do not damage fabrics etc. Suitable products include sodium hypochlorite (1–10 dilution household bleach) and enilconazole.
- Fogging may be useful in catteries and environments where fabrics cannot be treated with liquid disinfectant, e.g. enilconazole foggers.

Cattery management of dermatophytosis
General points:
This is an expensive procedure if performed adequately. Costing should be based on loss of revenue through cessation of breeding programme and selling of cats/kittens as well as treatment costs. It is sensible to prepare an estimate for your client before starting.

Fungal skin disease 63

Table 5.1 Dermatophyte colony and microscopic morphology.

Species	Culture characteristics on SBA			Appearance of macroconidia	Microconidia
	Form	Colour	Reverse pigment		
M. canis	Initial growth cotton wool like then powdery with central depression	White buff	Yellow/orange later orange brown	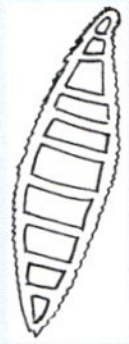 Abundant spindle-shaped, curved tip. Thick spinous wall contains 6–15 cells. Often terminal knob. **Figure 5.21** Line diagram macroconidia M. canis.	Uncommon
M. gypseum	Flat, powdery-granular, central umbo with irregular fringe	White-cinnamon brown	Pale yellow tan	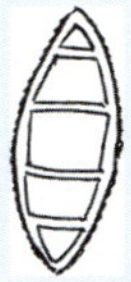 Abundant ellipsoid-shaped, round tip, relatively thin spinous walls contain 4–6 cells. No terminal knob. **Figure 5.22** Line diagram macroconidia M. gypseum.	Abundant
T. mentagrophytes (zoophilic form)	Flat powdery	Cream-light buff	Yellow buff tan occasionally dark red brown	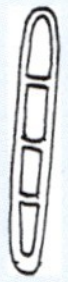 Rare structures, cigar shaped with thin smooth walls. **Figure 5.23** Line diagram macroconidia T. mentagrophytes.	Abundant
M. persicolor	Folded granular, fringed periphery	Light buff	Peach rose/deep ochre	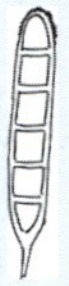 Sparse elongated, thin, smooth walls with spinous tips on short stalk. Multicellular. **Figure 5.24** Line diagram macroconidia M. persicolor.	Abundant

Table 5.2 Drugs suitable for topical therapy of dermatophytosis.

Local lesions	Generalised lesions
1% terbinafine cream	2% miconazole shampoo
1% clotrimazole cream, lotion, solution	2% ketoconazole shampoo
2% enilconazole cream	0.2% enilconazole
1–2% miconazole cream, spray lotion	2–4% lime sulphur
	2% boric acid shampoo

Estimation of costs should include the following:

- Systemic drug therapy for all cats over the age of 12 weeks (except pregnant individual who cannot be treated until after kittening) for up to 12–16 weeks for short-haired cats, more in long haired.
- Topical therapy ± clipping.
- Routine ectoparasitic control.
- Laboratory tests – multiple fungal culture initially to assess degree of cattery contamination and then at least three per cat before cessation of therapy.
- Treatment of the environment with liquid disinfectants/foggers.

Table 5.4 Protocol for therapy of dermatophytosis using pulse itraconazole.

Alternate week protocol	Weekend protocol
Itraconazole is given once daily at a dose of 10 mg/kg for 2 weeks then given for a week on and a week off	Itraconazole is given once daily at a dose of 10 mg/kg for 2 weeks then each Saturday and Sunday as a weekend treatment
Continue until 2 negative cultures 3 weeks apart	Continue until 2 negative cultures 3 weeks apart

Options for therapy
- Aim for complete eradication of dermatophytes from the cattery (Protocol 1).
- Depopulation of the cattery (Protocol 2).
- Treatment of only those cats leaving the premise (Protocol 3).

Protocol 1: Complete eradication of dermatophytes from the cattery (see Table 5.5)
- Assessment of degree of infection:
  - Toothbrush cultures performed on all cats.
  - Toothbrush cultures from environment, e.g. soft furnishings, window ledges, heating vents.

Table 5.3 Systemic therapy for dermatophytosis in dogs and cats.

Systemic drug	Dogs	Cats	Comments
Griseofulvin (microsized)	50 mg/kg/day po sid	50 mg/kg/day po sid	Best given with fatty meal
Ketoconazole	10 mg/kg po sid/bid	10 mg/kg/ po sid/bid	Best given with acid solution, e.g. tomato juice. Rarely tolerated in cats due to G.I. upsets. Hepatotoxic, effects cortisol and sex hormone levels
Itraconazole	5–10 mg/kg po sid	5–10 mg/kg po sid	Well tolerated in cats. Best given with food, can be used as pulse therapy (see Table 5.3 below)
Terbinafine	30–40 mg/kg po sid	30–40 mg/kg po sid	
Lufenuron	Not shown consistent efficacy in treating dermatophytosis in dogs or cats		

Table 5.5 Treatment groups used in therapy of dermatophytosis in a cattery.

Group 1	Group 2	Group 3	Group 4
Cats Weekly treatment with lime sulphur If any cats develop lesions move to Group 4 Continue to monitor this group with cultures whilst treating other groups	**Queens** Topical therapy with an anti-fungal rinse or shampoo until kittening then as Group 4	Positive cultures as Group 4	**Cats** Topical therapy with lime sulphur every 5–7 days Systemic therapy pulse itraconazole (see Table 5.3) Sample cats after 3 weeks, then every 2 weeks until 2 negative cultures 3 weeks apart; negative cats move to Group 1
Environment Weekly treatment with enilconazole and 5% sodium hypochlorite Continue to monitor with environmental samples	**Kittens** Topical therapy until at least 12 weeks of age when systemic therapy can be started as Group 4	Negative cultures as Group 1	**Environment** Liquid disinfection (enilconazole or 5% sodium hypochlorite) and enilconazole foggers twice weekly

- Close the cattery to all visitors, stop-breeding programmes, sale of kittens, etc.
- Isolate all cats that are culture negative in a culture negative environment (Group 1).
- Isolate all pregnant queens (Group 2).
- Isolate all breeding males (Group 3). Two separate groups, e.g. Group 3a (negative culture) and Group 3b (positive culture) can be created if necessary.
- Isolate all other positive cats (Group 4).
- To prevent cross-contamination to non-infected groups. All grooming equipment, feeding bowl, utensils, etc. should be confined to each group. Where possible specific persons should be allocated to the care of each group.
- All cats should have routine ectoparasitic control used on them throughout the treatment period.

Protocol 2: Depopulation of the cattery
- Rehoming or euthanasia (at owners request) of all infected animals.
- Thorough decontamination of environment (liquid disinfection/foggers).
- Repopulation after three negative cultures from the environment 2 weeks apart.

Protocol 3: Treatment of only those cats leaving the premise
- No attempt is made to treat any cats in the cattery that are accepted as having endemic ringworm.
- Isolation facilities should be made available for outgoing cats and kittens.
- The isolation facility allows any cat to be separated and treated with systemic and topical therapy to resolve the dermatophytosis before leaving the cattery.
- Pregnant queens may be treated with lime sulphur topically once weekly, during pregnancy. Once kittens are born, start the queen on itraconazole pulse treatment.
- At 4 weeks of age, culture the kittens and begin topical therapy as queens. Any positive kittens can be started on itraconazole at 12 weeks.
- No cat should leave the cattery until three negative cultures have been obtained 2 weeks apart.
- This can be used for queens wishing to go out to stud and for kittens to be sold.

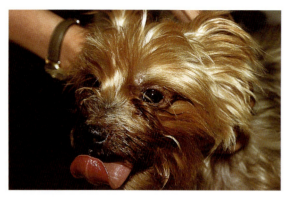

Figure 5.25 Mucocutaneous candidiasis of the periocular skin in a dog with hyperadrenocorticism.

Candidiasis

Candidiasis is an opportunistic cutaneous infection due to the dimorphic fungus *Candida* spp. Rare infection in both dogs and cats.

Cause and pathogenesis

- Infection is caused by *Candida* spp., especially *Candida albicans*, *Candida parapsilosis*.
- Opportunistic infection caused by loss of integrity of skin and mucocutaneous areas, due to, e.g. trauma, burns, skin maceration.
- Predisposing factors.
- Immunosuppression through
  - disease, e.g. diabetes mellitus, hyperadrenocorticism, neoplasia,
  - drug therapy, e.g. glucocorticoids, long-term antibiotics.

Clinical signs

- Lesions found at moist macerated areas of skin and mucous membranes, e.g. ear, intertriginous areas, oral cavity (Figure 5.25).
- Mucous membranes lesions appear as single to multiple malodorous shallow ulcers covered in thick grey/white plaques with erythematous margins.
- Skin lesions appear as non-healing, oozing erythematous plaques and ulcers. Crusted lesions can be seen around nail beds.

Differential diagnosis

Mucocutaneous form:

- Pemphigus vulgaris
- Bullous pemphigoid
- Erythema multiforme
- Leishmaniasis
- Systemic lupus erythematosus
- Necrolytic migratory erythema
- Vasculitis
- Epitheliotropic lymphoma

Skin:

- Pyotraumatic dermatitis
- Intertrigo
- Erythema multiforme
- Leishmaniasis
- Epitheliotropic lymphoma

Diagnosis

- History and clinical signs.
- Cytology of exudates by smear or acetate tape reveals mixed inflammatory infiltrate with typical budding yeasts and rare pseudohyphae.
- Culture on Sabouraud's dextrose agar not diagnostic as this is a normal mucosal inhabitant.
- Biopsy of lesions useful to confirm diagnosis. Shows parakeratotic hyperkeratosis, budding yeast with occasional hyphae in surface keratin.

Treatment

- Correction of underlying factors essential.
- Mucocutaneous lesions and generalised disease:
  - Systemic therapy is needed for at least 4 weeks and until complete resolution of lesions.
  - Systemic treatment ketoconazole 5–10 mg/kg po sid, itraconazole 5–10 mg/kg po sid, fluconazole 5 mg/kg po bid.

Cutaneous lesions

- Local lesions:
  - Clipping and application of topical treatment three times daily (see Table 5.6).
  - Lesions should be treated until complete clinical cure.

Fungal skin disease

Table 5.6 Topical therapy suitable for local lesions of candidiasis.

Drug	Administration
Nystatin	100,000 u/g cream, ointment tid–qid
Miconazole	1–2% cream, spray, lotion bid–sid
Clotrimazole	1% cream, lotion or solution qid–tid
Amphotericin B	3% cream, lotion or ointment tid–qid

Malasseziasis

Malasseziasis is a surface infection, principally of moist skin folds and the external ear canal. It is very common in dogs and rare in cats.

Cause and pathogenesis

In dogs the disease is caused by the skin commensal *Malassezia pachydermatis*, in cats *M. pachydermatitis* is involved but *M. sympodialis* and *M. globosa* have also been implicated.

Cutaneous overgrowth of *Malassezia* spp. on the skin leads to disease.

Invasion of superficial epidermal layers occurs due to changes in surface microclimate by

- increased sebum/cerumen production,
- moist maceration of skin,
- trauma especially licking.

In some animals a hypersensitivity reaction to Malassezia has been identified. It is controversial if this is a separate disease entity or merely production of antibody in atopic animals in response to cutaneous colonisation with yeast.

Predisposing factors:

- Allergy – atopy, food allergy.
- Bacterial infection.
- Viral disease – FIV, FeLV, FIP.
- Endocrine disease – hypothyroidism (dog), hyperthyroidism (cat) (Figure 5.26), hyperadrenocorticism.
- Internal disease, especially those affecting lipid metabolism, pancreatic disease, diabetes mellitus.

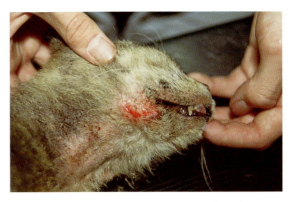

Figure 5.26 *Malassezia* secondary to hyperthyroidism.

- Chronic glucocorticoids therapy especially in allergic dogs.
- Keratinisation disorders.
- Neoplasia – thymoma (cat), paraneoplastic alopecia (cat).

Clinical signs

- No age or sex incidence.
- Predisposed breeds – West Highland white terrier, basset hound, English Setters, poodle, cocker spaniel, Jack Russell terrier, Shih-Tzu, springer spaniels, German shepherd dogs.
- Seasonality depends on underlying factors.

Dogs:

- Lesions found most commonly on ears, lip folds, interdigital spaces (Figure 5.27), ventral

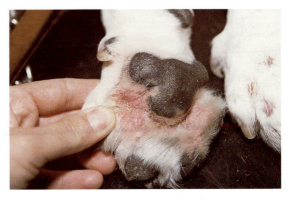

Figure 5.27 Malassezia of the interdigital spaces in a West Highland white terrier.

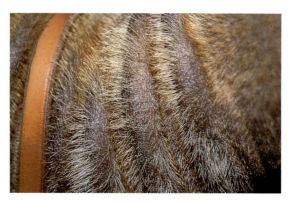

Figure 5.28 Malassezia in the body skin folds of a shar-pei.

neck, intertriginous areas (Figure 5.28), medial thighs, axillae (Figure 5.29) and perianal areas.
- Pruritus variable but usually moderate to severe, typically poorly responsive to anti-inflammatory therapy.
- Acutely – malodorous erythematous, greasy, scaly plaques, macules and patches.
- Chronically – skin becomes lichenified, hyperpigmented and hyperkeratotic.
- Paronychia common with dark brown nail bed discharge (Figure 5.30).
- Concurrent otitis externa often seen.

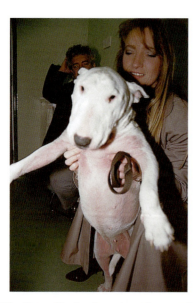

Figure 5.29 Generalised malassezia on the ventral abdomen of an English bull terrier.

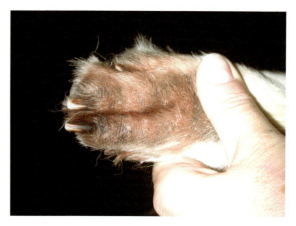

Figure 5.30 Malassezia affecting the nail bed producing a dark brown discharge.

Cats:
- Pruritus moderate to severe.
- Greasy seborrhoea with erythema and alopecia (Figure 5.31).
- Dark brown/black ceruminous otitis.
- Chronic chin acne.

Differential diagnosis

- Allergy (food, atopy, fleas)
- Staphylococcal folliculitis
- Ectoparasites – scabies, demodex
- Neoplasia (epitheliotropic lymphoma)

These diseases can occur concurrently with Malassezia dermatitis.

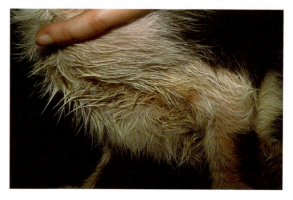

Figure 5.31 *Malassezia* secondary to hepatic carcinoma.

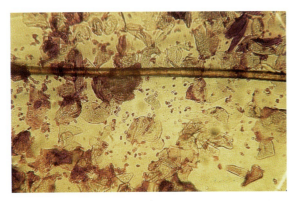

Figure 5.32 Purple staining peanut-shaped yeasts on tape strips stained with Diff-Quik.

Diagnosis

- History and clinical signs.
- Cytology of skin scrapings, direct smears or acetate tape impression smears stained with Diff-Quik reveal typical budding yeasts that appear as dark blue/purple peanut-shaped organisms (Figure 5.32). Organisms usually numerous but should be at least >2 per high power (100×) field. In hypersensitivity reactions yeast may be sparse.
- Serology available commercially to look for Malassezia IgE and intradermal allergy testing can be performed to identify dogs with 'Malassezia hypersensitivity'.
- Culture with special contact plates.
- Biopsy shows superficial perivascular to interstitial lymphohistiocytic dermatitis with yeasts in surface keratin.

Treatment

Therapy of predisposing factors is essential.
Topical treatment:

- Applied twice weekly to localised or generalised disease until a clinical improvement is seen, then reduced to every 10–14 days for maintenance.
- Shampoo containing miconazole, chlorhexidine, selenium sulphide, ketoconazole, tar, boric acid. Baths may be followed by a rinse or the rinse can be used alone.
- Rinses – enilconazole, lime sulphur.
- Creams/lotion containing miconazole, enilconazole, clotrimazole.

Systemic treatment:

Treatment should be given until lesions resolve and negative cytology is achieved:

- Ketoconazole 5–10 mg/kg po sid/bid for 7 days until clinical cure.
- Itraconazole 5–10 mg/kg po sid for 7 days until clinical cure or as pulse therapy (see the section on dermatophytosis).
- When predisposing factors cannot be identified or treated adequately, chronic therapy is indicated. Both ketoconazole and itraconazole can be given at a full dose rate twice weekly for maintenance therapy.
- Terbinafine 30 mg/kg po sid for 2–4 weeks has been successful in some cases.

Subcutaneous mycoses (intermediate mycoses)

Fungal infections of viable skin, usually caused by infection of traumatised skin by saprophytes:

(a) Pseudomycetoma
(b) Eumycotic mycetoma
(c) Phaeohyphomycosis
(d) Pythiosis
(e) Zygomycosis
(f) Sporotrichosis
(g) Lagenidiosis

Pseudomycetoma

Unusual form of dermatophytosis in which dermatophilic fungi form hyphae in dermal and subcutaneous tissue. Very rare in dogs and uncommon in cats.

Cause and pathogenesis

Nodular lesions formed by infection of deep tissue by dermatophytes. Differentiated from dermatophytosis by the fact that they are not restricted to superficial tissue. The dermatophyte most commonly involved in cat lesions is *M. canis*. Persian cats appear to be highly predisposed. Yorkshire terriers may also be at increased risk. *M. canis* and *T. mentagrophytes* most commonly isolated in canine cases.

Owners need to be aware of zoonotic risk, which can persist for months.

Clinical signs

- Lesions are usually non-painful, non-pruritic firm dermal or subcutaneous nodules.
- Commonly nodules ulcerate and produce purulent exudate.
- Lesions most commonly found on the trunk, flanks or tail.
- Animals commonly have concurrent dermatophytosis.

Differential diagnosis

- Other deep bacterial and fungal infection
- Foreign body reactions
- Neoplasia

Diagnosis

- Cytology of exudates or fine needle aspirate reveals pyogranulomatous inflammation with fungal hyphae.
- Biopsy of lesions shows nodular to diffuse pyogranulomatous dermatitis and panniculitis with septate hyphae, chains of pseudohyphae.
- Fungal culture of exudates, aspirate or tissue collected at biopsy. *M. canis* most commonly isolated.

Treatment

- Best response to therapy, and the best prognosis for clinical cure is if both surgical and medical therapies are used concurrently.
- Lesions need to be removed surgically if possible.
- Concurrent anti-fungal therapy is needed leading up to and for several weeks to months post-operatively until complete clinical cure.
- Systemic therapy most successful with itraconazole 10 mg/kg po sid.
- Ketoconazole and griseofulvin are generally not as effective in therapy (for dose rates, see the section on dermatophytosis).

Eumycotic mycetoma

Skin infection caused by a range of saprophytic environmental and pathogenic plant fungi. Uncommon to rare disease in dogs and cats.

Cause and pathogenesis

- Lesions are caused by wound contamination by soil saprophytes especially *Pseudoallescheria boydii*.
- Fungi form macroscopic colonies in the dermis and subcutis, which form tissue grains or granules.

Clinical signs

- Lesions usually solitary poorly defined nodules, especially on extremities (Figure 5.33), tend to be painful.
- Triad of signs typical of mycetoma:
  - Nodular swelling
  - Draining fistulas – serous, haemorrhagic or purulent
  - Granules – macroscopic fungal colonies
- Dematiaceous fungi – black-grained mycetoma, e.g. *Curvularia geniculata*, *Madurella* spp.
- Non-pigmented fungi – white-grained mycetomas, e.g. *P. boydii*, *Acremonium* spp.

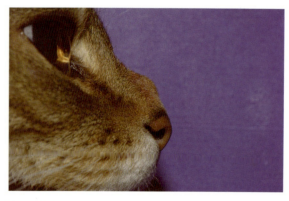

Figure 5.33 Mycetoma on a cat's nose. (Source: Copyright 2008, Dr. Stephen Shaw.)

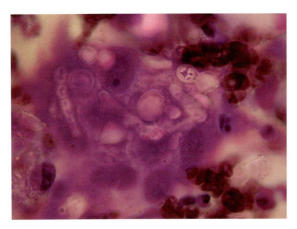

Figure 5.34 Cytology of mycetoma. (Source: Copyright 2008, Dr. Stephen Shaw.)

Differential diagnosis

- Sterile granulomas
- Infectious granulomas, e.g. bacteria, fungi
- Foreign body granuloma
- Neoplasia
- Cat bite abscess
- Plasma cell pododermatitis

Diagnosis

- History and clinical signs.
- Cytology of aspirates, direct smears or squashed preparations of grains reveal fungi; cell infiltrate tends to be pyogranulomatous (Figure 5.34).
- Culture of grains or biopsy material on Sabouraud's dextrose agar. To decide if fungi are acting as pathogens rather than contaminants, histopathological examination is required.
- Biopsy reveals nodular to diffuse pyogranulomatous dermatitis and panniculitis with irregularly shaped tissue grains. Tissue grains made up of broad, septate branching pigmented or non-pigmented fungal hyphae.

Treatment

- No zoonotic risk to humans or other animals.
- Wide surgical incision where possible; however, amputation of limb may be necessary.
- If the lesion cannot be completely excised then medical therapy may be used in combination.

Medical therapy alone produces a poor response, possible ketoconazole, itraconazole 5–10 mg/kg daily. Treatment should be continued for at least 2–3 months beyond clinical cure.

Phaeohyphomycosis

Cutaneous lesions formed by saprophytic fungi. Uncommon disease in cats and rare in dogs. No zoonotic risk to humans.

Cause and pathogenesis

Wound contamination by saprophytic fungi found in soil and organic materials. No granules, but fungi form pigmented hyphae. Causal organisms include *Alternaria* spp., *Bipolaris* spp., *Cladosporium* spp., *Curvularia* spp., *Exophiala* spp., *Monilia* spp., *Ochroconis* spp., *Phialemonium* spp., *Phialophora* spp., *Pseudo microdochium* spp., *Scolebasidium* spp., *Stemphilium* spp., *Fonsecaea* spp.

Clinical signs

Dogs:

- Single or multiple ulcerated subcutaneous nodules especially on extremities.
- Often underlying osteomyelitis.
- Disseminated disease has been reported.

Cats:

- Usually solitary subcutaneous nodules, abscess or cyst-like lesions that ulcerate and drain.
- Lesions most commonly identified on extremities (Figure 5.35) and face.
- Disseminated disease rare.

Differential diagnosis

As eumycotic mycetoma.

Diagnosis

- History and clinical signs.
- Cytology of aspirate or direct smear reveals pyogranulomatous inflammation. Pigmented

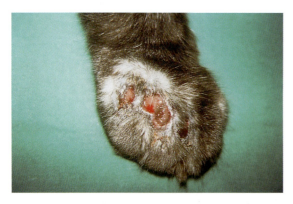

Figure 5.35 Skin disease caused by opportunistic fungus *Exophiala werneckii*. (Source: Picture courtesy R. Bond.)

fungi may be seen, but not a consistent finding.
- Culture preferably of biopsy material on Sabouraud's dextrose agar. Positive fungal culture should be confirmed by histopathology.
- Biopsy shows nodular to diffuse pyogranulomatous dermatitis and panniculitis, with thick-walled pigmented septate hyphae.

Treatment

- Wide surgical excision where possible; however, recurrence is common and the prognosis is poor.
- Systemic anti-fungal therapy is needed for weeks to months and should be continued for at least 4 weeks beyond clinical resolution.
- Some possible response to combinations of ketoconazole/itraconazole ± flucytosine or amphotericin B ± flucytosine.

Pythiosis

Deep tissue infection with aquatic protozoan, which has fungus-like features in mammalian tissue. Uncommon in dogs, large breed dogs especially German shepherd dog predisposed. Rare in cats. No zoonotic risk to humans and not contagious to other animals.

Cause and pathogenesis

- A disease mostly confined to tropical and subtropical swamp areas.
- Damaged skin or mucosa infected by aquatic fungi *Pythium insidiosum* usually through standing in stagnant water.

Clinical signs

Dogs:
Can present with either cutaneous lesions or gastrointestinal disease.

- Skin lesions:
  - Lesions solitary or multiple nodules that coalesce to form large masses of spongy, proliferative fistulating ulcerated tissue.
  - Lesions can be found at any site but usually correspond to the area that has been submerged in water, e.g. legs, tail base, ventral neck and head.
  - Pruritus variable.
- Gastrointestinal disease:
  - Clinical signs variable, depending on site of infiltrative lesions, e.g. granulomatous gastritis (vomiting), oesophagitis (regurgitation), enteritis (diarrhoea).
  - Dogs usually show signs of weight loss.

Cats:
Only the cutaneous form of the disease has been described.

- Skin lesions:
  - Single or multiple subcutaneous locally invasive, draining nodules and ulcerated plaques.
  - Lesions usually seen on extremities, e.g. feet, inguinal area, tail head or face.

Differential diagnosis

As eumycotic mycetoma.

Diagnosis

- History of water exposure and clinical signs.
- Cytology of aspirates or direct smear fungal element rarely seen. Cellular findings of granulomatous inflammation with eosinophils.
- Culture should be taken from biopsy material and special medium is required.

- Biopsy reveals nodular to diffuse granulomatous dermatitis with foci of necrosis with eosinophils. Visualisation of hyphae requires special stains.
- Immunohistochemistry can be used to detect *P. insidiosum* antigen.
- Polymerase chain reaction can identify *P. insidiosum* DNA.
- *P. insidiosum* serum antibodies can be detected by enzyme-linked immunosorbent assay (ELISA) or Western immunoblot analysis.

Treatment

- Wide surgical excision is the treatment of choice. Recurrence can occur; amputation of affected limb is often necessary. To monitor for recurrence serum anti-*P. insidiosum* antibody titres can be followed by ELISA every 3 months for a year.
- Immunotherapy with *P. insidiosum* vaccine may be useful in dogs with acute disease <2 months duration.
- Anti-fungal medication is rarely successful (<25% of cases). Progress can be monitored with serum anti-*P. insidiosum* antibody titres. Individual therapy with itraconazole or amphotericin B produces disappointing results. Best results reported with combination of itraconazole (10 mg/kg po sid) and terbinafine (5–10 mg/kg po sid).
- Chronic disease carries a poor prognosis.

Zygomycosis

Zygomycosis is a deep fungal infection caused by fungi from the class of fungi called *Zygomycetes*. Fungi in this class include *Rhizopus* spp., *Mucor* spp., *Absidia* spp., *Basidiobolus* spp., *Conidiobolus* spp. and *Mortierella* spp. Rare disease in both the dog and cat. No zoonotic risk to humans and not contagious.

Cause and pathogenesis

Ubiquitous soil saprophytes, also found as flora of skin and hair coat, produce infection through wound contamination. They can also gain entry into the body via the respiratory or gastrointestinal tract through the same route.

Clinical signs

- Clinical signs are usually those associated with gastrointestinal tract, respiratory system or disseminated disease.
- Generalised disease is usually fatal.
- Skin lesions ulcerated draining nodules especially extremities.

Differential diagnosis

As eumycotic mycetoma.

Diagnosis

- History and clinical signs.
- Cytology of aspirate or direct smear reveals pyogranulomatous inflammation with fungal elements.
- Culture of biopsy material to confirm the presence of bacteria must be confirmed on histopathology.
- Biopsy reveals nodular to diffuse pyogranulomatous dermatitis and panniculitis, with numerous broad, occasionally septate branching hyphae.

Treatment

- Wide surgical excision where possible or debulking therapy is essential. If complete surgical excision cannot be performed the prognosis is very poor.
- Anti-fungal therapy is needed for weeks to months and continued for at least 4 weeks beyond clinical resolution.
- Most suitable drug is amphotericin B 0.5 mg/kg, for dogs, or 0.25 mg/kg, for cats, given intravenously three times weekly up to 8–12 mg/kg, for dogs, and 4–6 mg/kg, for cats.
- Potassium iodide, benzimidazole and ketoconazole usually ineffective.

Sporotrichosis

Nodular skin disease caused by dimorphic fungus and environmental saprophyte. Uncommon in dogs and cats. Hunting dogs and intact male cats appear to be at increased risk. No zoonotic risk from dogs to humans; however cats highly contagious to man.

Cause and pathogenesis

- A common disease caused by ubiquitous soil saprophytes *Sporothrix schenckii*.
- Infection is caused by wound contamination usually through puncture wounds from splinters, thorn.

Clinical signs

Dogs:

- Cutaneous form – multiple ulcerated nodules and plaques especially head, pinnae and trunk. Lesions are non-pruritic and non-painful. No systemic signs.
- Cutaneolymphatic form – single nodule on limb leads to ascending lymphatic infection – regional lymphadenopathy.

Cats:

- Wide range of lesions including non-healing puncture wounds, abscesses, crusted nodules with draining sinus tracts, ulceration and tissue necrosis.
- Lesions usually found on head and extremities.
- Disseminated disease is common, cats systemically unwell, lethargic, anorexic and pyrexic.

Differential diagnosis

As eumycotic mycetoma.

Diagnosis

- History and clinical signs.
- Cytology of aspirate or direct smear reveals signs of suppurative or pyogranulomatous inflammation. Organisms usually difficult to find but when present typical intra- and extracellular oval cigar-shaped yeasts. Organism much more prevalent in cats than in dogs.

Table 5.7 Drugs used to treat sporotrichosis in the dog and cat.

Drug	Cat	Dog
Potassium iodide	20 mg/kg po with food bid	40 mg/kg po with food tid[1]
Ketoconazole	5–10 mg/kg po with food sid	5–15 mg/kg po with food bid
Itraconazole	5–10 mg/kg po with food bid/sid[1]	5–10 mg/kg po with food bid/sid

[1] Drug of choice in each species.

- Culture of both exudate and biopsy sample. Difficult to isolate organisms from canine cases, much easier to culture from cats.
- Biopsy reveals signs of nodular to diffuse suppurative to pyogranulomatous dermatitis. Fungal elements rarely seen in dogs, but common in cats.
- Immunofluorescent antibody test useful to identify *S. schenckii* in tissue or exudate.

Treatment

- Anti-fungal therapy is needed for weeks to months and should be given for at least 4 weeks after clinical resolution (see Table 5.7).
- Care should be taken when handling especially cats due to the zoonotic risk.
- Glucocorticoids are contraindicated in all cases. Even after apparent cure these can cause recurrence.

Lagenidiosis

Aquatic oomycetes that normally parasitise other water living organism such as fungi, algae, nematodes and crustaceans have been identified as causing cutaneous fungal infection in dogs. Rare in dogs; young/middle-aged dogs that swim in a lake or pond may be predisposed. Not recorded in cats. No zoonotic risk, no risk of contagion to other animals.

Cause and pathogenesis

Nodular ulcerative skin disease caused by *Lagenidium* spp. has recently been recognised in south-eastern United States.

Clinical signs

- Cutaneous lesions appear as firm dermal to subcutaneous nodules or erythematous masses with localised areas of necrosis.
- Fistulous tracts common, which drain a haemorrhagic mucopurulent exudate.
- Lesions are found most commonly on extremities and the trunk.
- Dissemination to lungs, mediastinum and great vessels has been recorded.

Differential diagnosis

As eumycotic mycetoma.

Diagnosis

- History and clinical signs.
- Cytology reveals evidence of granulomatous inflammation often with eosinophils and fungal elements.
- Fungal culture on conventional media usually unsuccessful, special media required.
- Biopsy typically shows nodular to diffuse eosinophilic pyogranulomatous dermatitis and panniculitis. Irregularly branching fungal hyphae found extracellularly and within giant cells.
- Western immunoblot analysis can be used to detect anti-*Lagenidium* serum antibodies.
- Polymerase chain reaction of infected tissue can be used to identify *Lagenidium* DNA.
- Radiography and ultrasound of thorax and abdomen essential if evidence of disseminated disease.

Treatment

- Wide surgical excision of affected area is treatment of choice. Limb amputation may be necessary in some cases.
- Unless radical excision is possible the prognosis is poor.
- Systemic anti-fungal therapy with itraconazole, amphotericin B rarely of benefit.

Systemic mycoses

Fungal infections of internal organs caused by soil saprophytes.

Contagion usually occurs by inhalation; direct cutaneous inoculation is rare. Skin lesions usually develop after haematogenous spread to skin.

(a) Blastomycosis
(b) Coccidiodomycosis
(c) Cryptococcosis
(d) Histoplasmosis
(e) Aspergillosis
(f) Protothecosis

Blastomycosis

Systemic disease with cutaneous manifestations caused by inhalation of conidia of *Blastomyces dermatitidis*, an environmental saprophyte. A rare disease in cats and uncommon in dogs. Most often seen in young male outdoor dogs especially sporting breeds.

Blastomycosis is a zoonosis; however, it is the fungal cultures that are infectious not the infected animals.

Cause and pathogenesis

Rare disease caused by inhalation of the conidia of *B. dermatitidis*. It is found most commonly in areas with acidic or sandy soil close to water. Primarily found in North America along the rivers, i.e. Ohio, Mississippi, Missouri, St Lawrence and Tennessee. It is also seen in the southern mid-Atlantic states and Southern Great Lakes. Initially, inhalation of conidia leads to lung disease. The disease then disseminates to lymph nodes, eyes, skin, bone and other organs. In rare cases, conidia can be inoculated directly into the skin.

Clinical signs

- Systemic disease causes respiratory (dyspnoea, cough, exercise intolerance), ocular (uveitis, retinal detachment, glaucoma) and locomotor and central nervous system signs.
- Forty per cent of cases have skin disease including ulcerated draining nodules producing a serosanguineous to purulent exudates and plaques.
- Lesions multiple and can be found at any site, especially face, nasal planum and claw beds.

Differential diagnosis

Other systemic bacterial and fungal diseases: Neoplasia.

Diagnosis

- History and clinical signs.
- Cytology of aspirates or direct smear reveals suppurative or pyogranulomatous inflammation with oval broad-based budding yeast with thick double-contoured cell walls.
- Culture not recommended due to the zoonotic nature of the disease. If submitted, important to send sample to specialised laboratory.
- Biopsy shows signs of nodular to diffuse, suppurative to pyogranulomatous dermatitis with large thick double-walled broad-based budding yeast easily seen in sections.
- Agar gel immunodiffusion to detect serum antibodies may be useful. In early disease this test may be negative.
- General diagnostic tests may also be performed to assess for involvement of other organ systems.

Treatment

- Long courses of anti-fungal therapy are needed. A minimum of 2–3 months and for 4 weeks beyond clinical resolution.
- Drug of choice is itraconazole:
  - For cats, 5 mg/kg po bid for 2–3 months as above.
  - For dogs, 5 mg/kg po bid for 5 days then 5 mg/kg po sid for 2–3 months as above.
- Other possible therapies include the following:
  - Fluconazole 2.5–5.0 mg/kg po or iv sid.
  - Amphotericin B:
    - For dogs, 0.5 mg/kg iv three times weekly up to cumulative dose of 8–12 mg/kg.
    - For cats, 0.25 mg/kg iv three times weekly up to cumulative dose of 4–6 mg/kg.
  - Amphotericin B lipid complex 1.0 mg/kg iv three times weekly up to a cumulative dose of 12 mg/kg (dogs).
- Prognosis is good unless there is severe CNS or respiratory disease.
- Relapse is common within 12 months usually due to shortened course of therapy, which can be successfully restarted in most cases.

Coccidiodomycosis

Systemic disease with cutaneous manifestations caused by inhalation of conidia of *Coccidiodes immitis*, an environmental saprophyte. A rare disease in cats and uncommon in dogs. Most often seen in young male medium to large outdoor dogs.

Coccidiodomycosis is a zoonosis; however, it is the fungal cultures that are infectious not the infected animals.

Cause and pathogenesis

Rare disease caused by inhalation of the conidia of *C. immitis*. It is found most commonly in desert areas, primarily found in southwestern United States, Mexico, Central America and South America. Initially, inhalation of conidia leads to lung disease. The disease then disseminates to lymph nodes, eyes, skin, bone and other organs. In rare cases, conidia can be inoculated directly into the skin.

Clinical signs

- Systemic disease causing respiratory (cough, dyspnoea, tachypnoea) ocular, locomotor system signs, pyrexia.
- Cutaneous lesions include multiple ulcerated papules, nodules and subcutaneous abscesses with draining tracts, especially in dogs over infected long bones.
- In cats, abscesses and nodules occur without involvement of underlying bone.

Differential diagnosis

Other systemic bacterial and fungal diseases: Neoplasia.

Diagnosis

- History and clinical signs.
- Cytology of aspirates or direct smear reveals suppurative or pyogranulomatous inflammation; the organisms are rarely found.
- Culture not recommended due to the zoonotic nature of the disease. If submitted, important to send sample to specialised laboratory.
- Biopsy shows signs of nodular to diffuse, suppurative to pyogranulomatous dermatitis and panniculitis with few to several large round double-walled structures called spherules that contain endospores.
- A variety of methods are available to detect antibodies against *C. immitis*. This includes complement fixation, latex agglutination and ELISA. False negative can be found in early cases of the disease. False positives can be seen in healthy dogs in endemic areas.
- General diagnostic tests may also be performed to assess for involvement of other organ systems.

Treatment

- Long courses of anti-fungal therapy are needed. A minimum of 12 months in cases of disseminated disease and for 8 weeks beyond clinical resolution (cutaneous and pulmonary disease).
- Drug of choice is ketoconazole:
  - For cats, 5 mg/kg po bid or 10 mg/kg po sid with food.
  - For dogs, 5–10 mg/kg po bid with food.
- Other possible therapies include
  - fluconazole 5 mg/kg po bid with food,
  - itraconazole 5–10 mg/kg po bid with food.
- Prognosis is variable.
- Relapse is common usually due to shortened course of therapy, which can be successfully restarted in most cases. Once relapse has occurred, animals need to stay on long-term low dose therapy for lifetime maintenance.

Cryptococcosis

Systemic disease with cutaneous manifestations caused by inhalation of organisms of *Cryptococcus neoformans*, an environmental saprophyte. An uncommon disease in cats that is rare in dogs. Most often seen in young male dogs.

Cryptococcus-infected animals and cultures have no risk to humans.

Cause and pathogenesis

- Rare disease caused by inhalation of the organisms of *C. neoformans*.
- It is especially associated with pigeon droppings.
- Immunosuppressed animals are more susceptible to disease.
- Initially inhalation of organisms leads to establishment in the animal's nasal cavity, paranasal sinuses or lungs. The disease then disseminates to lymph nodes, eyes, skin, CNS and other organs.
- In rare cases, conidia can be inoculated directly into the skin.

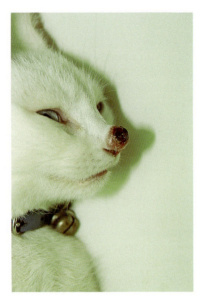

Figure 5.36 Ulcerated granuloma on the bridge of the nose in a cat with cryptococcosis.

Clinical signs

Cats:

- Most commonly present with respiratory disease (wheezing, snuffling, nasal discharge).
- CNS and ocular disease (dilated pupils, blindness) can occur.
- Skin signs are multiple non-painful papules and nodules that ulcerate (Figure 5.36).
- Typical lesion is a firm subcutaneous swelling over the bridge of the nose (Figure 5.37).
- Regional lymphadenopathy common.

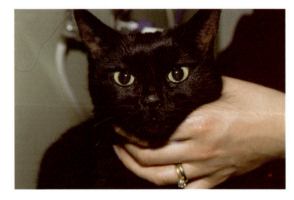

Figure 5.37 Typical lesion of cryptococcus over the bridge of the nose.

Dogs:

- Most commonly systemic disease usually CNS or ophthalmologic signs, also respiratory tract.
- Skin lesions less common and present as cutaneous ulcers on nose, lips, oral cavity or around the nail beds.

Differential diagnosis

Other systemic bacterial and fungal diseases: Neoplasia.

Diagnosis

- History and clinical signs.
- Cytology of aspirates or direct smear reveals pyogranulomatous inflammation with narrow budding thin-walled yeast surrounded by clear refractile capsule.
- Culture can be undertaken, samples best submitted to specialised laboratory.
- Biopsy shows signs of nodular to diffuse pyogranulomatous dermatitis and panniculitis with numerous organisms.
- ELISA or latex agglutination testing can be used to detect serum antibodies to cryptococcal capsular antigen. In localised disease this test may be negative.
- General diagnostic tests may also be performed to assess for involvement of other organ systems.

Treatment

- Cutaneous lesions should be removed surgically where possible.
- Long courses of anti-fungal therapy are needed. A minimum of 2–3 months and for 4 weeks beyond clinical resolution and ideally until negative serum cryptococcal antibodies.
- Drug regimes:
  - Itraconazole 5–10 mg/kg po sid/bid for 2–3 months as above.
  - Fluconazole 5–15 mg/kg po sid/bid for 2–3 months as above.

- □ Amphotericin B 0.5–0.8 mg/kg added to 0.45% saline /2.5% glucose:
  - For cats 400 ml; for dogs <20 kg, 500 ml and >20 kg, 1,000 ml sq 2–3 times weekly until cumulative dose of 8–24 mg/kg is reached.
- □ Ketoconazole 5–10 mg/kg po with food sid/bid.
■ Prognosis for cats is fair to good unless there is severe CNS disease. In cats with CNS disease and in dogs the prognosis is poor.

Histoplasmosis

Systemic disease with cutaneous manifestations caused by inhalation or ingestion of organisms of *Histoplasma capsulatum*, an environmental saprophyte. An uncommon disease in cats and a rare condition in dogs. Most often seen in young adult cats.

Histoplasmosis is a zoonosis; however, it is the fungal cultures that are infectious not the infected animals.

Cause and pathogenesis

■ Inhalation or ingestion of the conidia of *H. capsulatum* initially leads to infection in the lungs or gastrointestinal tract.
■ Worldwide distribution in both temperate and subtropical areas, especially moist humid environments often associated with birds and bat droppings.
■ The disease then disseminates to lymph nodes, eyes, skin, CNS and other organs.

Clinical signs

■ Systemic disease often vague and non-specific such as anorexia, pyrexia also respiratory (dyspnoea, tachypnoea), gastrointestinal, ocular signs.
■ Cutaneous lesions are uncommon multiple, ulcerated papules and nodules at any site.

Differential diagnosis

Other fungal and bacterial infections:
Neoplasia

Diagnosis

■ History and clinical signs.
■ Cytology of aspirate or direct smear reveals pyogranulomatous inflammation with numerous small round yeast like bodies with narrow halo.
■ Culture not recommended due to highly contagious nature of *H. capsulatum*.
■ Biopsy shows nodular to diffuse pyogranulomatous dermatitis with numerous intracellular organisms. Special fungal stains may be needed to help in identification of the yeast.
■ Serology is not a reliable test.
■ General diagnostic tests may also be performed to assess for involvement of other organ systems.

Treatment

■ Long courses of anti-fungal therapy are needed. A minimum of 4–6 months and for 8 weeks beyond clinical resolution.
■ Drug regimes:
  - □ Itraconazole 10 mg/kg po sid/bid.
  - □ Fluconazole 2.5–5 mg/kg po sid/bid.
  - □ Combination therapy with itraconazole or fluconazole with amphotericin B may be useful:
    - For cats, 0.25 mg/kg iv three times weekly until cumulative dose of 4–8 mg/kg is reached.
    - For dogs, 0.5 mg/kg iv three times weekly until cumulative dose of 5–10 mg/kg is reached.
■ Prognosis for cats is fair to good unless there is severe systemic disease. In dogs with GI or systemic disease the prognosis is poor.

Aspergillosis

Cutaneous disease caused by infection with the environmental and cutaneous saprophyte *Aspergillus* spp. Uncommon in cats and dogs. Does not represent a zoonotic risk to humans.

Cause and pathogenesis

- Caused by *Aspergillus* sp. especially *Aspergillus fumigatus*.
- Fungi are found as saprophytes in nature and as components of normal skin, hair coat and mucosae.
- Opportunistic invasion of mucosae or skin occurs, often seen in immunosuppressed animals.

Clinical signs

- Cutaneous and mucocutaneous aspergillosis presents most commonly as nasal disease with a haemorrhagic nasal discharge.
- Epistaxis is usually unilateral with secondary ulceration, crusting and depigmentation of external nares.
- Disseminated aspergillosis presents as mucosal ulcers and cutaneous ulcers and nodules.

Differential diagnosis

- Cutaneous lesions of nasal aspergillosis:
    - Discoid lupus erythematosus
    - Pemphigus foliaceus/erythematosus
    - Neoplasia especially epitheliotropic lymphoma
    - Drug eruptions

Diagnosis

- Clinical signs.
- Cytology of aspirates or direct smear inflammatory infiltrate unusual to find fungal elements. When cultured on Sabouraud's dextrose agar interpretation is difficult due to the fact that both false positives and negatives can be identified, as this organism is part of the normal skin flora.
- Biopsy reveals signs of numerous organisms that appear as septate branched hyphae.
- Serology using ELISA useful. Commercial testing is available for *Aspergillus fumigatus, niger, nidulus, terrus* and *flavus*.

Treatment

- Long courses of systemic medication are usually needed usually 2–3 months and for 3–4 weeks beyond clinical cure.
- Cutaneous and nasal lesions can be treated with systemic medication. Approximately 50% cure rate:
    - For dogs, ketoconazole 5–15 mg/kg po sid with food, itraconazole 5–10 mg/kg po sid with food, fluconazole 2.5–5 mg/kg po sid with food.
    - For cats, itraconazole 5 mg/kg po sid with food.
- Nasal aspergillus requires topical therapy usually with enilconazole flush.
- Disseminated disease treatment unsuccessful.

Protothecosis

Skin disease caused by a saprophytic, achlorophyllous alga found in Europe, Asia and North America. Rare disease in dogs and cats. No zoonotic risk to humans.

Cause and pathogenesis

- Rare disease caused by *Prototheca* spp. especially *Prototheca wickerhamii*.
- Infection can be via the gastrointestinal tract or through the skin and mucosa.
- *Protheca* sp. is an opportunistic invader of contaminated wounds and mucosa. Animals usually had contact with sewage or stagnant water.
- Disseminated disease usually seen in immunosuppressed animals.

Clinical signs

Cats:

- Cutaneous lesions appear as large firm nodules especially seen on the distal extremities, head or tail.
- Disseminated disease not reported.

Dog:

- Most commonly presents as disseminated disease. Usually gastrointestinal signs especially colitis also ocular and central nervous system signs.

- Skin lesions are rare, papules, nodules often on trunk, over pressure points and at mucocutaneous junctions.

Differential diagnosis

Other fungal and bacterial infections: Neoplasia.

Diagnosis

- History and clinical signs.
- Cytology of aspirate or direct smear reveals pyogranulomatous inflammation with numerous intracellular organisms. These appear as round, oval and polyhedral spherules that vary in size and contain endospores.
- Biopsy shows nodular to diffuse pyogranulomatous dermatitis and panniculitis with numerous intracellular organisms.
- Fungal culture is best performed by an experienced laboratory.

Treatment

- Wide surgical excision of lesions is the therapy of choice.
- Systemic anti-fungal therapy is rarely effective; possible drug combinations include the following:
  - Itraconazole 5–10 mg/kg po sid/bid with food.
  - Fluconazole 2.5–5 mg/kg po or iv bid.
  - Ketoconazole 10–15 mg/kg po sid/bid with food.
  - Combination therapy with tetracycline at 22 mg/kg po tid and amphotericin B may be useful:
    - For cats, 0.25 mg/kg iv three times weekly until cumulative dose of 4 mg/kg is reached.
    - For dogs, 0.25–0.5 mg/kg iv three times weekly until cumulative dose of 8 mg/kg is reached.

Prognosis is poor when disseminated disease is present and when lesions cannot be surgically resected.

Selected references and further reading

Bond, R. (2002) Pathogenesis of Malassezia dermatitis. In: Thoday, K.L. et al. (eds) *Advances in Veterinary Dermatology*. Vol. 4. pp. 69–75. Blackwell Science, Oxford

Campbell, K.L. (2004) Deep mycoses. In: Campbell, K.L. (ed) *Small Animal Dermatology Secrets*. pp. 170–177. Hanley and Belfus, Philadelphia

Foil, C.S. (1998) Dermatophytosis. In: Greene, C.E. and Kersey, R. (eds) *Infectious Diseases of the Dog and Cat*. pp. 262–270. WB Saunders, Philadelphia

Greene, C.E. and Chandler, F.W. (1998) Candidiasis, torulopsosis and rhodotorulosis. In: Greene, C.E. and Kersey, R. (eds). *Infectious Diseases of the Dog and Cat*. pp. 414–417. WB Saunders, Philadelphia

Hill, P.B. et al. (1995) A review of systemic antifungal agents. *Vet Dermatol*, **6**, 59

Medleau, L. and Hnilica, K. (2006) Fungal skin disease. In: *Small Animal Dermatology: A Color Atlas and Therapeutic Guide*. 2nd edn. pp. 63–97. WB Saunders, Philadelphia

Moriello, K.A. (1990) Management of dermatophytes infections in catteries and multiple cat households. *Vet Clin North Am Small Anim Pract*, **20**, 1457

Moriello, K.A. (2004) Superficial mycotic infections. In: Campbell, K.L. (ed) *Small Animal Dermatology Secrets*. pp. 157–169. Hanley and Belfus, Philadelphia

Moriello, K.A. and DeBoer, D.J. (1995) Efficacy of griseofulvin and itraconazole in the treatment of experimentally induced dermatophytosis in cats. *J Am Vet Med Assoc*, **207**, 439

Scott, D.W. et al. (2001) Fungal skin disease. In: *Muller and Kirk's Small Animal Dermatology*. 6th edn. pp. 336–422. WB Saunders, Philadelphia

Thomas, R.C. (2004) Principles of topical therapy. In: Campbell, K.L. (ed). *Small Animal Dermatology Secrets*. pp. 71–85. Hanley and Belfus, Philadelphia

Toboada, J. (2000) Systemic mycoses. In: Ettinger, S.J. and Feldman, E.C. (eds). *Textbook of Veterinary Internal Medicine*. 5th edn. pp. 453–477. WB Saunders, Philadelphia

Viral, rickettsial and protozoal diseases

Viral disease

(a) Canine distemper (CDV)
(b) Contagious viral pustular dermatitis (Orf)
(c) Pseudorabies ('mad itch')
(d) Papillomavirus
(e) Feline leukaemia virus (FeLV)
(f) Giant cell dermatosis
(g) Feline immunodeficiency virus (FIV)
(h) Feline pox virus
(i) Feline infectious peritonitis (FIP)
(j) Feline rhinotracheitis virus (FRV)
(k) Feline calici virus (FCV)
(l) Feline sarcoma virus (FSV)

Canine distemper

Cause and pathogenesis

Systemic disease caused by morbillivirus most commonly seen in young unvaccinated puppies. Rare in dogs; does not occur in cats.

Clinical signs

- Most common signs are systemic in the form of respiratory (mucopurulent oculonasal discharge, Figure 6.1), gastrointestinal (diarrhoea) and neurological signs.
- Cutaneous lesions:
    - Impetigo-like disease seen in young puppies.
    - Nasal and footpad hyperkeratosis (hard pad disease) (Figure 6.2).

Differential diagnosis

- Footpad and nasal signs:
    - Familial footpad hyperkeratosis
    - Hereditary nasal parakeratosis of the Labrador retriever
    - Pemphigus foliaceus
    - Lupus erythematosus
    - Drug eruption
    - Necrolytic migratory erythema
    - Zinc responsive dermatosis
    - Idiopathic nasodigital hyperkeratosis

Diagnosis

- History of lack of vaccination.
- Clinical signs and ruled out of other differentials.
- Immunocytology or PCR technique of blood, nasal, ocular discharge, saliva, conjunctival scrapings CSF to detect viral antigens.

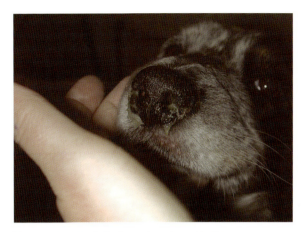

Figure 6.1 Nasal discharge in a dog with distemper.

- Biopsy of footpads reveals non-specific signs including orthokeratotic hyperkeratosis, mononuclear perivascular infiltrate. Rarely typical signs of balloon degeneration and eosinophilic intracytoplasmic viral inclusions are seen.
- Immunohistochemistry of skin of footpad or planum nasale to detect viral antigen.

Treatment

- Symptomatic treatment to make the dog comfortable with fluids and broad spectrum antibiotic cover.
- No specific antiviral therapy is available.
- Prognosis is guarded.

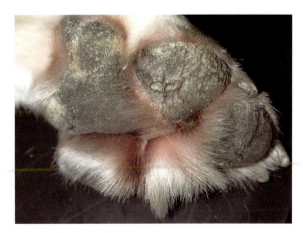

Figure 6.2 Footpad hyperkeratosis in a dog with distemper.

Contagious viral pustular dermatitis (Orf)

Cause and pathogenesis

Rare dermatitis of dogs and cats caused by parapox virus. A common disease of sheep and goats, which are the usual source of infection. Virus carried in infected scabs and crusts. Dogs contract infection through eating infected material; only isolated cases in cats. It is a zoonotic disease.

Clinical signs

- Lesions present as areas of acute moist dermatitis with ulceration and crusting.
- Predilection sites are contact areas especially the face and mouth.

Differential diagnosis

Other causes of acute moist dermatitis.

Diagnosis

- History and clinical signs especially farm dogs, which have contact with sheep/goats.
- Electron microscopy of scabs reveals signs of virus.
- Skin biopsy reveals signs of epidermal hyperplasia, balloon degeneration, acantholysis within the stratum spinosum and neutrophil accumulation.

Treatment

- Symptomatic therapy with antibacterial shampoo and creams and broad spectrum antibiotic cover.
- Clinical signs are usually self-limiting.
- Glucocorticoids contraindicated.

Pseudorabies ('mad itch')

Cause and pathogenesis

Severely pruritic skin disease caused by alpha-herpes virus, which results in the death of the animals. Very rare disease in dogs and cats. Pigs act as reservoirs of infection. Pets are infected by contact with infected animals or by eating infected carcasses. On oral or oronasal infection, the virus is spread by way of the cranial nerves to the central nervous system. The incubation period is short: from 1 to 6 days. Mortality in dogs and cats is 100%. In rural areas, infection is caused by consumption of uncooked pork or offal from pigs.

Clinical signs

- Excessive salivation, restlessness, neurological signs.
- Dogs approximately 50% – intense pruritus of upper body especially head.
- Cats mostly present with neurological signs; pruritus is rare.

Differential diagnosis

- Ectoparasites especially scabies
- Allergy – atopy, food allergy
- Neuritis
- Rabies

Diagnosis

- History and clinical signs especially contact with infected animals.
- Diagnosis is usually retrospective at postmortem.
- Histopathology of the brain reveals non-suppurative encephalitis located in the brain stem, mainly near the floor of the IV ventricle.
- Aujeszky's disease virus (ADV) antigen and ADV nucleic acid distribution can be identified using immunohistochemistry and in situ hybridization coincided with the histopathological lesions.

Treatment

- Source of infection should be identified.
- Prevention is possible by avoiding exposure to pigs or fresh pig products.
- Unrewarding to treat dogs; elective euthanasia once diagnosis has been made.

Papillomavirus

Cause and pathogenesis

Cutaneous lesions in the form of benign tumours induced by papillomavirus. Different cutaneous manifestations are thought to be caused by distinct papilloma viruses. At least five different papilloma viruses have been identified in dogs and eight in cats. Majority of lesions will regress in normal individual as a cell-mediated immune response develops. Regression can take 4–6 months for oral lesions and 6–12 months for cutaneous lesions. Transmission is by direct and indirect contact. The incubation period can be 1–2 months.

Clinical signs

Dogs:

- Oral papillomatosis:
  - Papillomas found in oral cavity (Figure 6.3), lips, conjunctiva and external nares.
  - Lesions appear as multiple smooth white papules and plaques.
  - Especially seen in immunosuppressed animals, e.g. puppies.
  - Lesions regress in 3 months.
- Cutaneous exophytic papillomas:
  - Lesions affect the head (Figure 6.4), eyelids and feet (Figure 6.5).
  - Usually solitary lesions; elevated smooth to papilliferous growths may be flesh coloured or pigmented on narrow base.

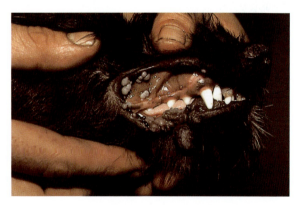

Figure 6.3 Papilloma lesions found in the oral cavity of a young puppy.

Viral, rickettsial and protozoal diseases 85

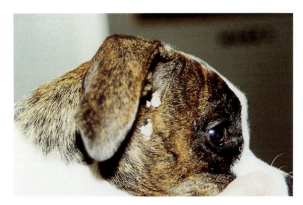

Figure 6.4 Cutaneous papillomas on the face of a young Boxer puppy.

- Usually <0.5 cm in size.
- Most commonly seen in older dogs, especially cocker spaniels and Kerry blue terrier.
■ Inverted papilloma:
- Most commonly seen on ventral abdomen and inguinal area.
- Lesions are single to multiple endophytic masses, 1–2 cm across extending into crater-like invagination.
■ Footpad papillomas:
- Usually seen in adult dogs as 'horn-like' projections on multiple pads.
- Interdigital lesions have been reported in greyhounds.
- Dogs commonly present with lameness.

■ Multiple pigmented epidermal plaques:
- Non-regressing lesions on the ventrum and medial thighs.
- Usually multiple pigmented macules and plaques.
- Possible genetic predisposition, especially young adult pugs, miniature schnauzers.
- Some lesions can undergo malignant transformation into squamous cell carcinoma.
■ Genital papilloma:
- Lesions appear as papillomatous plaques on penile or vaginal mucosa.

Cats:

■ Oral papilloma:
- Lesions found in oral cavity, especially on the ventral aspect of tongue.
- Multiple raised oval flat-topped lesions, 4–8 mm in size.
■ Multiple viral papilloma:
- Middle age to old cats.
- Lesions found on haired skin of head, neck, trunk and proximal limbs (Figure 6.6).
- Usually multiple lesions, 3 mm to 3 cm pigmented macules and plaques.
- Some lesions can undergo malignant squamous cell carcinoma.

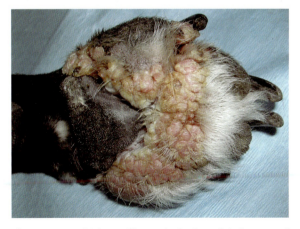

Figure 6.5 Multiple papillomas in the interdigital spaces of a dog.

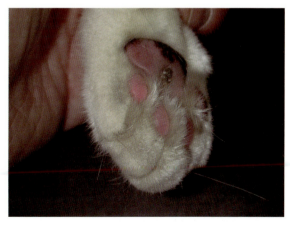

Figure 6.6 Pigmented viral papillomas on the footpad of a cat.

- Solitary cutaneous papilloma:
  - Rare disease; seen in adult cats.
  - Any site appears as small pedunculated masses <0.5 cm.
- Feline sarcoid (see Chapter 21).

Differential diagnosis

- Neoplasia especially squamous cell carcinoma
- Collagenous nevus
- Granulation tissue
- Eosinophilic granuloma

Diagnosis

- Clinical appearance of lesions.
- Biopsy reveals epidermal hyperplasia and papillomatosis with balloon degeneration. Intranuclear inclusions are an inconsistent finding.
- Immunohistochemistry or PCR techniques can be used to identify papilloma virus antigen in tissue.

Treatment

- Spontaneous regression occurs in many cases but can take many months.
- Surgical excision can be undertaken on persistent lesions, but care should be taken not to seed the infection to other sites.
- Ablation using laser or cryotherapy may be successful but multiple treatments are usually required.
- Topical therapy may be useful. An Elizabethan collar should be used to prevent animals licking off the medication.
  - Dogs:
    - 5-fluorouracil 0.5% solution can be used on cutaneous lesions every 24 hours for 5 days, then once weekly for 4–6 weeks.
  - Dogs and cats:
    - 5% imiquimod cream applied every 24–48 hours until lesion regression.
- Autogenous (wart) vaccines can be prepared by some laboratories, but are of questionable benefit.
- Immunomodulating drugs such as levamisole and thiabendazole show unproven benefit.

Feline leukaemia virus

Cause and pathogenesis

FeLV is an oncogenic retrovirus that causes immunosuppression leading to the formation of skin tumours and chronic infection.

Virus is contagious to other cats but not dogs or humans.

Clinical signs

- Skin tumours lymphoma, fibrosarcoma (see Chapter 21).
- Cutaneous horns, which present as firm horn-like projections usually seen on footpads, occasionally on face. Often seen as a cutaneous marker for FeLV.

Immunosuppression can lead to the following:

- Bacterial infection such as gingivitis, folliculitis, paronychia (Figure 6.7), abscesses (Figure 6.8) especially in cases of atypical mycobacterium, nocardia; may present as non-healing wounds.
- Yeast or fungal infection especially dermatophytosis, malassezia, cryptococcus; infection often poorly responsive or relapsing.
- Viral infection especially cow pox (Figure 6.9).
- Parasites especially demodicosis.

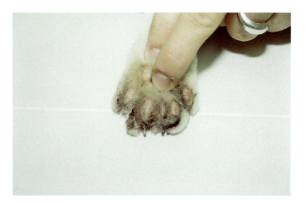

Figure 6.7 Bacterial paronychia in cat with FeLV.

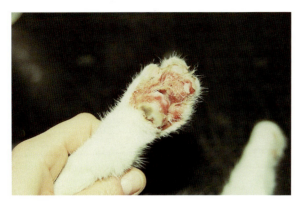

Figure 6.8 Abscess on paw in FeLV positive cat.

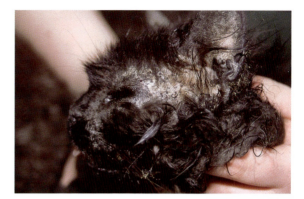

Figure 6.10 Lesions of giant cell dermatosis affecting the face.

Differential diagnosis

Any bacterial, fungal, viral or ectoparasitic disease, which is poorly responsive to appropriate therapy or where unusual organisms are isolated.

Diagnosis

- Serological tests to confirm FeLV.
- Specific investigations of dermatological lesions as appropriate.

Treatment

- Usually palliative and symptomatic treatment only.
- The response to therapy for secondary bacterial infection should be based on appropriate culture and sensitivity.

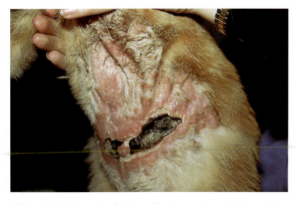

Figure 6.9 Extensive lesions of cat pox in an FeLV positive cat.

- Bactericidal and fungicidal therapy offers the best chance of success.
- Some cases respond completely and therapy can be withdrawn, others require long-term treatment.
- Immunosuppressive therapy in the form of glucocorticoids and cyclosporine should be avoided.

Giant cell dermatosis

Cause and pathogenesis

Infection with FeLV is thought to cause neoplastic alteration of keratinocytes by recombination with host's oncogenes, leading to skin disease.

Clinical signs

- No breed or sex predilection is seen.
- All reported cases have been less than 6 years of age.
- Lesions present as crusting and scaling with diffuse alopecia.
- Variable distribution, ears and periauricular skin commonly involved (Figures 6.10 and 6.11).

Differential diagnosis

- Dermatophytosis
- Neoplasia especially lymphoma, thymoma
- Primary keratinisation disorder
- Cheyletiella

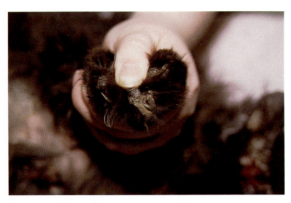

Figure 6.11 Lesions of giant cell dermatosis affecting the nail beds.

Diagnosis

- Rule-outs including fungal culture and skin scrapings.
- Serology to confirm the presence of FeLV.
- Biopsy reveals signs of typical syncytial-type giant cells in the epidermis and outer root sheath of the hair follicle.
- Immunohistochemistry may be used to identify FeLV antigen in skin samples.

Treatment

- No response to antibacterial or antifungal therapy.
- Poor prognosis; most cats euthanised.

Feline immunodeficiency virus

Cause and pathogenesis

A retrovirus capable of producing cytosuppression. Clinical signs overlap with those of FeLV infections. Virus is contagious to other cats but not dogs or humans.

Clinical signs

- See FeLV. The clinical signs associated with FIV infection are clinically similar to those of FeLV and can only be differentiated by serological identification of the virus involved (Figure 6.12).
- The two viruses can occur concurrently leading to synergistic immunosuppression.

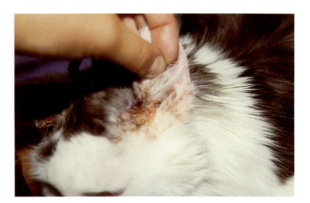

Figure 6.12 Pyoderma in an FIV positive cat.

Differential diagnosis

As FeLV.

Diagnosis

Serological tests for FIV.

Treatment

As FeLV.

Feline pox virus

Cause and pathogenesis

Cutaneous disease caused by poxvirus, which is a member of the *Orthopoxvirus* genus.

Uncommon disease only found in cats, rural hunting cats predisposed. Small wild rodents are thought to be the reservoir for infection. Cats become infected through a bite wound. Disease is seen in Western European countries, including the United Kingdom and Asia. No sex, breed or age incidence recognised, although most cases occur in the autumn when the rodent population is highest. It is a zoonotic disease.

Clinical signs

- Initial lesion is an infected bite wound usually on head (Figure 6.13) or forelimb.
- Viraemia after local replication leads to the formation of multiple secondary lesions, which are usually seen 1–3 weeks later.

Viral, rickettsial and protozoal diseases

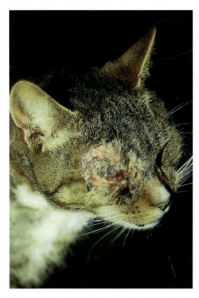

Figure 6.13 Primary bite wound thought to be from a rodent in the case of cat pox.

- Secondary lesions appear as ulcerated papules and nodules leading to crusted sores (Figure 6.14).
- Lesions are larger than those of miliary dermatitis and up to 1 cm in diameter.
- Pruritus variable but can be intense.

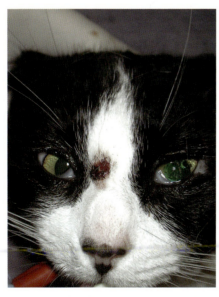

Figure 6.14 Secondary lesions of cat pox on the face of a cat.

- Less common manifestations include oral vesicles and ulcers.
- Lesions are self-limiting in a fit animal and will dry and exfoliate over the next 4–6 weeks.
- Systemic signs (pyrexia, diarrhoea) rare unless cat immunosuppressed or anti-inflammatory therapy is used.

Differential diagnosis

- Dermatophytosis
- Eosinophilic granuloma complex/miliary dermatitis
- Neoplasia (lymphoma, mast cell tumour)
- Superficial pyoderma
- Pemphigus foliaceus

Diagnosis

- Clinical signs and history.
- Electron microscopy of scabs for virus.
- Virus isolation from tissue or scabs (submitted to an appropriate laboratory in viral transport medium).
- Biopsy reveals epidermal hyperplasia, balloon and reticular degeneration, microvesicles occasionally with characteristic eosinophilic intracytoplasmic inclusions in keratinocytes.
- Serology (specialised laboratories only).

Treatment

- Lesions heal slowly over 3–4 weeks without therapy in uncomplicated cases.
- When secondary infection is present antibiotics should be prescribed based on culture and sensitivity. Empirical therapy can be undertaken with cephalexin, clindamycin or clavamox.
- Symptomatic therapy of pruritus should be with antihistamines:
    - Chlorpheniramine 4 mg/cat po bid/tid.
    - Promethazine 12.5 mg/cat po bid.
- An Elizabethan collar can be used to prevent self-traumatisation.
- Glucocorticoids are contraindicated.
- In immunosuppressed or systemically ill cats, supportive therapy is also required.
- Euthanasia is often necessary in severe cases.

Feline infectious peritonitis

Cause and pathogenesis

- A multi-systemic viral disease caused by a coronavirus. Systemic disease can be effusive (exudate found in body cavities) and/or non-effusive (pyogranulomatous lesions in various sites).
- Virus is contagious to other cats but not dogs or humans.

Clinical signs

Systemic disease:

- Usually affects abdominal organs often abdominal distension, also ocular and neurological signs.

Cutaneous lesions:

- Usually associated with debilitation and ataxia.
- Ulcerative lesions around the head and neck have been seen in experimentally infected cats.

Diagnosis

- History and clinical signs.
- Positive FIP titre in combination with supportive serum chemistry, haematology and fluid analysis.
- Histopathology in reported cases experimentally induced showed signs of a vasculitis.

Treatment

- Symptomatic and supportive therapy.

Feline rhinotracheitis

Cause and pathogenesis

Very common disease caused by a herpes virus (feline herpes virus 1, FHV1). Route of infection is intranasal, oral or conjunctival. Most commonly seen in boarding facilities and catteries.

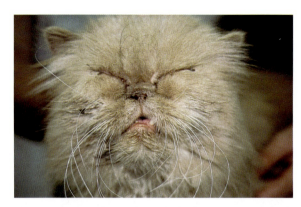

Figure 6.15 Ocular and nasal discharge in a cat with herpesvirus.

Upper respiratory tract signs most common, especially seen in young and immunosuppressed cats. Virus is contagious to other cats but not dogs or humans.

Clinical signs

Systemic signs:

- Depression, anorexia.
- Mucopurulent ocular and nasal discharge (Figure 6.15) leading to crusting of external nares and eyelids.
- Conjunctivitis and ulcerative or interstitial keratitis.
- Oral ulceration leading to hypersalivation.
- Sneezing and in severe cases dyspnoea and coughing.

Cutaneous signs – uncommon:

- Superficial ulcers can occur anywhere on the body especially footpads (Figure 6.16), face and trunk.
- Periocular alopecia with erythema and erosions.
- Ulcers can be precipitated by stress or trauma.

Differential diagnosis

Respiratory tract disease:

- FCV, *Bordetella*, *Chlamydia*, *Mycoplasma*

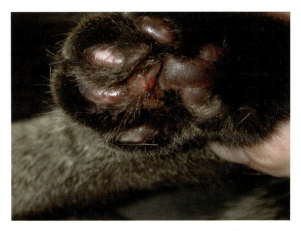

Figure 6.16 Ulcers on footpads of cat with feline herpes virus.

Cutaneous signs:

- Vasculitis
- Drug eruptions
- Contact irritant/allergy
- Erythema multiforme
- Neoplasia (lymphoma)
- Bacterial infection

Diagnosis

- History and clinical signs in an unvaccinated cat.
- Oropharyngeal or skin swabs in viral transport medium.
- Biopsy reveals ulcerative and necrotic dermatitis with mixed inflammatory cell infiltrate. In some cases epidermal cells may contain basophilic intranuclear inclusions.
- Electron microscopy to identify virus in keratinocytes.
- Fluorescent antibody or PCR techniques on conjunctival smears to detect viral antigen.

Treatment

- No specific anti-viral therapy is available.
- Symptomatic therapy using broad spectrum systemic and ophthalological antibiotics for secondary infection.
- Topical anti-viral eye preparations for ocular signs.
- Combinations of alpha-interferon, lysine and imiquimod may be useful:
  - Alpha-interferon 30 U po sid for a week on and a week off.
  - Lysine 200–400 mg/cat po sid.
  - Imiquimod cream initially applied to cutaneous lesions daily for 3 days then twice weekly until lesions resolve.
- Glucocorticoids are contraindicated.
- Prognosis is good; most cats recover in 2–3 weeks.

Feline calici virus

Cause and pathogenesis

- Common viral disease caused by a calici virus. Infection occurs by the oral, intranasal or conjunctival routes. Endemic in many catteries and rescue centres where chronic shedders are present.
- Upper respiratory and oral cavity signs occur most commonly.
- Three forms of infection are recognised:
  - Acute FCV infection
  - Chronic FCV infection
  - Virulent systemic FCV infection
- Acute and chronic infections are caused by vaccine sensitive strains of virus. Virulent systemic FCV is caused by one of at least two non-vaccine sensitive strains (FCV-ARI, FCV-KAOS) that have been identified.

Clinical signs

Acute FCV infection:

- Transient self-limiting disease.
- Most commonly cats present with oral lesions. Usually on the tongue (Figure 6.17) but also soft palate, lips, nasal philtrum.
- Primary lesions are vesicles (Figure 6.18) that rupture to form ulcers.
- Cutaneous ulceration has also been reported on feet and perineum.
- Ocular, nasal, conjunctival and pulmonary disease less severe than FVR1.

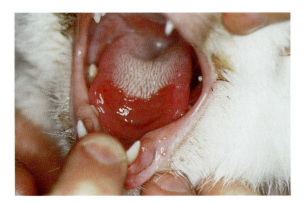

Figure 6.17 Oral ulceration in a cat with calicivirus infection. (Source: Picture courtesy of D. Crossley.)

- Systemic signs include depression, pyrexia, sneezing, conjunctivitis, oculonasal discharge; rarely arthropathy and pneumonia.

Chronic FCV infection:

- Clinical signs confined to the mouth.
- Proliferative or ulcerative gingivitis and stomatitis (plasmacytic/lymphocytic in nature).
- Animals often have halitosis, dysphagia, hypersalivation, inappetence and weight loss.

Virulent systemic FCV infection:

- Range of presentations from asymptomatic carrier to severe disease and death.
- Incubation period ~7 days.

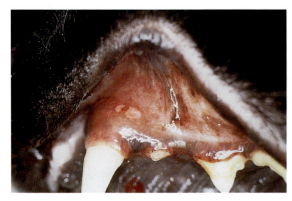

Figure 6.18 Vesicles on the gums of a cat with calicivirus infection. (Source: Picture courtesy of D. Crossley.)

- Skin lesions include oral ulcers, alopecia, crusting and ulceration of face, ear pinnae, footpads and nares; oedema of face and limbs reported.
- Systemic signs include pyrexia, nasal and ocular discharge, dyspnoea, arthropathy, jaundice, gastrointestinal signs and death.

Differential diagnosis

Respiratory tract disease:

- FCV, *Bordetella*, *Chlamydia*, *Mycoplasma*

Other causes of oral ulceration;

- Other viral infections
- Pemphigus vulgaris
- Bacterial stomatitis
- Drug eruption
- Systemic lupus erythematosus
- Renal disease
- Neoplasia especially lymphoma

Diagnosis

- Clinical signs in an unvaccinated cat, especially where oral ulceration predominates.
- Oropharyngeal or skin swabs in viral transport medium for culture; PCR technique to isolate FCV.
- Serology for FCV antibodies.
- Fluorescent antibody testing on conjunctival smears to look for calici virus antigens.
- Biopsy reveals in cases of virulent systemic FCV epithelial necrosis with ulceration. Inflammation usually minimal. Superficial oedema or vasculitis may be present.

Treatment

- Supportive nursing care with systemic broad spectrum antibiotic therapy for secondary infection.
- In outbreaks of virulent systemic FCV the establishment should be closed and disinfected.
- Prognosis:
    - For acute disease prognosis is good in fit mature animals. Can be fatal in young kittens and immunosuppressed cats.

- Chronic disease prognosis is guarded because the disease is progressive and difficult to treat.
- Virulent disease caries worst prognosis for adult cats who are most likely to develop severe disease and die.

Feline sarcoma virus

Sarcoma virus has been associated with the formation of cutaneous fibrosarcomas in young cats (see Chapter 21).

Rickettsial disease

Canine Rocky Mountain spotted fever

Cause and pathogenesis

Necrotising vasculitis caused by *Rickettsia rickettsii*. Only recognised to date in the United States. Disease is transmitted by ticks in eastern United States, *Dermacentor variabilis* (American dog tick), and western United States, *Dermacentor andersoni* (Rocky Mountain wood tick). *R. rickettsii* picked up by tick from small rodents and passed onto humans or dogs. It multiplies in vascular endothelium and vascular smooth muscle to produce vasculitis and thrombosis. A zoonotic disease. Most common in dogs in endemic areas and outdoor types. High incidence is during March to October during tick feeding times.

Clinical signs

Systemic signs of fever, anorexia, lethargy are seen ~ 5 days after the initial tick bite.
Other signs include the following:

- Abdominal pain, myalgia, polyarthritis, dyspnoea, neurological disease (vestibular disease, coma, seizures).
- Occasionally melaena, epistaxis and haematuria.

Cutaneous lesions:

- Acute disease:
  - Erythema, petechiation, oedema, ulceration and necrosis of mucus membranes and extremities, often with retinal haemorrhages.
  - Vesicles and macules are seen on buccal mucosa.
- Chronic/recovering disease:
  - Necrosis of the extremities can occur.

Differential diagnosis

Other causes of vasculitis:

- Infectious agents
- Immune-mediated disease
- Toxins

Diagnosis

- History and clinical signs.
- Blood profile reveals signs of thrombocytopaenia, leukocytosis and hypoalbuminaemia.
- Biopsy reveals signs of necrotising vasculitis and thrombosis.
- Indirect immunofluorescent assay for *Rickettsial rickettsii* antigen looking for fourfold increase in paired samples 3 weeks apart.
- Direct immunofluorescent or immunohistochemistry assay for *R. rickettsii* antigen from acute skin lesions.
- PCR technique on skin biopsies to look for *Rickettsia* DNA.

Treatment

- Careful removal of all ticks, taking care not to puncture their bodies, which will release infectious organisms.
- Supportive care for 1–2 weeks with antibiotics and fluids if needed.
- Antibiotic therapy with one of the following in order of preference:
  - Doxycycline 10–20 mg/kg po or iv bid 1–2 weeks.
  - Tetracycline 25–30 mg/kg po or iv qid 1–2 weeks.
  - Chloramphenicol may be useful in pregnant animals and puppies <6 months of

age; 15–30 mg/kg po, sq, im or iv qid 1–2 weeks.
- Enrofloxacin (adult dogs only) 5–10 mg/kg po or sq bid for 1–2 weeks.
- Topical therapy to prevent dogs in endemic areas; picking up ticks is important.
- Prognosis is good if the disease is identified and treated early. In chronic disease debilitating disfigurement can occur.

Canine ehrlichiosis

Cause and pathogenesis

Worldwide tick-borne disease caused by *Ehrlichia* spp. most commonly *Ehrlichia canis*. Ehrlichia rickettsial organisms infect mononuclear, granulocytic or thrombocytic cells.

Not a zoonosis, but humans can become infected by ticks.

Clinical signs

- Systemic signs include
  - depression, lethargy, anorexia;
  - commonly splenomegaly, hepatomegaly;
  - less commonly uveitis, polymyositis, polyarthritis and CNS signs.
- Cutaneous lesions:
  - Dermal petechiae and ecchymoses

Differential diagnosis

- Other causes of vasculitis and thrombocytopaenia including
  - immune-mediated disease,
  - infections especially Rocky Mountain spotted fever,
  - drug eruptions.

Diagnosis

- Blood profile reveals signs of normochromic, normocytic non-regenerative anaemia. Often thrombocytopaenia and/or leukopaenia also present.
- Indirect immunofluorescent antibody or ELISA to detect serum anti-Ehrlichia antibodies:
  - False negative can occur in acute disease <3 weeks duration.
  - False positive results can occur as natural titres in dogs in endemic areas.
- PCR technique on blood, bone or splenic aspirate to detect Ehrlichia antigen.

Treatment

- Supportive therapy with fluids as appropriate.
- Antibiotic therapy with one of the following in order of preference:
  - Doxycycline 10 mg/kg po bid for 4 weeks.
  - Tetracycline 22 mg/kg po tid 2–3 weeks.
  - Chloramphenicol may be useful in pregnant animals and puppies (<6 months of age); 15–30 mg/kg po, sq or iv qid 2–3 weeks.
  - Imidocarb dipropionate 5 mg/kg im given twice 2–3 weeks apart.
- Topical therapy to prevent dogs in endemic areas; picking up ticks is important.
- Dogs usually show a rapid response to treatment once it is started. Platelet counts should start to improve within 48 hours, taking 2 weeks to recover completely.
- Prognosis is good if the disease is identified and treated early. Dogs with chronic disease carry a guarded prognosis.

Protozoal diseases

(a) Caryosporosis
(b) Neosporosis
(c) Sarcocystosis
(d) Babesiosis
(e) Leishmaniasis

Caryosporosis

Nodular skin lesions caused by coccidia of genus *Caryospora* spp.

Cause and pathogenesis

A rare disease of dogs. Life cycle of the parasite is complex, involving rodents, reptiles and raptors. Infection of the dog occurs by ingestion of infected host containing the coccidia.

Clinical signs

- Systemic disease includes
  - anorexia, inappetence and diarrhoea.
- Cutaneous lesions include
  - nodules and plaques usually found on the trunk.

Differential diagnosis

- Infectious granulomatous disease – fungal and bacterial infection
- Neoplasia
- Sterile nodular panniculitis
- Sterile pyogranuloma and pyogranuloma
- Leishmaniasis

Diagnosis

- History and clinical signs.
- Skin biopsy reveals a pyogranulomatous tissue reaction with eosinophils and numerous protozoa. Immunohistochemistry useful for positive identification.

Treatment

- Supportive and symptomatic therapy where appropriate.
- Antibiotic therapy with either of the following:
  - Clindamycin 12.5 mg/kg po bid or 10 mg/kg po tid until complete resolution of lesions, which can take 4–6 weeks. Medication may need to be extended for a further 4 weeks in immunosuppressed animals.
  - Trimethoprim–sulphadiazine 15 mg/kg po bid until resolution of lesions as above

Neosporosis

Ulcerative skin disease caused by cyst forming protozoal parasite *Neospora caninum*.

Cause and pathogenesis

Disease can affect many different species including dogs, cattle, sheep, goats and horses. Life cycle is not completely understood but transplacental infection thought to occur. It is most commonly identified in young dogs with neuromuscular disease.

Clinical signs

- Systemic signs most commonly seen in young dogs; cutaneous lesions are rare and have only been recorded in middle aged to older dogs with immunosuppressive disease.
- Young dogs:
  - Neuromuscular dysfunction especially hind leg paralysis, also meningoencephalitis.
- Older dogs:
  - Cutaneous signs appear as multiple firm pruritic, ulcerative fistulous nodules ranging from 0.5 to 2.0 cm in diameter.
  - Can be found at any site but commonly on perineum, eyelid, neck and thorax.
  - Systemic signs include myocarditis and pneumonia.

Differential diagnosis

- Infectious granulomatous disease – fungal and bacterial infection
- Neoplasia
- Sterile nodular panniculitis
- Sterile pyogranuloma and pyogranuloma
- Leishmaniasis

Diagnosis

- History and clinical signs.
- Cytology shows signs of mixed inflammatory infiltrate; organisms can occasionally be seen in neutrophils and macrophages.
- Biopsy reveals diffuse pyogranulomatous dermatitis with deep dermal nodular infiltrates of plasma cells and lymphocytes. Neospora organisms appear as ovoid intracellular tachyzoites within keratinocytes, macrophages and endothelial cells.
- Indirect fluorescent antibody or Neospora agglutination test looking for serum antibody levels.
- Immunohistochemistry of skin biopsies to identify *N. caninum* tachyzoites.

Treatment

- Supportive and symptomatic therapy where appropriate.
- Antibiotic therapy with either of the following:
  - Clindamycin 12.5 mg/kg po bid or 10 mg/kg po tid until complete resolution of lesions, which can take 4–6 weeks. Medication may need to be extended for a further 4 weeks in immunosuppressed animals.
  - Trimethoprim–sulphadiazine 15 mg/kg po bid until resolution of lesions as above.
  - Pyrimethamine 1 mg/kg po sid.
- Prognosis is poor if the disease is rapidly progressive or not identified early. Treated animals may be left with permanent gait and conformational abnormalities.

Sarcocystosis

Vasculitis caused by protozoan parasite *Sarcocystis canis*. Life cycle of *Sarcocystis* spp. is unknown.

Cause and pathogenesis

Infection occurs by ingestion of tissue cysts within tissue of the host.

Clinical signs

- Usually non-pathogenic.
- Usually seen in hunting dogs and wild dogs due to scavenging for wild meat.
- Cutaneous lesions when occur multifocal abscesses.

Diagnosis

- History and clinical signs.
- Histopathology of skin reveals signs of protozoa seen in sections.
- Immunohistochemistry and PCR techniques can be used to identify the organisms in tissue.
- Transmission electron microscopy revealed merozoites consistent with *Sarcocystis* spp.

Treatment

- Usually unsuccessful and animals tend to be euthanised.
- Trimethoprim–sulphadiazine 15 mg/kg po bid until resolution of lesions, which can take 2–4 weeks then prolonged course for a further 4 weeks.

Babesiosis

Cause and pathogenesis

Babesiosis is caused by an intracellular parasite of the red blood cells inoculated by *Ixodes* ticks. *Babesia canis* is the most common cause of this disease and has a worldwide distribution. Seasonal incidence spring and autumn to correspond to tick feeding times. Parasite causes intravascular and extravascular haemolysis, thrombocytopaenia, disseminated intravascular coagulation. There are three forms of the disease, per acute, acute, and chronic.

Clinical signs

- Per acute disease:
  - Dogs present with inappetence, depression, weakness and pyrexia.
  - Examination reveals jaundice and anaemia.
  - Animals often die before a diagnosis can be confirmed.
- Acute and chronic disease:
  - Systemic signs:
    - Pyrexia, anaemia, icterus, gastrointestinal, renal, respiratory, neuromuscular signs.
  - Cutaneous lesions:
    - Babesia causes clinical signs of a vasculitis.
    - Oedema, petechiation, necrosis of axilla, groin, scrotum, lower limbs and ear tips.

Diagnosis

- History and clinical signs especially exposure to ticks.
- Blood smear taken from peripheral blood in per acute and some acute and chronic cases reveal 'bullseye' appearing red blood cells that contain low levels of haemoglobin. Babesia organisms are present as small, usually single, pleomorphic organisms.

- Where parasites are not seen on smears, blood may be submitted for indirect fluorescent antibody test.
- Skin biopsy reveals signs of leukocytoclastic vasculitis with or without epidermal necrosis.
- Serological tests for Babesia.

Treatment

- Symptomatic treatment with intravenous fluids and good nursing care.
- Antiparasitic treatment:
  - Imidocarb dipropionate at 5 mg/kg body weight by deep muscular injection every 2 weeks for two treatments.

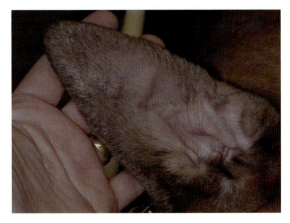

Figure 6.19 Scaling on the ear pinna of a dog with leishmaniasis.

Leishmaniasis

Dermatitis caused by protozoan parasite *Leishmania* spp. Disease is seen in Mediterranean countries, Central America, parts of Africa, Middle East and dogs imported from or holidaying in endemic areas. It is a common disease in dogs in endemic areas, rare in cats. Zoonotic disease, although direct transmission from dogs to humans is very rare. Infected animals in a household can act as a potential reservoir of infection.

Cause and pathogenesis

Disease transmitted by blood sucking sand flies usually *Phlebotomus*. In the Mediterranean areas *L. donovani* is recognised as being the most important vector. Incubation period is prolonged and can be from weeks to years.

Clinical signs

Dogs:

- Visceral signs include
  - weight loss, lethargy, exercise intolerance, muscle wasting, pyrexia, hepatosplenomegaly, lameness and conjunctivitis.
- Cutaneous lesions:
  - Most common clinical signs are of an exfoliative dermatitis with fine scaling; usually starts on the head but spreads to ear pinnae (Figure 6.19) and extremities before generalising. Periocular scaling and alopecia common (Figure 6.20).
  - Nasodigital hyperkeratosis can occur concurrently (Figure 6.21).
  - Ulcerative dermatitis especially at pressure points, mucocutaneous junctions (Figure 6.22), footpads and pinnae less common signs.
  - Onychogryposis and paronychia may be seen.
  - Sterile ventral pustular dermatitis (Figure 6.23).

Cats:

- Visceral signs very rare.
- Cutaneous lesions:
  - Single to multiple often ulcerated nodules on ear pinnae, eyelids, lips and nose.

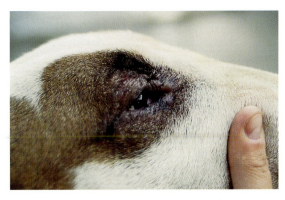

Figure 6.20 Periocular scaling caused by leishmaniasis.

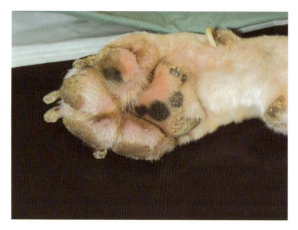

Figure 6.21 Digital hyperkeratosis in a dog with leishmaniasis.

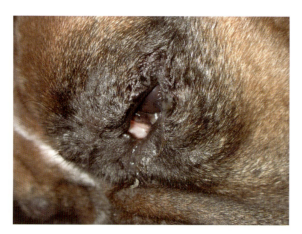

Figure 6.22 Ulceration at the mucocutaneous junction in a dog with leishmaniasis.

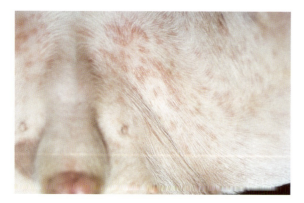

Figure 6.23 Ventral pustules on abdomen of a dog with leishmaniasis.

Differential diagnosis

Due to wide variety of presenting signs leishmaniasis can mimic almost any other disease.

Diagnosis

- History especially dogs in or from endemic areas and clinical signs.
- Cytology taken from lymph nodes or bone marrow reveals Leishmania amastigotes usually within macrophages.
- Indirect immunofluorescent assay or ELISA looking for high anti-Leishmania antibodies, false positive and negative results can be seen in dogs; false negatives common in cats.
- Biopsy reveals variable findings ranging from orthokeratotic hyperkeratosis and parakeratosis to granulomatous perifolliculitis, superficial perivascular dermatitis. Leishmania amastigotes appear as round to oval basophilic organism usually within macrophages. Organism can be identified in approximately 50% of cases.
- Immunohistochemistry of skin biopsies can be used to identify Leishmania antigen.
- PCR technique can be used to detect Leishmania DNA in skin biopsies or bone marrow.

Treatment

- The disease is not curable and carries a guarded prognosis. Relapses are common requiring repeat courses of treatment.
- In dogs without renal disease a good quality of life is possible with periodic retreatments. When concurrent renal disease is present the prognosis is very poor and euthanasia should be considered.
- Dogs drugs therapy can be undertaken with the following:
    - Protocol 1:
        - meglumine antimonate 100 mg/kg iv or sq sid for 3–4 weeks, or
        - sodium stibogluconate 30–50 mg/kg iv or sq sid for 3–4 weeks.
    - Protocol 2:
        - Allopurinol 6–8 mg/kg po tid or 15 mg/kg po bid for 6–9 months.

- Other drugs that have been used with variable success rate include amphotericin B, ketoconazole and itraconazole.
- Prevention should be practiced where possible to avoid endemic areas; use insect repellents and keep dogs indoors during high risk periods from 1 hour before sunset to 1 hour after dawn. Repellent collars containing 4.0% deltamethrin are available.

■ Cats:
- No treatment protocols have been reported in cats.

Selected references and further reading

Lappin, M.R. (2000) Protozoal and miscellaneous infections. In: Ettinger, S.J. and Feldman, E.C. (eds). *Textbook of Veterinary Internal Medicine*. 5th edn. pp. 408–417. WB Saunders, Philadelphia

Matousek, J.L. (2004) Miscellaneous infections. In: Campbell, K.L. (ed). *Small Animal Dermatology Secrets*. pp. 183–187. Hanley and Belfus, Philadelphia

Medleau, L. and Hnilica, K. (2006) Viral, rickettsial and protozoal diseases. In: *Small Animal Dermatology: A Color Atlas and Therapeutic Guide*. 2nd edn. pp. 139–158. WB Saunders, Philadelphia

Nagata, M. (2000) Canine papillomaviruses. In: *Kirk's Current Veterinary Therapy XIII Small Animal Practice*. p. 569. WB Saunders, Philadelphia

Scott, D.W. et al. (2001) *Viral, Rickettsial and Protozoal Diseases Muller and Kirk's Small Animal Dermatology*. 6th edn. pp. 517–542. WB Saunders, Philadelphia

Slappendel, R.J. et al. (2000) Leishmaniasis. In: Greene, C.E. (ed). *Infectious Diseases of the Dog and Cat*. 2nd edn. pp. 450–458. WB Saunders, Philadelphia

Sundberg, J.P. et al. (2000) Feline papillomas and papillomavirus. *Vet Pathol*, 37, 1–10

Parasitic skin disease 7

Arthropod parasites

Arachnids

Mites

(a) *Otodectes cynotis*
(b) Cheyletiellosis
(c) Demodicosis
(d) Sarcoptic mange
(e) Notoedric mange
(f) Trombiculiasis
(g) *Dermanyssus gallinae*
(h) *Lynxacarus radosky*

Otodectes cynotis

Cause and pathogenesis

Otodectes cynotis is a psoroptiform mite. It is a non-burrowing mite that lives and feeds on the surface of the skin especially in the ears (see Table 7.1). A common disease in dogs and cats,

Table 7.1 *Otodectes cynotis.*

Otodectes cynotis	Distinguishing features
	Oval mite, four pairs of legs, all except rudimentary fourth pair of female extend beyond body margin
	Male all legs short unjointed pedicles with suckers
	Female first two pairs of legs pedicles with suckers
	Terminal anus
	Active mite and will move about in samples collected into liquid paraffin
	Eggs found within ear wax Figure 7.2

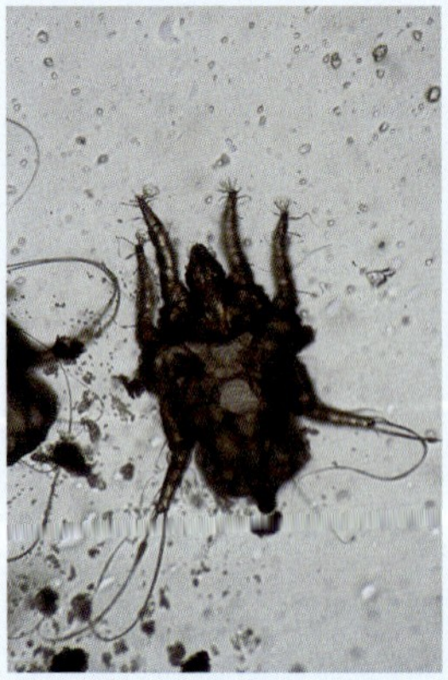

Figure 7.1 *Otodectes cynotis* mite.

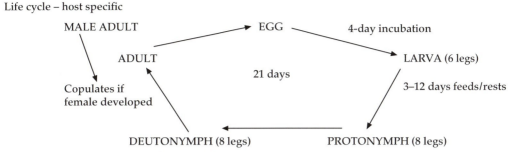

Life cycle – host specific

Can exist in environment for short periods

especially in kittens. It is highly contagious between animals, potential zoonosis.

Clinical signs
- Otitis externa:
  - Ceruminous discharge from ear canal – 'coffee ground' appearance (Figures 7.3 and 7.4).
  - Discharge can become purulent if secondary infection occurs.
  - Pruritus variable, but usually marked and not uncommon to see areas of self-inflicted trauma and 'hot spots' on side of faced over external ear canal.
  - Aural haematomas can occur as a result of head shaking.
- Ectopic infestation:
  - Usually seen in cats.
  - Tend to occur on the neck, rump and tail, can be asymptomatic or pruritic.
  - Lesions present as papular crusted eruptions.

Differential diagnosis
- Other causes of otitis externa.
- Ectopic infestation:
  - Other ectoparasitic diseases especially flea allergic dermatitis.
  - Allergic diseases.

Diagnosis
- History and clinical signs.
- Direct otoscopic observation of mites which can be seen with the naked eye as white moving specks.
- Examination of ear wax in liquid paraffin or potassium hydroxide for identification of eggs, nymph, larvae and adult *Otodectes cynotis*.
- Ectopic infestation both superficial skin scrapings or acetate tapes can be used to identify mites.

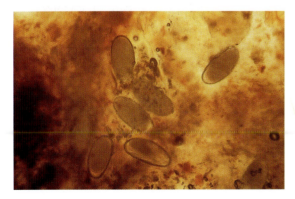

Figure 7.2 *Otodectes cynotis* eggs.

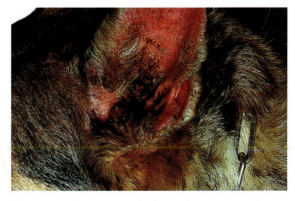

Figure 7.3 Ceruminous discharge from ear canal in a German shepherd dog.

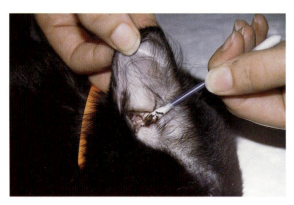

Figure 7.4 Coffee ground discharge typical of *Otodectes cynotis*.

Treatment
- Important to treat not only affected animal but all in contact.
- Cleaning of canals should be undertaken with a mild ceruminolytic cleaner to ensure good penetration of other topical medication.
- Medication should be directed at treating the aural infestation and also any ectopic mites. When topical treatment is used, it should be combined with a whole body treatment such as fipronil or pyrethrin powder (dogs).
- Topical therapy with a parasiticidal otic preparation.
- Most proprietary ear drops have a miticidal claim although most do not contain a specific anti-miticidal drug.
- Other preparations that may be used constitute an extra-label usage:
  - 10% fipronil solution 2 drops into the ear twice weekly for 3–4 weeks.
  - 1% injectable ivermectin diluted 1:9 with propylene glycol 2–4 drops into the ear daily for 3–4 weeks.
- Systemic therapy can be undertaken with propriety spot on preparation. Many products have miticidal claims:
  - Selamectin 6 mg/kg applied every 2 weeks for 4 applications.
  - Moxidectin 2.5 mg/kg applied every 2 weeks (dogs), 1.0 mg/kg (cats) for 4 applications.
- Oral miticidal drops also constitute an extra-label usage:
  - Ivermectin 0.3 mg/kg po every 10 days for 3 applications.
  - Moxidectin (dogs) 0.2 mg/kg po every 10 days for 3 applications.
- Where pruritus is severe a short course of anti-inflammatory therapy is indicated with prednisolone 1 mg/kg po sid 7–10 days.

Cheyletiellosis
Cause and pathogenesis
- Common disease caused by *Cheyletiella* spp. These are non-burrowing surface living and feeding parasites (Table 7.2). They are most commonly seen on puppies and kittens from 'breeding farms' and rescue centres. These are large mites that lead to the typical appearance of 'walking dandruff'. *C. yasguri* is considered the species to be found on the dog; *C. blakei* the cat species and *C. parasitovorax* the rabbit species. However, cross-infestation can occur.
- Highly contagious.
- Zoonoses: Human lesions appear as pruritic papules at contact sites with animal. Often arranged in groups of three.

Clinical signs
- Young and immunosuppressed animals are predisposed.
- Variable presentation; some animals can act as asymptomatic carriers.
- Marked scaling usually on the dorsum giving the coat a powdery appearance (Figure 7.7).
- Animals are usually pruritic leading to self-inflicted trauma (Figure 7.8).
- Primary lesions inconsistent finding but present as crusted papules.

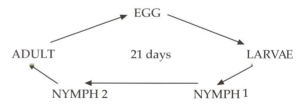

Can live for a short period in the environment, females up to 10 days

Table 7.2 *Cheyletiella* spp.

Cheyletiella	Distinguishing features
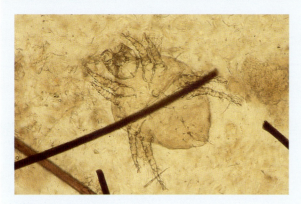 **Figure 7.5** *Cheyletiella* mite.	Large saddle shaped mite Four pairs of legs bear combs Accessory mouth part terminate in hooks. Figure 7.6 Sensory organ on genu 1 • Heart shape *C. yasguri* • Comb shape *C. blakei* • Global shape *C. parasitovorax* Egg attached to hair at one end only by filaments Fast moving mite in liquid paraffin

Differential diagnosis
- Flea allergic dermatitis
- *Sarcoptes scabiei*
- Ectopic otodectes
- Pediculosis
- Food allergy
- Atopy

Diagnosis
- History and clinical signs.
- Identification of parasite (adult cheyletiella mites, nymphs, larvae and ova):

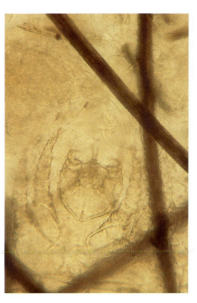

Figure 7.6 Close-up of *Cheyletiella* head showing hooks on accessory mouth parts.

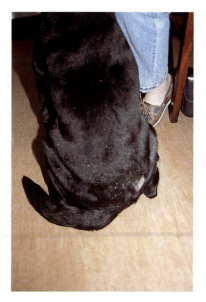

Figure 7.7 Dorsal scaling on a Labrador with cheyletiellosis.

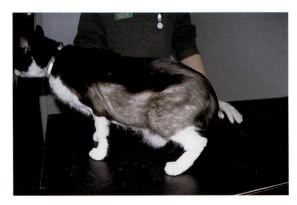

Figure 7.8 Flank alopecia secondary to *Cheyletiella*.

- Coat brushing onto dark paper or into a Petri dish, then direct examination with magnifying glass.
- Superficial skin scrapings into mineral oil or potassium hydroxide (10%).
- Acetate tape impression smears examined microscopically.
- Faecal examination for cheyletiella eggs.
■ Therapeutic trial with a topical miticidal drug.
■ Biopsy is usually non-diagnostic revealing non-specific pattern of superficial perivascular dermatitis with variable numbers of eosinophils.

Treatment
■ Important to treat all in contact animals as well as those showing clinical signs.
■ Topical sprays and shampoos are available; these should be applied once weekly for 4 applications; suitable products include 2–3% lime sulphur, 1% selenium sulphide, 1% permethrin.
■ Topical spot on preparations with licensed indication include those containing fipronil 7.5–15 mg/kg, selamectin 6 mg/kg, moxidectin 2.5 mg/kg (dog) 1.0 mg/kg (cat), which should be applied every 2 weeks for 3 applications.
■ Topical sprays that are suitable with licensed application include fipronil which is applied at a concentration of 6 ml/kg body weight twice at 2 weekly intervals.

■ Oral medication that can be used; extra-label is ivermectin 0.2–0.3 mg/kg po on 3 occasions at 10 day intervals.
■ Environmental treatment can be undertaken using any flea insecticidal sprays.

Demodicosis (demodectic mange/red mange)
Canine demodicosis
Cause and pathogenesis Common skin disease of dogs caused by increased number of demodex mites.

Demodex is a normal skin commensal. Three forms have been identified in the dog (see Table 7.3):

■ *Demodex canis* – inhabitant of canine pilosebaceous unit (hair follicle, sebaceous duct and gland) (Figure 7.9, Table 7.3).
■ *Demodex injai* – inhabitant of canine pilosebaceous unit (hair follicle, sebaceous duct and gland) (Figure 7.11, Table 7.3).
■ *Demodex cornei* – inhabitant of the stratum corneum (Figure 7.12, Table 7.3).

Demodex canis mites are passed from mother to pup during first 2–3 days after birth. The mode of transmission of the other two mites is unknown.

Development of the disease is associated with immune deficiency. A hereditary T cell defect of varying severity is thought to predispose certain dogs. T lymphocyte depression is induced by the parasite itself and is proportionate to the number of mites.

Concurrent pyoderma contributes to the immunosuppression.

Predisposed breeds:
Pure bred dogs have increased susceptibility, especially shar-pei, West Highland white terriers, English bulldogs, Scottish terriers, Old English sheepdogs, German shepherd dogs.

Types of demodex:

■ Localised (squamous):
  - Cutaneous – less than 5 patches
  - Pododemodicosis – single foot
  - Demodectic otitis
■ Generalised:
  - Juvenile onset – greater than 5 patches

Table 7.3 *Demodex* spp. in the dog.

Demodex canis

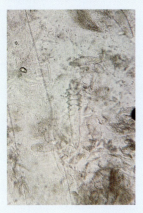

Figure 7.9 Photograph of *Demodex canis* adult mite.

Distinguishing features

Long cigar shaped mites

Adults and nymphs have eight legs, larvae six legs

Eggs typical fusiform shape Figure 7.10

Demodex cornei

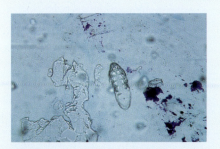

Figure 7.11 Photograph of adult *D. cornei*.

Distinguishing features

Short cigar shaped mites

Adults and nymphs have eight legs, larvae six legs

Eggs typical fusiform shape

Demodex injai

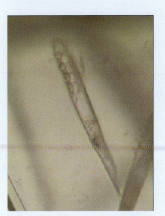

Figure 7.12

Distinguishing features

Very long cigar shaped mites

Adults and nymphs have eight legs, larvae six legs

Eggs typical fusiform shape

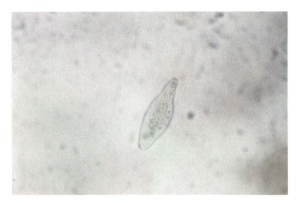

Figure 7.10 Photograph of *D. canis* egg.

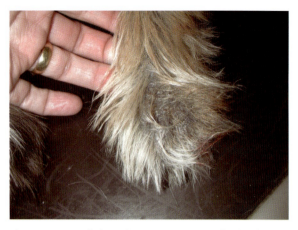

Figure 7.14 Pododemodicosis in a German shepherd dog.

- Pododemodicosis – 2 or more feet involved
- Adult onset

Clinical signs

- Localised demodicosis:
  - Cutaneous:
    - Age of onset usually 3–6 months.
    - Less than 5 patches.
    - Lesions present with erythema, alopecia often with fine scaling.
    - Pruritus variable, usually mild.
    - Commonly face affected especially the periocular skin (Figure 7.13).
  - Pododemodicosis:
    - Can be remnant of generalised disease or as the only area involved (Figure 7.14).
    - Usually secondary pyoderma leading to variable degrees of pruritus with oedema and pain.
  - Demodectic otitis:
    - May occur in isolation or as part of generalised disease.
    - Erythematous, ceruminous otitis, pruritus variable.
- Generalised:
  - Juvenile onset:
    - Caused by *Demodex canis* and *Demodex cornei*.
    - Age of onset 3–18 months.
    - Usually an extension of localised disease due to failure of spontaneous remission or glucocorticoid usage.
    - Numerous lesions especially head, legs and trunk (Figure 7.15).

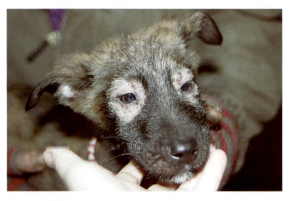

Figure 7.13 Localised demodectic mange showing periocular scaling.

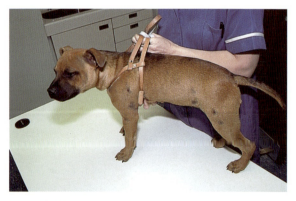

Figure 7.15 Generalised squamous demodicosis showing numerous alopecic patches over the trunk and legs.

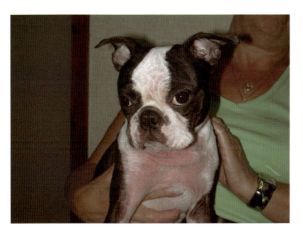

Figure 7.16 Puppy with generalised demodicosis.

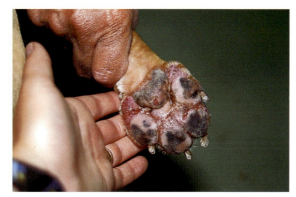

Figure 7.18 Chronic pododemodicosis in a Staffordshire bull terrier.

- Erythema, alopecia, scaling with comedones (Figure 7.16) progresses often to crusted, haemorrhagic lesions.
- Secondary pyoderma is common, usually caused by *Staphylococcus intermedius*, although *Proteus mirabilis* and *Pseudomonas aeruginosa* can be involved (Figure 7.17).
- Infection leads to folliculitis/furunculosis, generalised lymphadenopathy.
- Dogs with secondary infection tend to be depressed, lethargic, inappetent.
  □ Pododemodicosis:
- May be caused by all three forms of the mite (Figure 7.18).
- As localised except more than one foot involved.

- Predisposed breeds – Old English sheepdogs, Shih-Tzu, giant breeds.
- Often poorly responsive to treatment.
  □ Adult onset:
- Rare disease caused by all three forms of demodex mite.
- Age of onset usually greater than 3 years.
- Lesions and distribution as juvenile onset disease. When *D. injai* is present, lesions may be more dorsal with secondary seborrhoea.
- Dogs with secondary infection tend to be depressed, lethargic, inappetent.
- Usually secondary to internal disease (hypothyroidism (Figure 7.19), hyperadrenocorticism, diabetes mellitus) malignant neoplasia or immunosuppressive treatment.
- Underlying trigger can occur >2 years after cutaneous lesions.
- Prognosis dependent on identification of underlying problem.

Differential diagnosis

- Localised demodex:
  □ Dermatophytosis
  □ Canine acne
  □ Allergy especially atopy
- Generalised demodex:
  □ Pyoderma

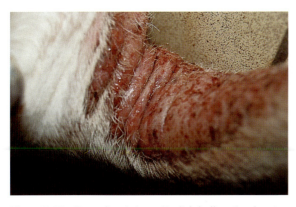

Figure 7.17 Demodicosis in an English bull terrier showing severely infected haemorrhagic lesions.

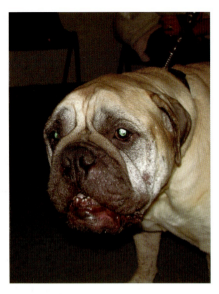

Figure 7.19 Adult onset demodicosis in a dog with hypothyroidism.

- Dermatophytosis
- Pemphigus complex
- Drug eruption
- Seborrhoea
- Dermatomyositis

Diagnosis

- History and clinical signs.
- Skin scrapings from predilection areas, i.e. areas of comedone formation to reveal the mites, larvae, nymphs and ova.
  - Deep scrapings from areas of comedones.
  - Squeeze skin to extrude mites from follicles before scraping.
  - Any dogs with pyoderma or seborrhoea should be scraped.
- Acetate tape impression smears:
  - Useful to identify superficial non-follicular mites
- Hair plucking:
  - Useful for follicular mites in pododemodicosis, which are pulled out with the hairs.
- Biopsy reveals perivascular dermatitis with mites present in stratum corneum and follicles. Varying degrees of perifolliculitis, folliculitis and furunculosis can be seen. Biopsies are essential in
  - shar-peis, where scrapings are often not adequate,
  - fibrotic interdigital lesions, where biopsy is the only way to rule out demodex.
- Examination of ear wax in cases of demodectic otitis will reveal mites as well, often evidence of secondary infection.
- Adult onset disease – investigation of internal disease is essential; diagnostic tests dependent on clues from history. A useful minimum database may include
  - blood samples including endocrine function tests,
  - radiography, ultrasonography.

Treatment

- Localised form:
  - Most cases resolve spontaneously after 6–8 weeks provided that glucocorticoids are not prescribed.
  - Where pyoderma is identified this must be treated.
  - No difference is seen in the healing between treated and untreated cases.
  - Topical therapy may be used in the form of gentle anti-parasitic treatments, e.g. lime sulphur, selenium sulphide or follicular flushing agents, e.g. benzoyl peroxide.
  - Anti-parasitic therapy is rarely required but any of the therapies for generalised disease may be used if necessary.
  - Monitor cases with repeat skin scrapes to ensure resolution.

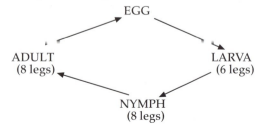

Life cycle – host specific

- Deterioration of condition indicates progression to generalised demodicosis.
- Otitis – amitraz in mineral oil 1:9 dilution daily (extra-label indication).
- Pododemodicosis can be very difficult to treat. Any of the therapies for generalised disease can be used. In addition, amitraz foot soaks may be useful using 0.125% solution every 1–3 days.
- Generalised forms:
  - Difficult disease to treat – good owner compliance is essential.
  - Check dog's general health and management; intact bitches should be neutered as oestrous or pregnancy will result in relapse of the disease.
  - In adult onset disease important to identify and treat the underlying condition where possible.
  - Any form of glucocorticoid contraindicated.
  - When secondary pyoderma is present, antibiotic therapy is needed for a minimum of 4 weeks for superficial infection and up to 12 weeks for deep infection and for at least 10 days after clinical resolution.
  - Antiparasitic therapy:
    5% amitraz:
    - Clip dog down to short stubble all over, and keep dog clipped throughout treatment (sedation may be necessary for clipping).
    - Bath dog in antiseborrhoeic shampoo to remove crust and scale, e.g. benzoyl peroxide or sulphur/salicylic acid containing products.
    - Apply amitraz at dilution of 1:100 (0.05%) in water to whole body. Applicators should be warned to wear gloves, protective clothing and work in a ventilated area. Allow the solution to dry on the dog.
    - Repeat every 7 days until 2 weeks after mites can no longer be identified on scrapings (6–12 weeks).
    - Side effects in dogs include sedation 12–24 hours duration, pruritus, allergic reactions (rare), weakness, ataxia (very rare).
- All of the drugs below are unlicensed for demodicosis and constitute an extra-label use for therapy. They should be used when amitraz treatment has failed or considered unsuitable:
  - *Ivermectin*:
    - Contraindicated in collie's and related breeds.
    - Administered orally at 0.2–0.6 mg/kg po sid until 30 days beyond clinical cure (60–200 days).
    - Dose should be started at 0.1 mg/kg daily and increased daily by 0.1 mg/kg up to 0.6 mg/kg to minimise the risk of side effects.
    - Side effects include incoordination, weakness, dilated pupils, blindness, ataxia and in rare cases collapse and coma.
  - *Milbemycin*:
    - Administered orally at 0.5–2 mg/kg po sid until 30 days beyond clinical cure (course may be prolonged).
    - Side effects uncommon, but if they occur are similar to those for ivermectin.
    Doramectin:
    - Administered orally at 0.6 mg/kg sq once weekly until 30 days beyond clinical cure (course may be prolonged).
    - Side effects are uncommon but similar to ivermectin.
    1% moxidectin:
    - Injectable cattle solution can be administered at a dose of 0.4 mg/kg po every 24–72 hours until 30 days beyond clinical cure (course may be prolonged).
    - Side effects similar to those for ivermectin are reported to be common.
- No dog should be considered cured until 12 months after treatment has stopped.
- Monitor treatment by scrapings into mineral oil will assess numbers of dead and live mites. Face and feet usually clear the last. These should always be scraped.
- Immunostimulants have been reported to have a variable benefit. Drugs that have been investigated include vitamin E, levamisole and thiabendazole.

Feline demodicosis

Cause and pathogenesis Rare skin disease of cats caused by increased number of demodex mites.

Demodex mites are commensals of normal feline skin. Two different species of demodex mites have been identified: *Demodex cati* and *Demodex gatoi* (see Table 7.4).

Demodex cati is usually associated with underlying disease:

- Viral infection FIV, FeLV
- Endocrine disease diabetes mellitus, hyperadrenocorticism
- Immune mediated disease, systemic lupus erythematosus

Demodex gatoi not known if this is a true commensal; thought to be contagious.

Clinical signs

- Localised and generalised forms of the disease are recognised.
- Pruritus is variable in both forms of disease.
- Localised disease:
  - Patchy alopecia with erythema and scale.
  - Affects face (Figure 7.21) and head especially eyelids and periocular skin.
  - Can occur as ceruminous otitis externa.
- Generalised form:
  - Lesions presents with multifocal variably pruritic macules, alopecic patches, hyperpigmentation, erythema and scaling (Figure 7.22).
  - Affects head also neck, trunk, limbs and ventrum.
  - Ceruminous otitis can also be present.

Table 7.4 *Demodex* spp. in the cat.

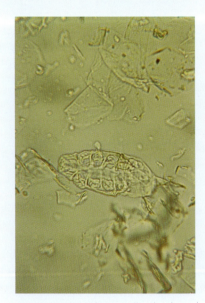

Figure 7.20 Short non-follicular demodex; *Demodex gatoi*. (Source: Picture courtesy of A. Foster.)

***Demodex cati*: Distinguishing features**

Long cigar shaped mites

Adults and nymphs have eight legs, larvae six legs

Eggs slim oval shape

***Demodex gatoi*: Distinguishing features**

Short mite with blunt rounded abdomen

Adults and nymphs have eight legs, larvae six legs

Eggs slim oval shape

Parasitic skin disease

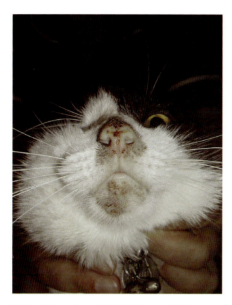

Figure 7.21 *Demodex cati* lesions on cat's face.

Differential diagnosis

- Generalised disease:
  - Dermatophytosis
  - Ectoparasitic diseases, especially *Otodectes*, *Cheyletiella*
  - Cutaneous neoplasia
  - Allergy (atopy, food 'allergy')
  - Scabies
  - Flea allergic dermatitis

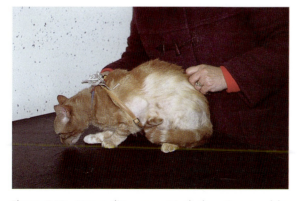

Figure 7.22 Non-scaling symmetrical alopecia caused by *Demodex gatoi*. (Source: Picture courtesy of J. Henfrey.)

Diagnosis

- History and clinical signs.
- Microscopy:
  - Deep and superficial scrapings to look for adult mites, eggs, larvae and nymphs of *D. cati*. *D. gatoi* may be difficult to find.
  - Acetate tape impression smears to identify surface mites of *D. gatoi*.
- Trial therapy with weekly lime sulphur dips together with history and clinical signs are often indicated for *D. gatoi*.
- Biopsy reveals suppurative perivascular dermatitis with mites present in stratum corneum and follicles Varying degrees of perifolliculitis, folliculitis and furunculosis can be seen.

Treatment

- No drug is licensed for treatment of demodectic mange in the cat.
- Clinical response is dependent on immune status of the cat. Any predisposing factors should be identified and treated.
- *D. gatoi*:
  - 2–4% lime sulphur:
    - Applied every 3–7 days for 4–8 weeks. Cats usually improve during the first 4 weeks but treatment must be continued for a total of 6–8 weeks.
  - Ivermectin and milbemycin:
    - There have been suggestions that this drug may also be effective, but reports are anecdotal.
- *D. cati*:
  - For both forms of disease treatment needs to be applied for 3–4 weeks and until clinical resolution of signs is seen and negative skin scrapes obtained.
  - Localised lesions:
    0.015–0.025% amitraz:
    - May be effective when applied to localised lesions daily until clinical resolution.
  - Generalised lesions:
    2% lime sulphur:
    - Applied as a whole body dip once weekly

Table 7.5 Sarcoptes scabiei.

Sarcoptes scabiei	Distinguishing features
Figure 7.23	Oval mite Length Two pairs anterior legs long unjointed stalks with suckers Two pairs posterior legs do not extend beyond the borders of the body Terminal anus Eggs round Very active mite in liquid paraffin

Amitraz 0.015–0.025%:
- Applied to whole body every 7–14 days; n.b.: amitraz should not be applied to diabetic cats.

Doramectin:
- Administered by injection at a dose rate of 0.6 mg/kg sq once weekly.

- Prognosis:
  - Localised demodicosis carries a good prognosis.
  - Generalised demodicosis carries a good to guarded prognosis depending on any immunosuppressive factors that are present and whether they are amenable to therapy.

Sarcoptic mange (canine scabies)
Cause and pathogenesis
Non-seasonal contagious ectoparasitic disease caused by *Sarcoptes scabiei var canis*, a superficial burrowing mite (see Table 7.5). Commonly seen in animals from large breeding farms and rescue shelters, also in areas with high fox populations, which act as a reservoir for infection to domestic pets. Common disease in dogs; very rare in cats. A zoonotic disease, which is passed from dogs to man. Human lesions appear as papular eruptions on arms and trunk. Disease in man (unlike human scabies) is self-limiting unless there is repeat contact with infected animals. Mites induce allergic reaction that leads to severe pruritus.

Clinical signs
- Predilection areas are those areas of skin with little hair.
- Acute disease lesions are found on ear tips (Figure 7.24), elbows (Figure 7.25), ventral abdomen and hocks:
  - Pruritus poorly controlled with glucocorticoids.
  - Crusted papules, with generalised scale.
  - Self-inflicted trauma leads to excoriation (Figure 7.26).

Parasitic skin disease

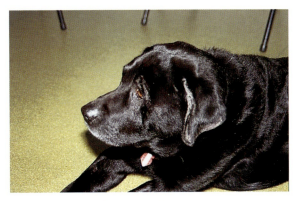

Figure 7.24 Typical crusting along the margins of the ear pinna in a Labrador.

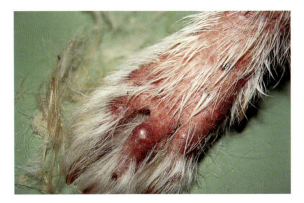

Figure 7.26 Severe self-inflicted trauma on the feet of a dog with scabies.

- In chronic disease, lesions will become generalised although dorsum is often spared (Figure 7.27):
  - Chronic lesions present with hyperpigmentation, lichenification.
- Norwegian scabies is a rare variant seen in immunosuppressed animals where there is intense pruritus, massive hair loss and scale and mites are numerous.

Differential diagnosis
- Allergy (contact, atopy, food)
- Malassezia dermatitis
- Cheyletiellosis
- Pelodera dermatitis
- Pediculosis

Diagnosis
- History and clinical signs.
- Pinnal – pedal reflex seen when the dog attempts to scratch with its back foot when the edge of the ipsilateral pinna is rubbed (70–90% of cases).
- Microscopy in the form of deep skin scrapings (important to scrape to achieve capillary ooze) from non-excoriated predilection sites, e.g. ear margins, elbows, hocks (clip hair before scraping). Mites, eggs or faecal pellets are difficult to find but are diagnostic.

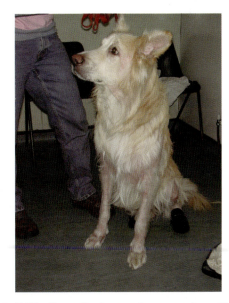

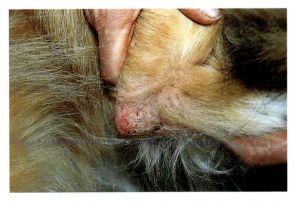

Figure 7.25 Erythema and crusting on the elbows of a dog with scabies.

Figure 7.27 Generalised sarcoptic mange in a German shepherd dog.

Life cycle

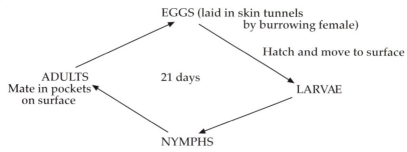

Survival of the host approximately 7 days

- Biopsy reveals a non-specific pattern of superficial perivascular dermatitis often with heavy eosinophilic infiltrate with epidermal hyperplasia. Mites are a rare finding in the stratum corneum.
- Therapeutic trial is useful where mites have not been identified by other diagnostic tests. An improvement in clinical signs after treatment with an appropriate scabicide allows a retrospective diagnosis.
- Serology by ELISA can be used to detect circulating IgG antibodies against Sarcoptes antigen. False negative can be seen early in the disease and in young animals. False positives can be seen in animals recovering from the disease.
- In Norwegian scabies, attempts should be made to identify any concurrent immunosuppressive factors.

Treatment
- Animal treatment – affected and all in contact animals need to be treated:
  - Antiparasitic therapy:
    Selamectin:
    - Selamectin is licensed for the treatment of canine scabies. It should be applied topically at 6–12 mg/kg. The best results are seen when it is applied on 3 occasions at 2 weekly intervals.
    Moxidectin:
    - Moxidectin is licensed as a spot on preparation for treatment of sarcoptic mange. It should be applied topically at 2.5 mg/kg for dogs and 1.0 mg/kg for cats. The best results are seen when it is applied on 3 occasions at 2 weekly intervals.
    5% amitraz:
    - Clip dog down to short stubble all over, and keep dog clipped throughout treatment (sedation may be necessary for clipping).
    - Bath dog in antiseborrhoeic shampoo to remove crust and scale, e.g. benzoyl peroxide or sulphur/salicylic acid containing products.
    - Apply amitraz at dilution of 1:100 (0.05%) in water to whole body. Applicators should be warned to wear gloves, protective clothing and work in a ventilated area. Allow the solution to dry on the dog.
    - Repeat every 7 days for 6 weeks.
    - Side effects in dogs include sedation 12–24 hours duration, pruritus, allergic reactions (rare), weakness, ataxia (very rare).
- Drugs detailed below are unlicensed for sarcoptic mange and constitute an extra-label use for therapy:
  2–3% lime sulphur:
  - Applied topically to whole body every 5–7 days as a leave on solution for 4–6 weeks. Useful in very young animals.
  - Side effects uncommon, and can be irritant on ulcerated skin.
  Fipronil spray:
  - Applied topically at a concentration of 3.0 ml/kg to whole body on 3

occasions at 2 week intervals. Useful in very young animals.
- Side effects uncommon; may be irritant on ulcerated skin.

Ivermectin:
- Contraindicated in collie's and related breeds.
- Administered at 0.2–0.4 mg/kg po once weekly or sq every 2 weeks for 4–6 weeks.
- Side effects – see demodicosis.

Milbemycin:
- Administered at 0.75 mg/kg po sid for 30 days or 2 mg/kg po every 7 days for 4–6 weeks; beyond clinical cure.
- Side effects – see demodicosis.

1% moxidectin:
- Injectable cattle solution can be administered at a dose of 0.2–0.25 mg/kg po or sq every 7 days for 4–6 weeks.
- Side effects similar to those for ivermectin are reported to be common.

- Environmental treatment is important especially in kennel situations:
  - Infested bedding should be disposed of and antiparasitic sprays should be used in the environment, e.g. permethrin.
- Glucocorticoids may be useful in severely pruritic animals but should not be given until a diagnosis is made. Prednisolone 1 mg/kg po sid for 7–10 days can be given.
- Pyoderma can occur as a rare secondary complication. Appropriate systemic antibiotics should be given for 3–4 weeks. In such cases glucocorticoids should be withheld.
- In cases of Norwegian scabies, underlying immunosuppressive factors should be treated where possible.
- Prognosis is good for uncomplicated cases, provided adequate therapy is given. In Norwegian scabies, the prognosis is guarded unless an underlying trigger can be identified and treated successfully.

Notoedric mange (feline scabies)
Cause and pathogenesis
Non-seasonal contagious ectoparasitic disease caused by *Notoedres cati* a superficial burrowing mite (see Table 7.6). Rare disease in cats; can also

Table 7.6 *Notoedres cati*.

Notoedres cati: Distinguishing features
Oval mite, eggs round (smaller than *Sarcoptes*)
Two pairs anterior legs long medium length unjointed stalks with suckers
Two pairs posterior legs do not extend beyond the borders of the body
Body obvious striations
Dorsal anus (terminal anus *Sarcoptes*)

infest foxes, dogs and rabbits. A zoonotic disease; can be passed from infested hosts to man. Disease has a worldwide distribution but is very rare in the UK foxes, dogs and rabbits. *N. cati* is an obligate parasite that survives off the host only a few days. Infested cats carry large numbers of mites, which are easily found on scrapings.

Clinical signs
- Severely pruritic skin disease that is poorly controlled with glucocorticoids.
- Disease initially starts on the medial edge of ear pinna, spread rapidly to rest of face and neck (Figure 7.28).
- Cats grooming activities lead to further spread to feet and perineum.
- Skin appears thickened and alopecic, covered with thick yellow/grey crusts with papules.
- Self-inflicted trauma leads to excoriation.

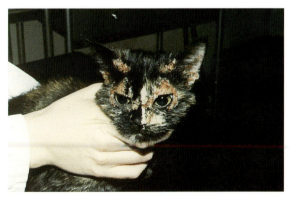

Figure 7.28 Facial excoriation due to *Notoedres cati*. (Source: Picture courtesy of J. Henfrey.)

- Chronic disease will generalise and debilitated animals with severe disease can die.

Differential diagnosis
- Allergy – atopy, food, fleas
- Cheyletiellosis
- *Otodectes cynotis*
- Pediculosis
- Autoimmune skin disease especially pemphigus foliaceus

Diagnosis
- History and clinical signs.
- Microscopy in the form of deep scrapings. Mites easier to find than scabies mites but are small and best identified under low power with reduced light.
- Biopsy will occasionally reveal signs of mites. Pattern is non-specific of superficial perivascular dermatitis often with heavy eosinophilic infiltrate. Areas of focal parakeratosis are common.
- Therapeutic trial rarely indicated as mites can be easily found. However, a significant improvement seen after treatment with matricide allows retrospective diagnosis.

Treatment
- Animal treatment – affected and all in contact animals need to be treated:
    - Antiparasitic therapy:
        2–3% lime sulphur:
        - Clip cat down to short stubble all over, and keep the coat clipped short throughout treatment (sedation may be necessary for clipping).
        - Bath cat in a mild antiseborrhoeic shampoo to remove crust and scale, e.g. sulphur/salicylic acid.
        - Apply lime sulphur topically to whole body every 5–7 days as a leave on solution for 2–3 weeks.
        5% amitraz:
        - Clip and shampoo cat as for lime sulphur therapy.
        - Apply amitraz at concentration of 0.015% in water to whole body. Applicators should be warned to wear gloves, protective clothing and work in a ventilated area. Allow the solution to dry on the dog.
        - Repeat every 7 days for 3 weeks.
        Selamectin:
        - May be applied topically at 6.0 mg/kg. The best results are seen when it is applied on 3 occasions at 2 weekly intervals.
        Ivermectin:
        - Administered at 0.2–0.3 mg/kg po or sq every 2 weeks for 4–6 weeks.
- Environmental treatment is important especially in catteries:
    - Infested bedding should be disposed of and antiparasitic sprays should be used in the environment, e.g. permethrin.
- Glucocorticoids may be useful in severely pruritic animals but should not be given until a diagnosis is made. Prednisolone, 2 mg/kg po sid for 7–10 days, can be given.
- Pyoderma can occur as a rare secondary complication. Appropriate systemic antibiotics should be given for 3–4 weeks. In such cases glucocorticoids should be withheld.
- Prognosis is good for uncomplicated cases, provided adequate therapy is given.

Trombiculiasis
Cause and pathogenesis
Seasonal pruritic skin disease caused commonly by harvest mite *Neotrombicula autumnalis*, also *Walchia americana* in the USA and chiggers *Eutrombicula* spp. (see Table 7.7, Figure 5.29). They are worldwide in distribution and found in a wide range of different environmental habitats. The mites are free living and it is larval form that is parasitic on animals. The usual hosts are wild animals but domestic pets, e.g. dog and cat, as well as man can be affected. Harvest mites are seen in grassland areas in late summer/early autumn especially chalky soils in temperate climates but can be seen all year round in warm regions. Trombiculiasis is uncommon in dogs and cats. Not a zoonotic disease but humans can be infested from the same source as dogs and cats.

Parasitic skin disease

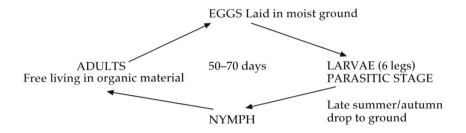

Clinical signs
- Larvae found in areas of skin in contact with the ground, e.g. between paws, ear pinnae (Figure 7.30).
- Larvae are visible to the naked eye as bright red dots, 'paprika' in appearance.
- Pruritus directed at sites where larvae feed especially the feet.
- Lesions are papulocrustous eruptions, occasionally wheals and vesicles.
- Secondary lesions are caused through self-inflicted trauma, i.e. excoriations and alopecia.

Differential diagnosis
- Allergy especially atopy, contact allergy
- Sarcoptic mange
- Pelodera dermatitis
- Hookworm dermatitis
- Demodicosis

Table 7.7 *Neotrombicula autumnalis.*

Neotrombicula autumnalis	Distinguishing features
	Larvae are found on animal have six legs
	Length 0.6 mm
	Bright red/orange in colour when engorged
	Long whip like appendages on legs
	Size of a pin head

Figure 7.29

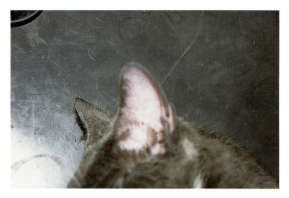

Figure 7.30 Bright red *Trombicula* larvae on ear pinna.

Diagnosis
- Microscopy in the form of skin scrapings into mineral oil and directly mounted tape strips from areas where mites are visible. Larvae can be seen with naked eye as bright orange/red dots approximately 0.6 mm in length.
- Biopsy reveals a non-specific pattern that is usually an eosinophil-rich superficial perivascular dermatitis.

Treatment
- Pets should be kept away from high risk areas where larvae are known to be a problem.
- Many of the anti-flea therapies have been shown to be effective.
- Fipronil spray 0.25% is the preferred method of treatment at a concentration of 6 mg/kg applied every 2 weeks. It may also be used as a preventative treatment in animals in high risk environments.
- Glucocorticoids at anti-inflammatory dosage, i.e. prednisolone 1 mg/kg po sid (dogs) or 2 mg/kg po sid (cats) for 2–3 days, may be used where severe pruritus is present.

Dermanyssus gallinae
Cause and pathogenesis
The poultry mite *Dermanyssus gallinae* caused non-seasonal pruritic skin disease in dogs and cats (see Table 7.8, Figure 7.31). Non–host-specific ectoparasite whose main host is poultry but will also attack dogs, cats and man. Adult mite lives in nests and cracks in poultry cages/houses. Animals are infected through environmental contamination. Rare disease in both dogs and cats. Non-zoonotic but humans can be infested from the same source as dogs and cats.

Clinical signs
- Clinical signs are usually confined to the extremities and the dorsum.

Table 7.8 *Dermanyssus gallinae*.

Dermanyssus gallinae	Distinguishing features
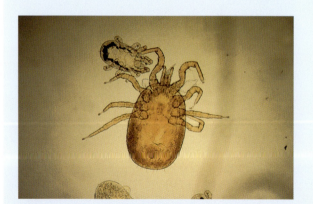	Eight-legged white/grey/black mite; becomes red when engorged
	Length up to 1.0 mm
	First pair of appendages (chelicerae) whip-like
	Anus posterior half of anal plate

Figure 7.31 *Dermanyssus gallinae* mite.

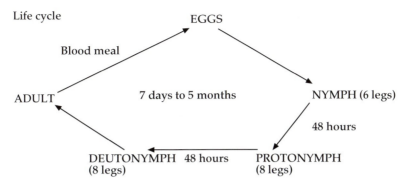

- Lesions appear as areas of erythema with papulocrustous eruptions.

Differential diagnosis
- Other ectoparasitic diseases especially
  - Trombiculiasis
  - Flea allergic dermatitis
  - Cheyletiellosis
- Contact allergy/irritants
- Allergy (atopy/food)

Diagnosis
- History and clinical signs.
- Microscopy in the form of skin scrapings into mineral oil and directly mounted tape strips reveal the typical red mites.
- Biopsy reveals a non-specific pattern of eosinophil-rich superficial perivascular dermatitis.

Treatment
- Avoidance of the infested premise is important to prevent continual re-infestation.
- Dogs/cats antiparasitic therapies as cheyletiella.
- Environmental treatment with permethrin- or pyrethrin-based sprays.

Lynxacarus radosky
Cause and pathogenesis
Lynxacarus radosky is a small cat fur clasping mite that has been primarily reported in Australia, Fiji, Puerto Rico and parts of America (Hawaii and Florida) (see Table 7.9). In the United Kingdom, it may be found on imported animals. It is poorly contagious. Infections occur through direct contact or via fomites.

Similar in appearance to other fur mites; identification requires a competent parapsychologist. Very rare disease of cats. Can cause a papular rash in humans.

Clinical signs
- Cats may be infested asymptomatically, only showing signs of a dull coat.
- Mites usually attach to the ends of hairs on the dorsum to give the coat a 'salt-and-pepper' appearance.
- Damaged hair can be easily epilated.
- May present with signs of multiple papulocrustous eruptions. Often pruritus may be minimal.

Differential diagnosis
- Other ectoparasitic diseases:
  - Cheyletiella
  - Pediculosis
  - *Otodectes cynotis*

Table 7.9 *Lynxacarus radosky*.

***Lynxacarus radosky*: Distinguishing features**

Elongated body 430–520 μm in length

Flap-like sternal extensions contain first two grasping legs

All legs have terminal suckers

- Allergy (fleas, atopy, food)
- Dermatophytosis

Diagnosis
- History and clinical signs.
- Microscopy in the form of superficial skin scrapes, tape strippings from hair or hair plucks. Mites can be identified attached to hairs.
- Biopsy of no benefit, often no skin changes present.

Treatment
All in contact cats must be treated.
Topical ectoparasiticides as cheyletiella.

Ticks

(a) Argasid – soft ticks
(b) Ixodid – hard ticks

Argasid ticks
Cause and pathogenesis
The most important of the soft ticks affecting dogs and cats in the spinous ear tick, *Otobius megnini*. It is principally found in warm arid climates such as North and South America. The adult form is not parasitic; it is the larvae and nymph that can infest the external ear canals of domestic pets leading to acute otitis externa. They uncommonly cause disease in dogs and rarely in cats. This is not a zoonosis but humans can be infested as a result of the same environmental contamination as pets.

Clinical signs
- Animals present with acute onset otitis externa with shaking and rubbing of the head.
- There is severe inflammation of the external ear canal with a ceruminous discharge

Differential diagnosis
- Other causes of otitis externa, especially *Otodectes cynotis*.

Diagnosis
- Microscopy of ear wax and superficial scrapes of skin from external ear canal reveal larvae, nymphs and adult spinous ear ticks.

Treatment
- Where possible, ticks should be removed manually with fine forceps. It is essential to ensure that the tick is not squashed as its body fluids may be infectious. There is, however, a risk of incomplete removal and the production of 'tick head' granulomas.
- Topical acaracides should be used on the animal to remove the ticks; suitable products include those containing fipronil, amitraz (dog) and permethrin (dogs), pyriprole (dogs).
- Preventative therapy with topical spot on or collars containing acaracides may be useful to prevent re-infestation, e.g. collar impregnated with 4.0% deltamethrin.
- Environmental therapy with permethrin- or pyrethrin-based sprays may be useful in kennels or the immediate environment.

Ixodid ticks
Cause and pathogenesis
Ixodid or hard ticks contain several genera. These are *Rhipicephalus* spp., *Dermacentor* spp., *Ixodes* spp., *Amblyomma* spp. and *Haemophysalis* spp. Ixodid ticks are large parasites up to 0.5 cm in size. Common ticks in the United Kingdom include *Ixodes ricinus* (caster bean tick, Figure 7.32) and *Ixodes hexagonus* (hedgehog tick,

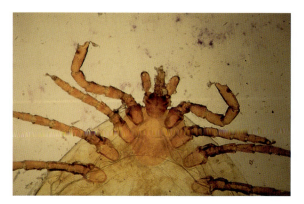

Figure 7.32 Head of *Ixodes ricinus* tick.

Parasitic skin disease

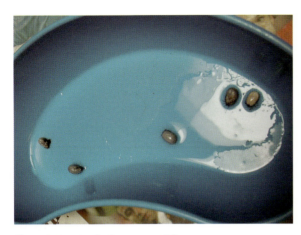

Figure 7.33 *Ixodes hexagonus* ticks.

Figure 7.33). Both dogs and cats can be infested. It is a common disease of dogs and rare in cats. This is not a zoonosis but humans can be infested from the same environmental source as the dogs and cats.

Clinical signs
- In many cases dogs act as asymptomatic carriers.
- Local irritation or hypersensitivity reactions can occur at the site of tick attachment.
- Ticks tend to attach to sites in contact with the ground, e.g. feet, neck, head (Figure 7.34), ears.
- A 'tick head' granuloma can form, especially if the tick is scratched out by the pet or the tick is removed by an owner and the head remains embedded.

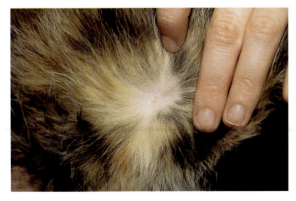

Figure 7.34 *Ixodes ricinus* tick on the head.

- Ticks can be vectors of bacterial, rickettsial, viral and protozoal diseases. Examples of tick-borne disease include ehrlichiosis, Rocky mountain spotted fever and Lyme disease and tick paralysis.

Diagnosis
- History and clinical signs.
- Identification of the tick in situ.

Treatment
- Where possible, ticks should be removed manually with fine forceps. It is essential to ensure that the tick is not squashed as its body fluids may be infectious. There is, however, a risk of incomplete removal and the production of 'tick head' granulomas.
- Topical acaracides should be used on the animal to remove the ticks; suitable products include those containing fipronil, amitraz (dog) and permethrin (dogs), pyriprole (dogs).
- Preventative therapy with topical spot on or collars containing acaracides may be useful to prevent re-infestation, e.g. collar impregnated with 4.0% deltamethrin.
- Environmental therapy with permethrin- or pyrethrin-based sprays may be useful in kennels or the immediate environment.

Insects

(1) Fleas
(2) Pediculosis
(3) Flies
    (a) Fly dermatitis
    (b) Mosquito bite hypersensitivity
    (c) Fly strike (Myiasis)
(4) Cuterebriasis
(5) Hymenoptera

Fleas

Fleas are small, wingless, blood-sucking insects. They are the most common cause of skin disease in dogs and cats worldwide. In temperate climates, they are generally only a problem during the warmer summer months. In warmer climates, fleas can cause disease for 12 months of the year.

122 Manual of Skin Diseases of the Dog and Cat

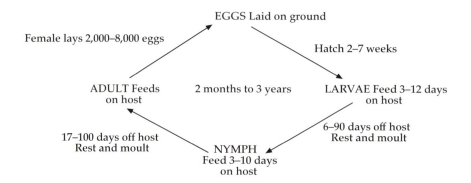

More than 90% of fleas found on dogs and cats are *Ctenocephalides felis felis* (see Table 7.10, Figures 7.35 and 7.36).

Other species that may also be found on dogs:

- *Ctenocephalides canis* (dog)
- *Echidnophaga gallinacea* (stick tight poultry)
- *Spilopsyllus cuniculi* (rabbit)
- *Pulex irritans* (human)
- *Archaeopsylla erinacei* (hedgehog)

Cause and pathogenesis

- A very common pruritic skin disease of dogs and cats that have been sensitised to flea saliva. Should be considered and ruled out of the differentials for any pruritic skin disease of the dog or cat.
- Flea saliva contains at least 15 potentially allergenic components, these are complete antigens not haptens.
- Non-allergic animals tolerate fleas and develop minimal clinical signs.
- Reactions occurring in flea allergic animals include the following:
  - Type I – immediate hypersensitivity
  - Type IV – delayed hypersensitivity
  - Cutaneous basophil hypersensitivity
- It is common that atopic animals have concurrent flea allergy.

Table 7.10 *Ctenocephalides felis*.

Ctenocephalides felis felis	Distinguishing features
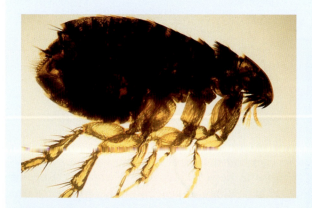 **Figure 7.35**	Small brown wingless insects, body laterally compressed Elongated head Both genal and pronotal combs present; 8–9 genal combs present the first comb same length as second Figure 5.36 Eggs oval

Parasitic skin disease 123

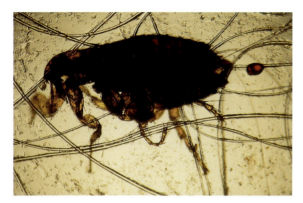

Figure 7.36 Head of *Ctenocephalides felis felis* showing both genal and pronotal combs.

Clinical signs
- Dogs:
  - Non-flea allergic animals:
    - May have fleas but show no dermatological signs (Figure 7.37).
    - May show any one of a range of anaemia (Figure 7.38), mild skin irritation, tape worms, acute moist dermatitis (hot spots) or acral lick granuloma.
  - Flea allergic animals:
    - Most commonly 3–5 years of age.
    - Acutely pruritic crusted papules with erythema, areas of acute moist dermatitis.
    - Chronically – alopecia, lichenification, hyperpigmentation usually dor-

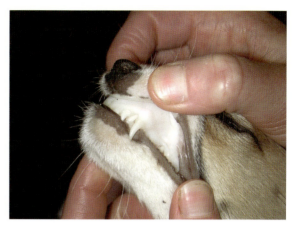

Figure 7.38 Anaemia in a puppy with severe flea infestation.

sal (Figure 7.39), lumbosacral area, caudomedial thighs, ventral abdomen.
- Fibropruritic nodules seen occasionally in dorsal lumbosacral area (Figure 7.40).
- Usually ears, feet, face spared.
- Cats:
  - Non-flea allergic animals:
    - May have fleas but show no clinical signs.
    - May show any one of a range of anaemia, mild skin irritation, tape

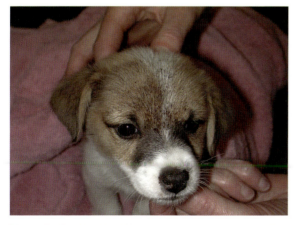

Figure 7.37 Non-flea allergic puppy with numerous adult fleas.

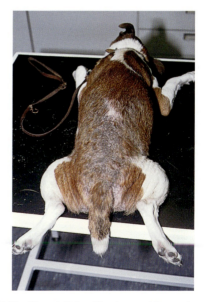

Figure 7.39 Dorsal lichenification and hyperpigmentation with secondary alopecia in the flea allergic dog.

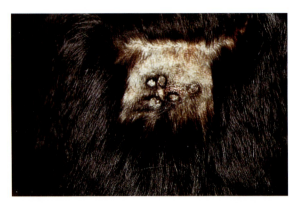

Figure 7.40 Fibropruritic nodules on the dorsum of a Retriever.

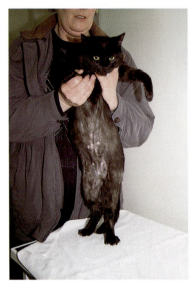

Figure 7.42 Ventral abdominal alopecia caused by flea allergy.

worms, acute moist dermatitis (hot spots).
- Flea allergic animals:
  - No age incidence.
  - Can present with many different clinical signs including the following:
    - Papulocrustous reaction especially on the dorsum – 'miliary dermatitis' (Figure 7.41).
    - Self-induced symmetrical alopecia on ventrum (Figure 7.42) or flanks.
    - Eosinophilic granuloma complex (Figure 7.43).
    - Facial pruritus.

Differential diagnosis
- Allergy especially food, atopy
- Pediculosis
- Cheyletiellosis
- Malassezia dermatitis
- Dermatophytosis
- Superficial pyoderma
- Demodicosis
- Psychogenic alopecia (cat)

Diagnosis
- History and clinical signs.
- Identification of fleas or flea 'dirt' may be difficult especially in a cat that is overgrooming or a dog that is being regularly shampooed. A wet paper test allows visualisation

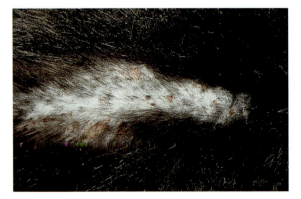

Figure 7.41 Miliary dermatitis caused by flea allergic dermatitis.

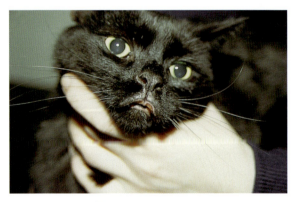

Figure 7.43 Indolent ulcer secondary to flea allergic dermatitis.

Life cycle

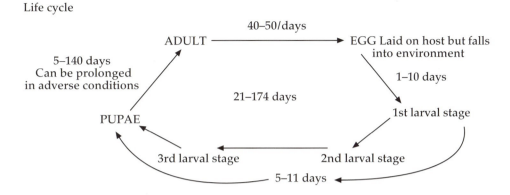

of pet's blood in flea faeces, which produces red streaks when coat is brushed onto wet paper (Figure 7.44).
- Tapeworm segments from *Dipylidium* spp. (the flea is the intermediate host of this tape worm) found in the perianal area or in faecal flotation samples indicate the presence of fleas.
- Human lesions pruritic papules usually on lower legs (Figure 7.45).
- Intradermal allergy or in vitro allergy testing with flea antigens. False-negative reactions can be seen due to limitation of the test to identify a type I hypersensitivity and the lack of specificity of same allergens, i.e. whole body flea extract versus flea saliva.
- Biopsy reveals signs of a non-specific pattern of superficial to deep usually eosinophil-rich perivascular to interstitial dermatitis.
- Response to strict flea control programme.

Treatment
(a) Flea control:
This should be tailored to the individual based on numbers and types of pet, ability of owner to use particular products and client finances. Affected and all in contact dogs and cats should be treated. It is important to use integrated flea control so that both an adulticide and insect growth regulator (juvenoid) are used in combination. This may be undertaken using different combinations, e.g. topical animal and environmental products, systemic animal products alone, or topical animal products alone.
Client education regarding flea life cycle essential:
- Environmental control:
  - Internal environment most important in temperate climate, both indoor and outdoor environments (yards,

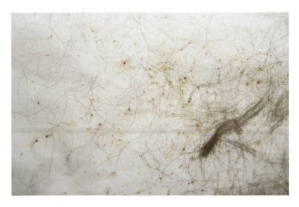

Figure 7.44 Flea dirt on wet paper.

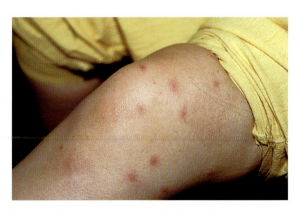

Figure 7.45 Pruritic papules on the leg of the owner.

pounds, etc.) need to be treated in warm climates.
- ☐ Thorough vacuuming plus disposal of bag is useful within the home.
- ☐ Pesticides applied to the environment as powders or sprays:
  - Desiccating agents, e.g. sodium borate.
  - Insect growth regulators – cyromazine, fenoxycarb, methoprene, permethrin, piriproxyfen.
- ☐ Animal spot on containing juvenoid, e.g. methoprene (dogs).
- ☐ Systemic treatment given to dogs or cats as tablets, liquids or injections:
  - Insect growth regulators, e.g. lufenuron
- ■ Animal:
  - ☐ Adulticide therapy may need to be used at an increased frequency in the early stages of the disease, first 4-6 weeks until environmental therapy becomes effective. Nitenpyram at 1 mg/kg may need to be used every other day in a dog and every third day in a cat. Topical spot on or spray therapy may be needed every 2 weeks. Examples of adulticides include the following:
    - Sprays – fipronil.
    - Systemic – nitenpyram.
    - Spot-on – fipronil (cat and dog), imidacloprid (cat and dog), metaflumizole (dog), pyriprole (dog), selamectin (cat and dog).
(b) Anti-inflammatories:
- ■ Glucocorticoid may be given to help control pruritus in the early stages of therapy, but if flea treatment is used as a therapeutic trial this may make interpretation of results difficult:
  - ☐ Prednisolone 0.5–1 mg/kg po sid (dogs) 1–2 mg/kg po sid (cats) for 7–10 days then tapering to lowest possible alternate day dosage. Only short courses should be required if flea control is rigorous.
  - ☐ Methylprednisolone acetate (cat only) 20 mg/cat or 4 mg/kg sq or im on two occasions 2–3 weeks apart. Prolonged use of this drug should be avoided.
  - ☐ Medroxyprogesterone acetate not suitable for therapy of this disease in the cat or dog.
    - ■ Antihistamines – limited usage.
(c) Antibiotics should be given for secondary pyoderma for 3–4 weeks. If pyoderma is present then glucocorticoids should not be given.
(d) Hypo-sensitisation – success questionable.

Pediculosis

Cause and pathogenesis
Pediculosis is an uncommon pruritic skin disease caused by lice (see Table 7.11). Lice tend to be host specific. They can be spread from dog to dog and from cat to cat but spread between species including man is uncommon.

Two suborders:

- ■ Mallophaga – biting lice:
  - ☐ *Trichodectes canis* (dog)
  - ☐ *Heterodoxus spiniger* (dog) (warm climates only)
  - ☐ *Felicola subrostratus* (cat)
- ■ Anoplura – sucking lice:
  - ☐ *Linognathus setosus* (dog)

Biting lice cause more irritation than sucking lice. Biting lice move rapidly through the coat and can be difficult to sample.

Disease seen especially in winter, tend to be seen in cold climates where they are a more common ectoparasite than fleas, lice killed by high skin temperatures.

Predisposing factors include systemic disease especially in cats immunosuppressed with viral disease and poor hygiene, poor levels of nutrition and overcrowding as seen in neglected animals.

Clinical signs
- ■ Lice usually found feeding at body openings (medial canthus eyes, perianal area), ear tips and matted areas of hair on body.
- ■ Sucking lice cause anaemia plus debilitation.
- ■ Pruritus may be variable; some animals can be asymptomatic carriers, other present with seborrhoea.

Table 7.11 Lice in the dog and cat.

Biting lice *Trichodectes canis*	*Felicola subrostratus*
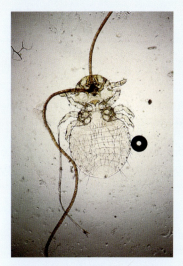 **Figure 7.46** Photograph of *Trichodectes canis* adult.	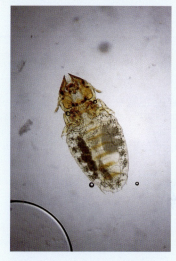 **Figure 7.47** *Felicola subrostratus* – biting louse.

Distinguishing features

Small dorso-ventrally flattened wingless insects 2–3 mm in length

Six legs, broad head, three segmented antennae at side of head

Large mouth parts designed for biting

Rapidly moving parasite

Operculate egg of louse cemented to hairs	**Sucking lice** ***Linognathus setosus*: Distinguishing features sucking lice**
	Small dorso-ventrally flattened wingless insects 2–3 mm in length
	Six legs, broad head, three segmented antennae at side of head
	Mouth parts adapted for sucking
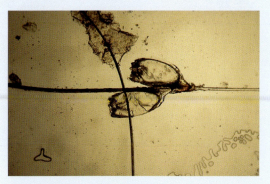 **Figure 7.48** Lice eggs cemented to hair shafts.	Slow moving parasite

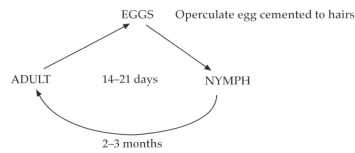

Life cycle – host specific

- Papular eruptions in sensitive animals leading to self-excoriation (Figure 7.49) and alopecia; may present with signs of military dermatitis or eosinophilic granuloma (Figure 7.50) in cats.

Differential diagnosis
- Flea allergic dermatitis
- Cheyletiellosis
- Scabies
- Dermatophytosis
- Allergy especially atopy, food

Diagnosis
- History and clinical signs.
- Microscopy to identify:
  - Lice by either acetate tapes or superficial skin scrapings:
    - Sucking lice – slow moving, easy to catch.
    - Biting lice – active, move rapidly.
  - Eggs (nits) stuck to hairs identified by hair pluckings or acetate tape of hairs.
- Biopsy reveals non-specific and non-diagnostic signs of superficial perivascular dermatitis often with eosinophilic component.

Treatment
- Identification and treatment of any underlying factors is important. Where anaemia is present this should be treated, which includes blood transfusion in severe cases.
- Treatment of affected animal and all in contacts is important.
- Animal treatment:
  - Clip coat to remove thick crusts and mats to allow penetration of treatment.
  - Insecticidal shampoo or leave on dips may be used on 3 occasions at 14 day intervals. Suitable products contain selenium sulphide 1%, lime sulphur 2%,

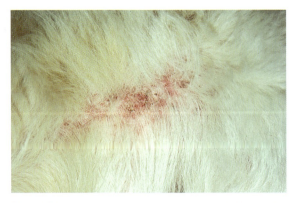

Figure 7.49 Papules and erythema from the flank of a dog with lice.

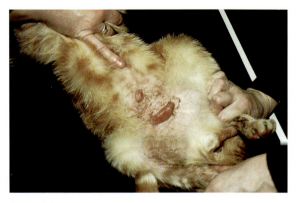

Figure 7.50 Eosinophilic granuloma secondary to lice infestation.

permethrin 1% (dogs). Selenium sulphide and lime sulphur have the advantage of being keratolytic to help remove the scale.
- Licensed topical insecticide spot on formulations include those containing fipronil, imidacloprid, pyriprole, metaflumizole, and selamectin have good activity against lice. These are probably most effective when used at the recommended dose rate (per label) but more frequently than recommended at 14 day intervals for 3 applications.
- Insecticidal sprays include fipronil 0.25% used at a dose of 6 mg/kg every 14 days for 3 applications.
- Systemic therapy with ivermectin constitutes an extra-label use at 0.2 mg/kg po or sq every 14 days for 3 applications.
■ Environmental treatment:
- This should be undertaken as part of therapy especially bedding and grooming equipment. Products suitable for environmental flea control may be used once or twice at 2 week intervals.

Flies

Fly dermatitis
Cause and pathogenesis
Uncommon pruritic skin disease caused by biting flies usually dogs housed outdoors. It is a rare disease in cats.

Important flies include the following:

- *Stomoxys calcitrans* (stable fly)
- *Simulium* spp. (black fly)
- *Tabanus* spp. (horse fly)
- *Chrysops* spp. (deer fly)

Clinical signs
■ Bites usually occur on the most exposed areas of the body. The most common site is the ear tip in prick-eared dogs but other areas can be involved especially the face, ventral abdomen and legs.
■ Lesions consist of haemorrhagic papules and crusts, overlying areas of erosions and ulcerations.
■ Pruritus is variable.

Differential diagnosis
■ Other ectoparasitic diseases especially
- Scabies
- Pediculosis
■ Vasculitis
■ Leishmaniasis
■ Autoimmune skin disease
■ Sunlight-induced neoplasia

Diagnosis
■ History (especially exposure to flies) and clinical signs.
■ Elimination of other causes by microscopy and biopsy.
■ Response to appropriate measures to control flies.

Treatment
■ Fly avoidance where possible. The source of flies should be identified, e.g. local dung heap, area of standing water (knowledge of fly life cycle important) and removed or the animals housing should be moved.
■ Fly repellents containing permethrin (dogs) may be applied daily, where small flies are thought to be important barrier cream/oils may be useful. Collars containing 4% deltamethrin may be useful in dogs.
■ Treatment of lesions with a topical antibiotics/glucocorticoid preparation may be used twice daily for up to 10 days. Prolonged use of such products can lead to skin changes and should be avoided.

Mosquito bite hypersensitivity
Cause and pathogenesis
An uncommon seasonal disease seen in cats that are hypersensitive to mosquito bites. Only occur in warm climates and any seasonality is related to the mosquito feeding times. Lesions are seen most commonly in outdoor cats. Lesions resolve without treatment when cats are confined to a mosquito-free environment.

Clinical signs
■ Lesions commonly affect the bridge of the nose, medial aspect of ear pinnae, also footpads, lips and chin.

- Acute lesions range from erythematous plaques and papules to ulcerated erosions with superficial crusting. They have a symmetrical distribution.
- Chronic lesions include scaling, alopecia and nodules often with pigment changes (hypo- or hyperpigmentation). Crusting and hyperkeratosis can be seen on the footpads.
- Systemic signs include lymphadenopathy and pyrexia.

Differential diagnosis
- Pemphigus foliaceus/erythematosus
- Allergy (atopy, food, flea)
- Dermatophytosis
- Demodicosis
- *Otodectes cynotis*
- Plasma cell pododermatitis

Diagnosis
- History of mosquito exposure and clinical signs.
- Resolution of lesions occurs when cat is hospitalised in a mosquito-free environment for 5–7 days.
- Response to therapy with insect repellents.
- Histopathology reveals non-specific changes of superficial perivascular dermatitis with eosinophilic infiltrates and collagen degeneration.

Treatment
- Prevention of mosquito bites by
  - hospitalisation or confinement during high risk periods especially dawn and dusk when mosquitoes feed;
  - insect repellents applied to short and sparsely haired areas; permethrin-based repellents should be used with care as many human insect repellent products are toxic to cats.
- Treatment of the bites:
  - Anti-inflammatory doses of prednisolone 3–5 mg/kg po sid may be used for 2–3 weeks to treat bites once they have occurred.
  - Courses of prednisolone can be extended and used on an alternate day basis for cats that have continual re-exposure for the remainder of the mosquito season.
  - Methylprednisolone acetate 20 mg/cat or 4 mg/kg sq or im on every 2–3 months during the mosquito period. Prolonged use of this drug should be avoided.

Fly strike (myiasis)
Cause and pathogenesis
Myiasis is the infestation of the skin of living animals with maggots from dipterous flies. The flies are attracted to lay their eggs on warm wet skin, especially urine and faecal stained areas as well as draining wounds. The maggots (larvae) that hatch secrete proteolytic enzymes that digest the tissue. Myiasis is a common disease in both dogs and cats. Predisposing factors include poor hygiene, debilitation due to age or illness and urinary or faecal incontinence. Three types of flies are important in the pathogenesis of the disease:

- Primary flies – initiate strike especially *Lucilia* spp. and *Calliphora* spp.
- Secondary flies – larvae extend lesions *Chrysomyia* spp., *Sarcophaga* spp.
- Tertiary flies – last to invade; cause further inflammation, e.g. *Musca* spp.

Clinical signs
- Lesions affect skin around nose, eyes, mouth, anus (Figure 7.51) and genitalia, as well as neglected wounds.

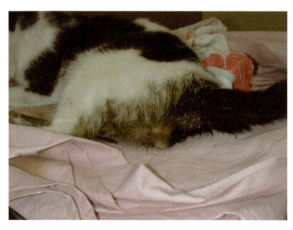

Figure 7.51 Debilitated cat with fly myiasis of perianal skin.

Parasitic skin disease

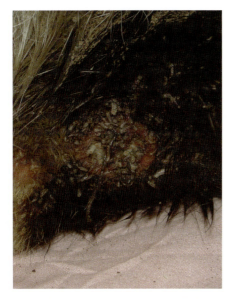

Figure 7.52 Close-up of the case in Figure 7.51.

- Typical appearance is of punched out ulcers with tissue necrosis containing larvae (Figure 7.52).
- Maggots will orientate vertically within the wounds to maximize use of the space.

Diagnosis
- Identification of larvae in wounds, on hair and skin.

Treatment
- Treatment of predisposing factors is important to prevent recurrence. Animal should be moved to a clean fly-free environment.
- Clip hair from lesions and clean the area thoroughly with an antibacterial wash, e.g. acetic acid, chlorhexidine, ethyl lactate to remove all larvae. Surgical debridement may be necessary in severe cases.
- Insecticidal wash or spray may be used on the rest of coat, e.g. pyrethrin or pyrethroid based (dogs) with care to avoid toxicity in a debilitated animal.
- Systemic larvicidal drugs (unlicensed) that may be of benefit include the following:
  - Nitenpyram 1 mg/kg po sid for 7 days.
  - Ivermectin 0.2–0.4 mg/kg sq on a single occasion.
- Antibiotics based on culture and sensitivity if necessary.
- Prognosis is variable depending on the underlying causes and the extent of tissue damage prior to therapy.

Cuterebriasis

Cause and pathogenesis
Infection of skin of living animals with larvae of *Cuterebra* spp. Generally, a disease seen in dogs and cats in warm climates in the late summer and autumn and imported dogs and cats in temperate climates, such as in United Kingdom.

Animals are contaminated by picking up eggs laid by adult flies in the environment usually close to burrows or nests of rabbits or rodents, which are their natural hosts (rabbits, chipmunks, squirrels, mice). Normally, the larvae crawl into the fur of the host, enter the body through a natural opening, and then migrate to a subcutaneous site.

Aberrant migration can occur, in unnatural host, to the central nervous system, trachea, nostrils, pharynx or intraocularly.

Clinical signs
- Lesions usually found as solitary nodules on the head, neck and trunk.
- Nodular swelling is approximately 1 cm across with a central air hole and fistula.
- Lesions are non-painful and non-pruritic.
- Other clinical signs can occur dependent on the site of aberrant migration.

Differential diagnosis
- Subcutaneous abscesses
- Myiasis
- Neoplasia

Diagnosis
- History of exposure and clinical signs.
- Identification of larvae in lesions as a variably coloured (white, cream, brown or black) larva with black spines covering its body.

Treatment

- Incision of the air hold, which needs to be carefully enlarged for gentle extraction of larvae using fine forceps. There is a risk of anaphylaxis if the larva is crushed or incompletely removed.
- Wound hygiene is important as the hole will tend to heal slowly. It must be kept clean with daily flushes with chlorhexidine ± edta-tris.
- Where secondary infection is present, appropriate antibiotics will be needed for 2–3 weeks.

Hymenoptera (bees, wasps, hornets)

Cause and pathogenesis

Hymenoptera are non-parasitic venomous insects that cause an acute inflammatory reaction in the skin of dogs and cats. Toxin released into the skin as insect stings leading to local or systemic signs. The severity of clinical signs depends on the number of stings and animal sensitivity. Common disease in dogs, uncommon disease in cats. Tends to be a seasonal problem found in the summer in temperate climates but is perennial in warm climates.

Clinical signs

- Lesions may be localised or generalised.
- Localised lesions in mild cases present with redness and oedema.
- Generalised disease can produce extensive areas of angioedema (Figure 7.53) with anaphylaxis leading to death; can occur in severe cases.

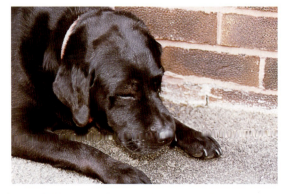

Figure 7.53 Angioedema on the face of a Labrador after a bee sting.

Differential diagnosis

- Other localised and generalised causes of urticaria and angioedema.

Diagnosis

- History of exposure to the insects and clinical signs.

Treatment

- Localised problem:
  - Remove sting if possible and give a single injection of a short-acting glucocorticoid injection, e.g. dexamethasone 0.05–0.1 mg/kg sq or im followed by antihistamines, e.g. chlorpheniramine po 0.2–1.0 mg/kg tid or qid.
  - Topical antihistamine cream may have some benefit.
- Anaphylaxis should be treated with intramuscular adrenaline and intravenous glucocorticoids.

Helminth parasites

Uncinariasis (hookworm dermatitis)

Cause and pathogenesis

Cutaneous lesions caused by the percutaneous penetration of the third stage larvae of the hookworm *Uncinaria stenocephala* in previously sensitised individuals. Hookworm rarely completes its life cycle by this route. *U. stenocephala* is the hookworm that causes disease in temperate and sub-artic climates and has been most commonly recorded in Ireland, England and United States. The dog is the natural host for *Uncinaria*. It is most commonly seen in dogs that live outdoors, especially in grassed or earthed runs, or damp contaminated kennels. It is a rare cause of skin disease.

Clinical signs

- Acute lesions appear as papular eruptions on contact sites with ground especially feet (interdigitally), sternum and ventral abdomen.

- Chronic lesions are erythematous with swelling and alopecia, which can be severe on the feet. Digital hyperkeratosis is a common finding.
- Pruritus variable, but lesions tend to be painful.
- Occasionally onychorrhexis may be seen and arthritis of the interphalangeal joints.

Differential diagnosis

- Contact dermatitis
- Pododemodicosis
- Pelodera dermatitis
- Dirofilariasis
- Dermatophytosis
- Strongyloidiasis

Diagnosis

- History especially of poor housing together with clinical signs.
- Rule out of other differentials.
- Faecal examination by floatation for hookworm eggs.
- Biopsy reveals non-specific signs of perivascular dermatitis, which is often eosinophil rich. On rare occasions, larvae can be seen in tissues surrounded by a mixed inflammatory cell infiltrate.
- Therapeutic trial with anthelmintics. Lesions will improve after appropriate treatment.

Treatment

- Animal treatment:
  - It is important to treat both the affected and all in contact animals immediately and then establish an anthelmintic protocol for future prophylaxis.
  - Anthelmintics suitable for use for treatment and prophylaxis include fenbendazole, mebendazole, and pyrantel. Initial therapy should be twice 3 weeks apart.
- Environmental treatment:
  - Improvement of hygiene by faeces removal in runs and frequent changes of bedding.
  - Remove earthed and grassed runs and replace with dry paved runs, or gravel treated, which may be treated with sodium borate 0.5 kg/m^2 periodically.

Ancylostomiasis

Cause and pathogenesis

Cutaneous lesions caused by the percutaneous penetration of the third stage larvae of the hookworm *Ancylostoma braziliense, A. caninum*. *Ancylostoma* sp. is the hookworm that causes disease in warm climates. The dog is the natural host for *Uncinaria*. It is most commonly seen in dogs that live outdoors especially in grassed or earthed runs, or damp contaminated kennels. It is a very rare cause of skin disease in dogs.

Clinical signs

As *Uncinaria stenocephala*.

Diagnosis

As *Uncinaria stenocephala*.

Treatment

As *Uncinaria stenocephala*.

Pelodera dermatitis

Cause and pathogenesis

Pelodera dermatitis is caused by cutaneous infestation with larvae of free living nematode *Pelodera strongyloides*. The adult nematodes, which are not parasitic, live in damp soil and decaying vegetation. The larval form is parasitic and will invade skin of dogs at points of contact with ground. Most commonly seen in dogs kept in poor sanitation on earth runs or dirty straw bedding. Uncommon condition of dogs.

Clinical signs

- Acute lesions present as papules with erythema and secondary alopecia on areas that are in contact with the ground especially feet, legs, perineum and sternum.
- Chronic lesions may lead to lichenification and hyperpigmentation of the skin.

- Pruritus very variable; may be mild to intense.
- Secondary pyoderma is present in some cases.

Differential diagnosis

As *Uncinaria stenocephala*.

Diagnosis

- History of environmental exposure and clinical signs.
- Microscopy in the form of superficial skin scrapings demonstrates small motile nematode larvae approximately 65 mm in length.
- Larvae and adults can be found in contaminated litter from environment.
- Biopsy reveals signs of a perifolliculitis, folliculitis and furunculosis, which is eosinophil rich. Nematodes can be seen within follicles and within dermal granulomas.

Treatment

- Animal treatment:
  - Antiseborrhoeic shampoo, e.g. sulphur/salicylic acid to remove crust and scale followed by a scabicidal dip, e.g. 0.025% amitraz or 2% lime sulphur.
  - Anti-inflammatory therapy with prednisolone 0.5–1 mg/kg po sid for 5–7 days.
  - Antibiotics may be necessary if secondary pyoderma is present.
- Environmental treatment:
  - Improvement of hygiene in kennels by removal and destruction of all bedding and treatment of the environment with a parasiticide, e.g. sodium borate (see *Uncinaria*).
- Prognosis is good, provided the environment is treated adequately.

Dracunculiasis

Cause and pathogenesis

Nodular cutaneous disease caused by *Dracunculus* spp., a nematode that parasitizes subcutaneous tissue. Dogs become infected by ingestion of *Cyclop* (a crustacean), the intermediate host, whilst drinking contaminated water. Adults develop over the subsequent 8–12 months in subcutaneous tissues of limbs. Females migrate to the surface of the skin to form a nodule. When the dog enters water again the nodule ruptures to expose females, which release L_1 stage. In North America *Dracunculus insignis* principally affects racoons, minks and other wild mammals. Infection in dogs and cats is uncommon. In Africa and Asia *D. medinesis* infests many different mammals including dogs and man.

Clinical signs

- Lesions present as single or multiple subcutaneous nodules on limbs, head and ventral abdomen.
- Nodules may be painful and show variable degrees of pruritus.
- Non-healing fistulae develop over the nodules.

Differential diagnosis

- Cuterebriasis
- Bacterial or fungal granuloma
- Neoplasia

Diagnosis

- History of exposure to the parasite and clinical signs.
- Microscopy in the form of cytology of exudates from the fistula demonstrates a mixed inflammatory infiltrate with 500 µm long nematode larvae with tapered ends.
- Biopsy reveals a subcutaneous pseudocyst that contains adult and larval nematodes surrounded by a pyogranulomatous infiltrate, which is eosinophil rich.

Treatment

- Environmental treatment:
  - Removal of contaminated water source or decontamination of the source.
- Animal treatment:
  - Worm can be removed from the nodule by winding up on a stick over several days.
  - Preferred treatment is excision of the nodule.

- ☐ Medical treatment may be undertaken with thiabendazole or metronidazole.
- Prognosis is good, provided the source of nematode and crustacean is removed from the environment.

Dirofilariasis (heart worm)

Cause and pathogenesis

- Dirofilariasis is a skin disease caused by either *Dirofilaria immitis* (heart worm) or *D. repens*. It is an uncommon disease of dogs seen principally in warm climates. Dogs are infected by intermediate host, a biting fly, usually a mosquito.
- *D. immitis* lives in right ventricle of the heart; its microfilaria rarely cause skin disease.
- *D. repens* lives in subcutaneous tissue, is of trivial veterinary importance, but causes lesions in cutaneous tissues due to microfilaria.

Clinical signs

- Lesions present as pruritic ulcerated papules, nodules and plaques.
- They are principally found on the head and limb.

Differential diagnosis

- Cuterebriasis
- Bacterial or fungal granuloma
- Neoplasia

Diagnosis

- History and clinical signs.
- Microscopy in the form of a direct examination of blood smear for microfilaria.
- Blood test – positive Knott's test for microfilaria.
- Biopsy reveals signs of microfilarial segments seen within dermal pyogranulomas often surrounded by an eosinophil-rich eosinophilic infiltrate.

Treatment

- Therapy for the heartworm will lead to a resolution of the cutaneous lesions.
- Suitable drugs include sodium thiacetarsamide or melarsomine dihydrochloride.

Selected references and further reading

Buerger, R.G. (1995) Insect and arachnid hypersensitivity disorders of dogs and cats. In: *Kirk's Current Veterinary Therapy XII Small Animal Practice*. pp. 631–634. WB Saunders, Philadelphia

Carlotti, D.N. and Jacobs, D.E. (2000) Therapy control and prevention of flea allergic dermatitis in dogs and cats. *Vet Dermatol*, **11**, 83–98

Curtis, C.F. (2004) Current trends in the treatment of Sarcoptes, Cheyletiella and Otodectes mite infestations in dogs and cats. *Vet Dermatol*, **15**, 108–114

Kennis, R. (2004) Arthropod parasites. In: Campbell, K.L. (ed) *Small Animal Dermatology Secrets*. pp. 126–131. Hanley and Belfus, Philadelphia

Kennis, R. (2004) Parasiticides in dermatology. In: Campbell, K.L. (ed). *Small Animal Dermatology Secrets*. pp. 64–68. Hanley and Belfus, Philadelphia

Medleau, L. and Hnilica, K. (2006) Viral, parasitic skin disorders. In: *Small Animal Dermatology: A Color Atlas and Therapeutic Guide*. 2nd edn. pp. 99–138. WB Saunders, Philadelphia

Mueller, R.S. (2004) Treatment protocols for demodicosis: an evidence based review. *Vet Dermatol*, **15**, 75–89

Scott, D.W. et al. (2001) Parasitic skin disease. *Muller and Kirk's Small Animal Dermatology*. 6th edn. pp. 423–515. WB Saunders, Philadelphia

Thomas, R.C. (2004) Helminth dermatoses. In: Campbell, K.L. (ed) *Small Animal Dermatology Secrets*. pp. 137–142. Hanley and Belfus, Philadelphia

Endocrine and metabolic skin disease

Canine hypothyroidism

Most common endocrine skin disease in the dog.

Cause and pathogenesis

Most cases of hypothyroidism in the dog are due to primary hypothyroidism, most of which are lymphocytic thyroiditis:

- Primary hypothyroidism caused by a direct deficiency of thyroid hormone:
  - Lymphocytic thyroiditis (90% of all cases) caused by autoimmune damage mediated through both humoral and cell mediated responses.
  - Idiopathic atrophy may possibly be the end stage of lymphocytic thyroiditis.
  - Neoplastic destruction.
- Secondary hypothyroidism caused by a deficiency of thyroid-stimulating hormone (TSH) from anterior pituitary:
  - Congenital defect – usually associated with pituitary dwarfism.
  - Pituitary destruction – expanding neoplasms.
  - Pituitary suppression – illness, e.g. hyperadrenocorticism, malnutrition.
  - Receptor defects.
- Tertiary hypothyroidism caused by a deficiency of thyrotropin-releasing hormone (TRH) from hypothalamus:
  - Congenital defects
  - Acquired destruction
  - Receptor deficits

Clinical signs

Adult onset hypothyroidism:

- Age incidence 6–10 years (earlier in giant breeds).
- Predisposed breeds include golden retriever, Labrador, Doberman, dachshund, Irish setter, Great Dane, English bull terrier but can be variable depending on local gene pool.
- Non-cutaneous signs:
  - Lethargy, obesity (Figure 8.1), heat seeking, aggression, anaemia.
  - Gastrointestinal signs – often vague intermittent diarrhoea.
  - Central nervous system – head tilt, nystagmus, hemiparesis, cranial nerve

Endocrine and metabolic skin disease

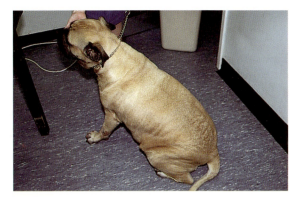

Figure 8.1 Obese hypothyroid Bullmastif.

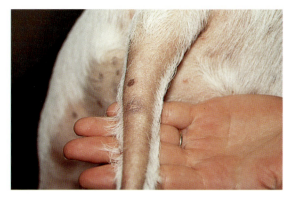

Figure 8.3 Rat tail in an English bull terrier with hypothyroidism.

dysfunction (facial, laryngeal nerve paralysis), hypermetria.
- Cardiovascular signs – exercise intolerance, bradycardia; cardiac arrhythmias ECG shows signs of flat T waves.
- Ocular signs – corneal lipidosis, keratoconjunctivitis sicca.
- Urogenital signs – infertility, abnormal seasons.
■ Cutaneous signs:
- Bilaterally symmetrical alopecia (Figure 8.2) spares the extremities; hairs easily epilated.
- Alopecia can also be seen on bridge of nose and tail (rat tail, Figure 8.3).
- Dry dull brittle hair coat.
- Myxoedema – cool puffy skin.
- Variable pigment changes to skin and coat.

- Seborrhoea generalised plus ceruminous otitis (Figure 8.4).
- Recurrent bacterial (*Staphylococcus* spp.) (Figure 8.5) and yeast (*Malassezia*) infections, plus demodicosis.
- Hypertrichosis – rare finding, especially Boxers and Irish setters.
- Pruritus mild except where secondary infection present.
- Delayed wound healing – poor hair regrowth after clipping.

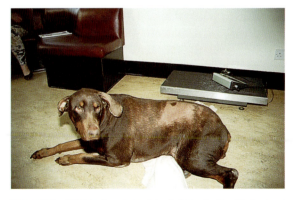

Figure 8.2 Bilaterally symmetrical alopecia in a Doberman with hypothyroidism.

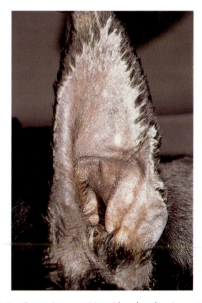

Figure 8.4 Ceruminous otitis with seborrhoeic casts around the periphery of the ear pinna in a hypothyroid Doberman.

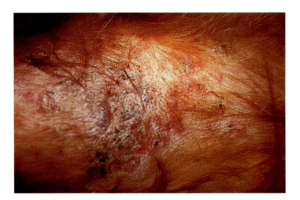

Figure 8.5 Recurrent bacterial infection in a hypothyroid dog.

Congenital hypothyroidism:

- Very rare condition seen in puppies from 4 weeks of age.
- Quiet, mentally retarded, disproportionate dwarves, i.e. short limbs and necks compared to the rest of their bodies.

Differential diagnosis

Hypothyroidism is a multisystemic disease that can mimic many other diseases. Other causes of endocrine alopecia, superficial pyoderma, Malassezia dermatitis and demodicosis should be considered.

Diagnosis

- History and clinical signs.
- Haematology and biochemistry show a range of non-specific signs including normochromic, normocytic non-regenerative anaemia (30%), elevations in cholesterol (50–75%), creatinine kinase (~ 50%), serum aspartate transaminase (SAT) and alanine transaminase (ALT).
- Skin biopsy reveals non-specific endocrine changes including orthokeratotic hyperkeratosis, follicular keratosis, follicular dilatation, telogenisation of hair follicles, epidermal melanosis, sebaceous gland atrophy and a thin dermis. Evidence of pyoderma, Malassezia and demodicosis may also be present.

Thyroid function tests:

- Basal levels of total thyroxine (TT4), free thyroxine (FT4), total triiodothyronine (TT3), and free triiodothyronine (fT3) can be misleading. They can be elevated or depressed in conditions other than thyroid disease (see Table 8.1).
- Endogenous TSH assay can be used in combination with TT4 and FT4:
    - TSH levels elevated in primary hypothyroidism.
    - TSH levels low or normal in secondary hypothyroidism.
- TSH and TRH stimulation tests are rarely used now in diagnosis of primary hypothyroidism. TRH stimulation test can be used to distinguish between primary, secondary and tertiary hypothyroidism:
    - Primary hypothyroidism low basal TT4/high basal TSH/unresponsive to TRH.
    - Secondary hypothyroidism low basal TT4/low basal TSH/unresponsive to TRH.

Table 8.1 Factors affecting total T4 levels (TT4).

Factors reducing TT4	Factors increasing TT4
Normal fluctuations	Normal fluctuations
Non-thyroidal illness	Recovery from disease
Age >7 years	Age <3 months
Autoantibodies	Autoantibodies
Drugs including phenobarbitone, frusemide, glucocorticoids, sulphonamides, non-steroidal anti-inflammatory drugs, phenylbutazone, mitotane, general anaesthetics	Drugs including oestrogen, progesterone, insulin, narcotic analgesics
Some breeds especially greyhounds	Dioestrous, pregnancy
Prolonged periods of inappetence	Obesity

- Tertiary hypothyroidism low basal TT4/low basal TSH/responsive to TRH.
■ Thyroid biopsy – not useful in practice.

Treatment

■ Therapy of any concurrent diseases, e.g. pyoderma, Malassezia, demodex needs to be addressed but may only be partially successful until thyroid treatment is started.
■ Therapy of hypothyroidism:
  - Lifetime treatment required in all cases. Supplementation with levothyroxine (T4) at a dose of 0.01–0.02 mg/kg po sid or bid. Dogs with cardiac disease should start at lower dose rate of 0.005 mg/kg po sid or bid increasing by 0.005 mg/kg increments every 2 weeks to maintenance.
  - Lethargy improves often within days.
  - Cutaneous lesions can take up to 5 months to respond.
  - Side effects rare due to the rapid metabolic turnover of the T4, faecal excretion, and poor absorption from gastrointestinal tracts. If these occur, signs of hyperthyroidism include anxiety, panting, polydipsia, polyphagia, diarrhoea.
  - Supplementation with liothyronine (T3) rarely indicated.
■ Post-pill monitoring should be undertaken 4–6 weeks after starting treatment. TT4 peaks 4–6 hours after T4 administration, therefore bloods at this time should show high normal or supranormal TT4 levels.
■ Prognosis for a full recovery is good in most cases except where central nervous system or muscular signs have been present for some time.

Feline hypothyroidism

Very rare endocrine skin disease in the cat.

Cause and pathogenesis

■ Adult onset hypothyroidism:
  - Spontaneously occurring hypothyroidism is a very rare disease; only a few cases recorded.
  - Iatrogenic disease most commonly seen secondary to radioactive iodine therapy or thyroidectomy for hyperthyroidism.
■ Congenital hypothyroidism seen in young kittens caused by a variety of mechanisms; all are thought to be inherited as an autosomal recessive trait.
  - Thyroid gland agenesis or dysgenesis
  - Dyshormonogenesis
  - Impaired organification of iodides (domestic short-haired cats and Abyssinians).
  - Inability of the gland to respond to TSH.

Clinical signs

Adult onset – spontaneous occurring:

■ Non-cutaneous signs – lethargy, obesity, heat seeking.
■ Cutaneous signs:
  - Dry, dull brittle hair coat.
  - Myxoedema – cool puffy skin.
  - Variable pigment changes to skin and coat.
  - Seborrhoea generalised.
  - Delayed wound healing – poor hair regrowth after clipping.
  - Alopecia not normally a feature; some cats may loose hair from their ears.

Adult onset – iatrogenic:

■ Non-cutaneous signs – initially lethargy but usually short lived, no changes in body weight or appetite.
■ Cutaneous signs:
  - Generalised seborrhoea.
  - Dorsal matting due to reduced grooming activity.
  - Alopecia of pressure points, pinnae, dorsal and lateral tail base region.

Congenital hypothyroidism:

- Very rare disease; recognised in kittens from 4 weeks of age.
- Often kittens will die at an early age before hypothyroidism is suspected.
- Non-cutaneous signs – lethargic and mentally dull, decreased rate of growth. Stunted kittens are disproportionate dwarves with short broad head, enlarged skull, shortened limbs, retained deciduous teeth, short round body, small ears.
- Cutaneous signs:
  - Hair coat is fine due to reduction in primary hairs; true alopecia is rare.
  - Seborrhoea commonly seen.
  - Thickened skin.

Differential diagnosis

- Traumatic alopecia, e.g. due to allergy, ectoparasites, psychogenic
- Dermatophytosis
- Demodicosis
- Hyperadrenocorticism
- Hyperthyroidism

Diagnosis

- History and clinical signs.
- Haematology and biochemistry reveal non-specific but inconsistent changes including normochromic, normocytic, non-regenerative anaemia and hypercholesterolaemia.
- Thyroid function tests:
  - Basal levels of TT4, FT4, TT3, and FT3 can be misleading.
  - In cases of congenital hypothyroidism TT4 should be within the range 52–72 nmol/l by 4 weeks of age.
  - Non-thyroidal illness – (euthyroid sick syndrome) and drug therapy (see Table 8.1) can influence these tests.
  - TSH stimulation tests – superior to basal thyroid levels. Contact laboratory for advice before performing the test. Protocol undertaken by measuring T4 level before and 6–7 hours after administration of 0.5–1.0 IU/kg of bovine TSH. Healthy cats double or treble their levels; hypothyroid cats show little or no response.
  - TRH stimulation test – most reliable test for diagnosis of hypothyroidism in the cat. Measure T4 levels before and 4 hours after the slow (may induce vomiting) intravenous injection 100 μg of TRH. Healthy cats demonstrate a 50–100% rise in T4; hypothyroid cats fail to respond.
- Thyroid biopsy – not useful in practice.

Treatment

- Lifetime treatment required in all cases. Supplementation is undertaken with levothyroxine (T4) at a dose of 0.05–0.2 mg/cat po sid.

  The response to therapy depends on the form of disease. Congenital hypothyroidism is often poorly responsive whereas acquired hypothyroidism usually responds well to therapy:
  - Lethargy improves often within days.
  - Cutaneous lesions can take up to 6 weeks to respond.
- Liothyronine (T3) supplementation rarely indicated.

Feline hyperthyroidism

Very common endocrine disorder caused by overproduction of thyroid hormone thyroxine (T4) and triiodothyronine (T3).

Cause and pathogenesis

In most cases hyperthyroidism can be attributed to a solitary thyroid adenoma or multinodular adenomatous hyperplasia of the thyroid. Carcinomas of the gland are rare in cats. Clinical signs are caused by the resulting acceleration in basal metabolic rate.

Clinical signs

- Age incidence 6–20 years with an average age 12 years.

Endocrine and metabolic skin disease

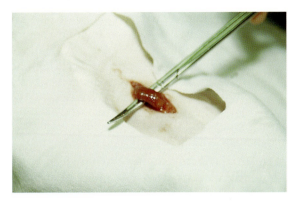

Figure 8.6 Enlarges thyroid gland – palpable in the conscious cat.

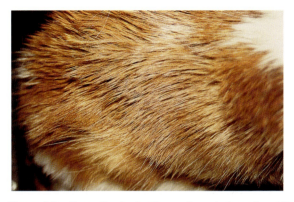

Figure 8.8 Generalised seborrhoea oleosa in hyperthyroid cat.

- No breed or sex predilection has been recognised.
- Onset of signs tends to be insidious.
- 95% of cats have a palpable enlarged cervical mass (Figure 8.6).
- Non-cutaneous signs include weight loss (Figure 8.7), polyphagia, polydipsia, diarrhoea and vomiting, hyperactivity, tachycardia and respiratory abnormalities. Occasionally lethargy, weakness and inappetence can be seen.
- Cutaneous signs seen in about 30–40% of cases and include the following:
  - Excessive shedding of hair coat, which can be easily epilated.
  - Seborrhoea oleosa leading to matting of hair coat (Figure 8.8).
  - Focal, often bilaterally symmetrical, alopecia (usually flanks) due to overgrooming. In severe cases self-inflicted trauma can occur (Figure 8.9).
  - Increased claw growth.
  - Secondary pyoderma (*Staphylococcus* spp.) and yeast (*Malassezia* spp.).

Differential diagnosis

- Hyperadrenocorticism
- Allergy (food, fleas, atopy)*
- Dermatophytosis*
- Psychogenic alopecia

Note: Asterisk (*) signifies that the condition can occur concurrently, exacerbated by hyperthyroid state.

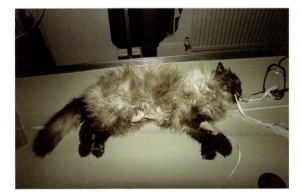

Figure 8.7 Severe weight loss in an untreated hyperthyroid cat.

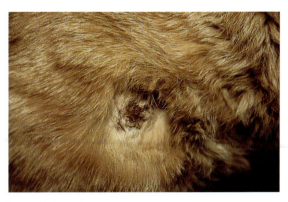

Figure 8.9 Acute moist dermatitis due to overgrooming in a hyperthyroid cat.

Table 8.2 Factors affecting TT4 level in cats.

Factors causing depression of elevated TT4 levels (false-negative reactions)	Non-thyroidal factors causing elevation of TT4 (false-positive reactions)
Concurrent disease, e.g. renal disease, diabetes mellitus	Overlap with normal cats
Concurrent therapy, e.g. glucocorticoids (methyl prednisolone acetate), hormones (megestrol acetate)	
Sedation where it is needed to take blood samples	

Diagnosis

- History and clinical signs especially palpable thyroid nodule.
- Haematology and biochemistry reveal a variety of non-diagnostic changes including increases in serum alkaline phosphatase (SAP), lactate dehydrogenase (LDH), alanine aminotransferase (ALT) and aspartate transaminase (AST).
- Thyroid function tests:
  - Elevations in basal levels of total T4 (TT4), and total T3 (TT3) are diagnostic; however, both false-negative and false-positive reactions can be seen (see Table 8.2).
  - T3 suppression test can be performed when 15–25 μg of liothyronine given orally every 8 hours for 7 doses. TT4 and FT4 levels are measured before drug administration and 2–4 hours after the last dose. Hyperthyroid cats show no change in their TT4 or FT4 levels. Normal cats show a 50% depression in TT4 and FT4.
  - TSH stimulation test is performed by giving 0.5 IU/kg intravenous injection of bovine TSH. Bloods are taken at 0 and 6 hours. Euthyroid cats show a 100% increase in TT4; hyperthyroid cats minimal or no increase.
  - TRH stimulation test is performed by giving 0.1 mg/kg TRH by slow intravenous injection. Bloods are taken at 0 and 4 hours. Euthyroid cats show a greater than 60% increase in TT4; hyperthyroid cats show less than 50% increase in TT4 levels.
- Radionuclide imaging can be useful to identify any ectopic thyroid tissue. Thyroid scanning is undertaken after the intravenous administration of a suitable radionuclide, e.g. technetium-99M (pertechnetate). Radionuclide is concentrated in a hyperactive glandular tissue.

Treatment

- Surgical excision has both advantages and disadvantages (see Table 8.3); see further reading list for suitable surgical texts for details of thyroidectomy.
- Oral anti-thyroid drugs can be used successfully to treat many cats (see Table 8.4). Suitable drugs include carbimazole 5 mg/cat po tid or methimazole 5 mg/cat po sid. These drugs may need to be used in combination

Table 8.3 Advantages and disadvantages of surgical therapy of hyperthyroidism.

Advantages	Disadvantages
Relatively inexpensive	Anaesthetic risk especially if cat is tachycardic or has renal dysfunction
Surgery that can normally be undertaken in first opinion practice without need for referral	Induction of thyrotoxic crisis
	Iatrogenic hypoparathyroidism
	Iatrogenic hypothyroidism
	Incomplete removal of abnormal tissue and recurrence
	Risk of damage to recurrent laryngeal nerve

Table 8.4 Advantages and disadvantages of medical therapy for hyperthyroidism.

Advantages	Disadvantages
Inexpensive therapy	Side effects of medication include anorexia, vomiting, anaemia, and thrombocytopaenia
Highly effective	Many hyperthyroid cats are difficult to medicate with oral drugs
Can be used on an outpatient basis	Iatrogenic hypothyroidism
Safe in high surgical risk patients	Monitoring is necessary of TT4 and FT4 levels every 2 weeks during induction period and every 3 months during maintenance

with propanolol to treat the tachycardia. They are used daily at this dose rate initially to decease TT4 than tapered down to the lowest dose rate to maintain normal thyroid function.

- Radioactive iodine can also be used to treat hyperthyroid cats. It also has advantages and disadvantages (see Table 8.5).

Table 8.5 Advantages and disadvantages of radioactive iodine therapy for hyperthyroidism.

Advantages	Disadvantages
Single treatment only in 70–80% of cats	Sophisticated facilities needed including hospitalisation and isolation cages
Anaesthesia and surgery not necessary safer for high risk animals	Expensive
Highly effective	Health and safety aspects of risk of medication to human contacts
	Iatrogenic hypothyroidism Re-treatment necessary in 20–30% of cats

Canine hyperadrenocorticism (Cushing's syndrome)

Canine Cushing syndrome has various causes, all of which lead to increased concentration of circulating cortisol.

Cause and pathogenesis

- Naturally occurring hyperadrenocorticism:
  - Pituitary-dependent hyperadrenocorticism (80–85% of naturally occurring cases):
    - Seen as a bilateral adrenocortical hyperplasia due to micro- or macro-adenoma/adenocarcinoma of pituitary, which leads to defective negative feedback of adrenocorticotrophic hormone (ACTH)
  - Adrenal-dependent hyperadrenocorticism:
    - Adrenocortical neoplasia (approx. 10–15% of naturally occurring cases) caused by a functional adenoma or adenocarcinoma.
- Ectopic ACTH syndrome (very rare):
  - Neoplasia other than those of pituitary or adrenal glands but are capable of producing ACTH, e.g. lymphosarcoma, bronchial carcinoma.
- Iatrogenic hyperadrenocorticism:
  - Chronic overuse of steroids by injection, tablet or topical application (eyes, ears, skin), especially in dogs with pruritic skin disease and immune mediated disorders (Figure 8.10).

Clinical signs

- Middle-old age; no sex predilection.
- Predisposed breeds include Boxers, poodles, dachshunds, small terriers (West Highland white, Boston terrier, Scottish terrier).
- Non-cutaneous signs:
  - Lethargy, poor exercise tolerance, behavioural changes, polydipsia, polyuria (>100 ml/kg/day).
  - Polyphagia – only seen in 50% of cases.

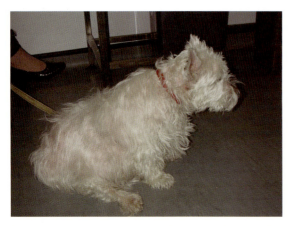

Figure 8.10 Iatrogenic Cushing's disease in a dog caused by prolonged glucocorticoid usage.

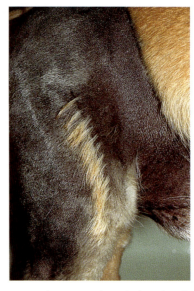

Figure 8.12 Poor hair regrowth on the leg of a Labrador (after cruciate surgery) secondary to hyperadrenocorticism.

- Neuromuscular signs – muscle atrophy, pot-bellied appearance (from hepatomegaly, fat redistribution and weakness of abdominal muscles) (Figure 8.11), osteomalacia, osteoporosis (rare), pseudomyotonia.
- Urogenital signs – anoestrus (entire bitches) testicular atrophy (entire dogs), clitoral enlargement, recurrent urinary tract infections, urolithiasis.
- Respiratory signs – panting, bronchopneumonia, coronary thrombosis, dystrophic mineralisation and fibrosis.
- Neurological signs – blindness, head pressing, Horner's syndrome, seizures.
- Ocular signs – exophthalmos, corneal ulcers, conjunctivitis.
- Pancreatic signs – acute pancreatitis, diabetes mellitus.
- Cutaneous signs:
  - Changes in coat condition and colour, slow hair regrowth after clipping (Figure 8.12).
  - Alopecia usually bilaterally symmetrical of the flanks, sparing of the extremities.
  - Thin skin with poor elasticity (Figure 8.13).
  - Hyperpigmentation, easy bruising, poor wound healing.
  - Seborrhoea.
  - Comedone formation especially on ventrum (Figure 8.14).
  - Calcinosis cutis is seen on dorsum especially neck and rump, axillary and inguinal areas. Appears as whitish, gritty, firm bone-like papules and more extensive plaques (Figure 8.15).
  - Striae – spontaneous or at site of scar (Figure 8.16).
  - Secondary infection with bacteria, yeast, dermatophytes or demodex – response to therapy is poor in these cases unless hyperadrenocorticism is treated concurrently.

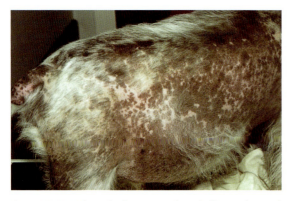

Figure 8.11 Bilateral alopecia and potbelly in dog with hyperadrenocorticism.

Endocrine and metabolic skin disease   145

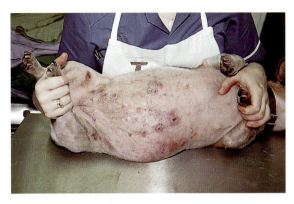

Figure 8.13 Thin skin with poor elasticity, prominent cutaneous blood vessels and haemorrhages due to trauma in dog with hyperadrenocorticism.

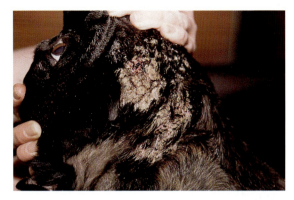

Figure 8.15 Calcinosis cutis on the neck of a Staffordshire bull terrier.

Differential diagnosis

- Cutaneous lesions:
    - Other endocrine diseases especially
        - Hypothyroidism
        - Testicular tumour (Sertoli cell tumours)
        - Hair cycle arrest alopecia

Diagnosis

- History and clinical signs.
- Haematology and biochemistry show typical 'steroid' pattern of a stress leucogram (eosinopaenia, lymphopaenia, neutrophilia). Seventy per cent of dogs show abnormalities in biochemical parameters (30% show no changes), notably elevations in SAP (90% of cases due to steroid-induced enzyme of hepatic origin, which is not specific for hyperadrenocorticism), also increases in cholesterol, alanine transaminase, aspartate transaminase and glucose.
- Thyroid levels, both TT4 and to a lesser degree FT4, are low; endogenous TSH is usually normal.
- Urine sample usually has a low specific gravity <1.012, often also proteinuria, glucosuria, bacteriuria.
- Imaging techniques:
    - Radiography reveals signs of hepatomegaly, osteoporosis, osteomalacia, dystrophic mineralisation, adrenocortical neoplasia (approximately 50% of adrenal tumours are calcified).

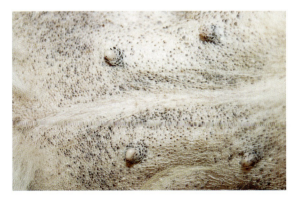

Figure 8.14 Comedone formation on the ventral abdomen of a dog with hyperadrenocorticism.

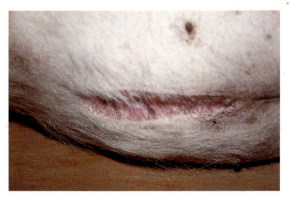

Figure 8.16 Cutaneous striae at site of old ovariohysterectomy scar in hyperadrenocorticism.

- Ultrasonography, computer tomography and magnetic resonance imaging can be used to identify adrenal or pituitary masses.
■ Skin biopsy reveals signs of non-specific endocrine changes (see hypothyroidism); however, other changes more typical of hyperadrenocorticism include dystrophic mineralisation, thin dermis and absence of erector pili muscles.
■ Adrenal function tests are important to make a diagnosis of hyperadrenocorticism after a high level of clinical suspicion has been raised by clinical signs and other tests. They can then be used to determine if it is adrenal or pituitary-dependent disease:
  - Urinary cortisol: creatinine ratio is not specific for hyperadrenocorticism and there is overlap with other causes of polyuria and polydipsia. False-positive tests are very common.
  - Endogenous plasma ACTH can be used to differentiate between adrenal- and pituitary-based disease. An elevated ACTH level is suggestive of pituitary disease, a depressed level suggestive of adrenal disease. False negatives can occur as not all dogs with hyperadrenocorticism have abnormal levels. Samples must be collected into cooled tubes and frozen immediately due to the short half life of ACTH then transported on ice to the laboratory.
  - ACTH stimulation test is useful to differentiate naturally occurring hyperadrenocorticism from iatrogenic disease. It is accurate in 50–60% of cases to identify naturally occurring hyperadrenocorticism:
    • Protocol should be performed on a starved dog. Plasma or serum cortisol levels are measured before and 1 hour after intravenous injection of 0.25 mg of synthetic ACTH (Synacthen).
    • Interpretation varies between laboratories; usually exaggerated response to ACTH is seen. Positive tests usually have levels at 1 hour greater than three times the basal. In iatrogenic disease an inadequate or flat response is seen.
  - Low dose dexamethasone suppression test is the test of choice to diagnose naturally occurring hyperadrenocorticism. It is accurate in 90–95% of cases:
    • Protocol should be performed on a starved dog. Plasma or serum cortisol levels are measured before, 3 hours and 8 hours after intravenous injections of 0.01 mg/kg of dexamethasone.
    • Cortisol levels suppressed consistently throughout the 8 hour period in normal dogs. Levels that fail to suppress or escape at 8 hours (see different laboratories for specific levels) are consistent with naturally occurring pituitary-dependent hyperadrenocorticism.
  - High dose dexamethasone suppression test is not suitable as an initial diagnostic test. It should only be used to differentiate pituitary- from adrenal-dependent disease:
    • Protocol should be performed on a starved dog. Plasma or serum cortisol levels are measured before, 3 and 8 hours after intravenous injection of 0.1–1.0 mg/kg dexamethasone. The higher dose range is recommended by some authors to ensure that maximum suppression occurs.
    • Precise interpretation depends on the laboratory – generally cortisol should suppress to less than 50% of basal level at time zero, by 4 hours in pituitary-dependent cases, no suppression is usually seen with adrenal neoplasia.
  - Corticotropin-releasing factor (CRF) stimulation test is not widely available commercially but could be used to differentiate pituitary-dependent from adrenal-dependent disease:
    • Protocol involves the intravenous injection of CRF leading to hyper-responsiveness of ACTH and cortisol in pituitary-dependent disease; no response is seen in adrenal disease.
  - Combined test using a combinations of ACTH with dexamethasone suppression tests is inferior to each individual test.

Treatment

Naturally occurring disease:

Start therapy of other conditions when start treatment for hyperadrenocorticism, e.g. diabetes mellitus, urinary tract infection, pyoderma.

- Pituitary-dependent disease:
  - Surgical treatment:
    - Bilateral adrenalectomy or transsphenoidal hypophysectomy requires an experienced surgeon and a lifetime of replacement treatment. Post-operative complication can occur so specialist post-operative nursing facilities are also important.
  - Radiation therapy available in specialist centres only.
  - Medical treatment:
    - Trilostane (inhibits steroidogenesis) is currently the licensed drug of choice for pituitary-dependent hyperadrenocorticism. It is well tolerated in most dogs but has been recorded to have caused sudden death in dogs with cardiac disease. It is contraindicated in pregnant/lactating animals and those with renal and hepatic disease. It is given at the following dose rate:
      ○ For dogs <5 kg, give 30 mg po with food sid.
      ○ For dogs 5–20 kg, give 60 mg po with food sid.
      ○ For dogs 20–40 kg, give 120 mg po with food sid.
      ○ For dogs >40 kg, give 240 mg po with food sid.
      ○ Monitoring can be undertaken with ACTH stimulation tests at 10 days, 4 weeks and 12 weeks after starting therapy then every 3 months. If a dog remains unstable then tests should be repeated every 10 days until a stable level is achieved. ACTH stimulation tests should be done 4–6 hours after trilostane therapy. For interpretation see Table 8.6.
  - Mitotane (o,p'-DDD, adrenolytic agent) has also been used successfully to

Table 8.6 Interpretation of ACTH test results in dogs on trilostane therapy.

Post-ACTH levels and health of dog	Interpretation and action
<20 nmol/l Irrespective of dogs health	Stop trilostane for 5–7 days and reinstitute at a lower dose rate; repeat tests as per protocol
>20 nmol/l and <150 nmol/l Dog well, normal thirst, appetite	Good control maintain the dose and repeat tests as per protocol
>20 nmol/l and <150 nmol/l Dog unwell, polyuria, polyphagia, polydipsia	Despite blood results animal health suggests poor control; dose rate too low; switch to twice daily dosing and retest before increasing the dose rate by 30 mg daily; repeat test as per protocol
>20 nmol/l and <150 nmol/l Dog unwell depression, inappetence, vomiting, diarrhoea	Despite blood levels suggesting good control dog showing signs of adrenal insufficiency; stop trilostane for 5–7 days and reinstitute at a lower dose rate; repeat tests as per protocol
>150 nmol/l and <250 nmol/l Dog well, normal thirst, appetite	Good control probable despite blood tests; maintain the dose and repeat tests as per protocol
>150 nmol/L and <250 nmol/L Dog unwell depression, inappetence, vomiting, diarrhoea	Despite blood levels suggesting moderate/good control dog showing signs of adrenal insufficiency Stop trilostane for 5–7 days and reinstitute at a lower dose rate; repeat tests as per protocol
>150 nmol/l and <250 nmol/l Dog unwell, polyuria, polyphagia, polydipsia	Poor control dose rate too low increase trilostane by 30 mg daily and repeat test as per protocol; dog may achieve better control with twice daily dosing

treat pituitary-dependent hyperadrenocorticism. Two different protocols are available for stabilisation:
- Low dose protocol should be used for dogs with concurrent diabetes mellitus where stabilisation should be undertaken more slowly:
  - Low dose Protocol 1: Mitotane 25–50 mg/kg po 7–10 days for induction. Prednisolone at a dose of 0.2 mg/kg po can be given concurrently to decrease signs of steroid withdrawal. Side effects during induction include lethargy, vomiting, diarrhoea, weakness. Monitor response to mitotane by water consumption decreasing from 100 ml/kg daily, eosinophil count returning and ACTH stimulation test (no steroids given on day of test). Once the disease has been stabilised maintenance dosage of mitotane 25–50 mg/kg orally every 7–10 days can be instituted.
- High dose Protocol 2 is used to create a state of hypoadrenocorticism:
  - High dose Protocol 2: Mitotane 50–100 mg/kg po. Start glucocorticoids and mineralocorticoid replacement treatment on day 3. Monitoring response is best by performing an ACTH after 25 days to ensure flat response, i.e. complete destruction of adrenal cortex.
- Ketoconazole (inhibits steroidogenesis) at a dose of 10–30 mg/kg/day po until a response is seen. A useful but expensive drug. Can be used to treat adrenal neoplasia.
- Other drugs that have not been shown to be very effective include the following:
  - Cyproheptadine hydrochloride (anti-serotonin agent) at a dose of 0.3–3.0 mg/kg/day po.
  - Bromocriptine mesylate (dopamine agonist) at a dose of 0.1 mg/kg/day po.
  - Selegiline hydrochloride (monoamine oxidase inhibitor) at a dose of 1–2 mg/kg po.

- Adrenal-dependent disease:
  - Surgical treatment:
    - Unilateral adrenalectomy is the therapy of choice. Post-surgery replacement therapy is required until atrophic gland recovers.
  - Medical treatment:
    - This is really only an option where the adrenal mass is inoperable, where there are metastases or an owner will not consent for surgery. Medical drugs that may give some palliation include the following:
      - Ketoconazole as for pituitary-dependent disease.
      - Mitotane as for Protocol 2 for pituitary disease.

Iatrogenic disease:
Withdrawal of steroids essential but replacement treatment indicated whilst hypothalamic–pituitary–adrenal cortex recovers.

Feline hyperadrenocorticism

A rare disease in the cat caused by increased levels of circulating cortisol.

Cause and pathogenesis

- Naturally occurring hyperadrenocorticism:
  - Pituitary-dependent hyperadrenocorticism (80% of naturally occurring cases):
    - Seen as a bilateral adrenocortical hyperplasia due to pituitary adenoma or adenocarcinoma.
    - Defective negative feedback of ACTH at level of hypothalamus.
  - Adrenal-dependent hyperadrenocorticism:
    - Adrenocortical neoplasia due to a functional adenoma or adenocarcinoma.
- Iatrogenic hyperadrenocorticism:
  - Chronic overuse of steroids by injection or tablet. Rare in the cat due to its high steroid tolerance.

Endocrine and metabolic skin disease 149

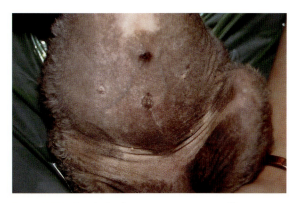

Figure 8.17 Pot-bellied appearance in naturally occurring hyperadrenocorticism.

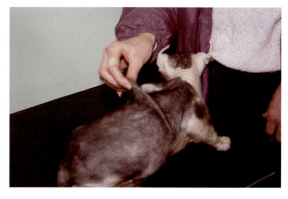

Figure 8.18 Thin alopecic skin on dorsum and flanks in cat with hyperadrenocorticism.

Clinical signs

Naturally occurring hyperadrenocorticism:

- Middle-old age cat; females are predisposed.
- No breed predisposition is recognised.
- Non-cutaneous signs:
  - Depression, anorexia, weight loss.
  - Polydipsia, polyuria, polyphagia.
  - Ninety per cent of cats are prediabetic or overtly diabetic (due to corticosteroid-induced insulin antagonism).
  - Neuromuscular signs – muscle atrophy, pot-bellied appearance (Figure 8.17).
  - Respiratory signs – recurrent respiratory infections.
- Cutaneous signs (in decreasing order of frequency):
  - Alopecia – partial or complete, involving dorsum, flanks or ventrum usually symmetrical (Figures 8.18 and 8.19).
  - Thin and fragile skin that tears often only with routine handling.
  - Easy bruising (Figure 8.20).
  - Poor hair coat and seborrhoea sicca.
  - Secondary infection with bacteria, yeast or demodex – response to therapy is poor in these cases unless hyperadrenocorticism is treated concurrently. Recurrent abscesses can be seen in some cases.
  - Comedones.
  - Hyperpigmentation.

Iatrogenic hyperadrenocorticism:

- Any age, sex or breed.
- Typically cats with pruritic skin disease or immune mediated disease. Rare to see this disease induced by prednisolone, more commonly more potent longer acting glucocorticoids.
- Clinical signs are similar to those for naturally occurring disease, except in addition typical medial curling of the ear tips is seen.

Differential diagnosis

- Cutaneous lesions especially where alopecia is present:
  - Traumatic alopecia (allergy, psychogenic alopecia, parasites, etc.)

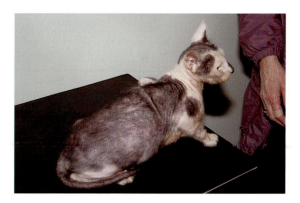

Figure 8.19 Same cat as in Figure 8.18 – skin remains tented after release, showing lack of elasticity.

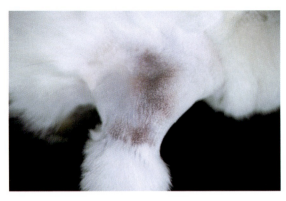

Figure 8.20 Bruising at the site of blood sampling in cat with hyperadrenocorticism.

- Diabetes mellitus
- Hyperthyroidism
- Cutaneous asthenia
- Pancreatic paraneoplastic alopecia
- Acquired skin fragility

Diagnosis

- History and clinical signs.
- Haematology and biochemistry rarely show any consistent findings other than hyperglycaemia. Other changes include elevations in cholesterol (~50%), serum alanine aminotransferase [ALT] (~40%) and alkaline phosphatase [ALP] (~20%).
- Urine sample often shows signs of glycosuria where concurrent diabetes mellitus is present. Urine cortisol: creatinine levels may be elevated but stress leads to false positives.
- Imaging techniques:
  - Radiography shows signs of hepatomegaly.
  - Ultrasonography, computer tomography and magnetic resonance imaging can be used to identify adrenal or pituitary masses.
- Skin biopsy reveals no specific changes other than a decrease in dermal collagen.
- Adrenal function tests – poorly described, always consult your laboratory for advice before performing these tests in the cat:
  - ACTH stimulation test. Many different protocols have been described:
    - Protocol – two separate cortisol peaks are seen in the cat after stimulation, therefore blood samples are taken to measure cortisol levels at time 0, then 1 and 2 hours after the intravenous administration of 125 µg synthacthen.
    - Most cats with naturally occurring hyperadrenocorticism show an exaggerated response to ACTH. Cats with iatrogenic disease fail to stimulate adequately.
  - Low dose dexamethasone suppression test:
    - Dexamethasone at a dose of 0.01–0.015 mg/kg intravenously will often not suppress cortisol in normal cats. Essentially, this screening test is a high dose suppression test.
    - Protocol – blood samples are taken to measure cortisol levels at time 0 and 8 hours after the intravenous administration of 0.1 mg/kg dexamethasone.
    - Cortisol levels in most cats with hyperadrenocorticism fail to suppress.
  - High dose dexamethasone suppression test:
    - Protocol as the low dose dexamethasone test except a dose of 1.0 mg/kg dexamethasone is used. Lack of cortisol suppression is suggestive of adrenal neoplasia.
  - Combined test:
    - Protocol – collect a baseline blood sample for serum cortisol. Administer a high dose of dexamethasone (0.1 mg/kg intravenously). Collect a post-dexamethasone sample for serum cortisol after 2 hours. At the same time administer 125 µg synthacthen intravenously. Collect a third sample for cortisol estimation a further 1 hour later.
    - Cortisol levels in cats with hyperadrenocorticism usually do not suppress after dexamethasone administration and overstimulate after synthacthen.
  - Endogenous ACTH measurement:

- This test is useful to differentiate between adrenal neoplasia and pituitary-dependent disease. An elevated level of ACTH suggests pituitary disease, a depressed level suggested adrenal disease.
- Test not widely available and difficult technically as sample needs to be taken into chilled blood tubes and transported immediately on ice to the laboratory.

Treatment

Naturally occurring disease:

Therapy of concurrent disease should be started at the same time as the treatment for the hyperadrenocorticism. However, control of these will be poor/incomplete until the hyperadrenocorticism is controlled.

- Medical therapy:
  - A poor response has been recorded to any medical therapy. Surgical management is preferable. However, if surgery is impossible then:
  - Metyrapone – blocks adrenal synthesis of steroids. It can be given at a dose of 65 mg/kg po bid. The response to treatment is monitored by a reduction in ACTH stimulation and improvement in clinical signs.
  - Other drugs such as ketoconazole (10–15 mg/kg po bid), trilostane (15–30 mg/cat po sid/bid) and mitotane have no recorded benefit in hyperadrenocorticism in the cat.
  - The use of other drugs such as bromocriptine, cyproheptadine and selegiline has not been documented in the cat.
- Surgical therapy:
  - Pituitary-dependent disease is best managed by bilateral adrenalectomy followed by life long therapy for hypoadrenocorticism. Alternative therapy for pituitary-dependent disease involves microsurgical trans-sphenoidal hypophysectomy. This can really only be undertaken by an experienced neurosurgeon with specialised aftercare facilities.
  - Adrenal-dependent disease caused by adrenal neoplasia is best treated by adrenalectomy (usually unilateral). This is usually curative.
- Radiotherapy has been used with partial success to treat some cats with pituitary-dependent disease. It has only a limited availability.
- Prognosis is fair to poor. Provided the hyperadrenocorticism is controlled, the diabetes should be manageable.

Pituitary dwarfism

Hereditary hypopituitarism leading to proportionate dwarfism.

Cause and pathogenesis

Usually cyst of Rathke's cleft leading to varying degrees of deficiency of anterior pituitary.

Clinical signs principally of growth hormone deficiency. However, the disease can lead to a deficiency of any one or more of the other anterior pituitary hormones, that is TSH, prolactin, ACTH, follicle-stimulating hormone and luteinising hormone. Very rare disease in cats and dogs, although more commonly seen in dogs especially German shepherd dogs as an autosomal recessive disease, although also described in the Weimaraner, Carnelian bear dog.

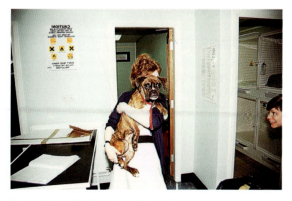

Figure 8.21 Pituitary dwarf Boxer dog.

Clinical signs

- Puppies and kittens are normal for the first 2–3 months, then fail to grow. They present as proportionate dwarfs (Figure 8.21). They have a reduced life expectancy of 3–8 years.
- Cutaneous signs:
    - Early signs – hair coat shorter, lack of primary hairs.
    - Puppy coat retains soft woolly, easily epilated hair, sparing of the extremities.
    - Within first year – bilaterally symmetrical alopecia with chronic hyperpigmentation.
    - Skin thin and scaly with comedones.
    - Often secondary pyoderma, Malassezia and seborrhoea.
- Non-cutaneous signs:
    - Mental dullness; dogs have a high pitched bark.
    - Signs associated with hypothyroidism, hypoadrenocorticism (although in German shepherd dogs ACTH secretion is not affected) and gonadal abnormalities may be present.
    - Muscular skeletal abnormalities as stunted growth, square chunky contour.
    - Reproduction – failure to cycle, testicular atrophy.

Differential diagnosis

- Congenital hypothyroidism
- Juvenile diabetes mellitus
- Congenital cardiovascular disease
- Congenital hepatic disease (portacaval shunts)

Diagnosis

- History and clinical signs, especially compared to litter mates.
- Laboratory tests to rule out thyroid and adrenocortical disease.
- Skin biopsy reveals non-specific endocrine changes especially decreased dermal elastin.
- Radiography mostly reveals skeletal abnormalities such as delayed closure of long bones, delayed eruption of permanent teeth.
- Advanced imaging techniques with MRI or CT scan may aid in detection of a pituitary cyst.
- Basal growth hormone levels not reliable as a diagnostic test.
- Dynamic function tests:
    - Clonidine/xylazine stimulation tests:
        - Injection of clonidine or xylazine leads to increases in growth hormone and glucose in a normal dog; no response is seen in pituitary dwarfs.
        - These are poorly documented in the cat, and are not widely available.
        - Consult your local laboratory for details.
    - Insulin-like growth factor – 1 (IGF-1):
        - A single basal sample can be used to assess pituitary function indirectly.
        - In dogs the IGF-1 level parallels body size; small dogs have lower levels than big dogs so detailed knowledge of laboratory normal values is essential to make a diagnosis.

Treatment

- Therapy of any secondary infection is important.
- Growth hormone replacement therapy with porcine or bovine growth hormone has produced increased hair growth but not skeletal changes. Therapy carries a risk of hypersensitivity and diabetes mellitus.
- Progestin therapy, which stimulates the mammary glands to produce growth hormone, has been used in some cases. Medroxyprogesterone acetate 2.5–5.0 mg/kg or proligesterone 10 mg/kg sq can be administered every 3–6 weeks. Risks include diabetes mellitus, acromegaly and in entire bitches reproductive abnormalities including pyometra.
- Thyroid, steroid replacement therapy, if appropriate.
- Castration or ovariohysterectomy are recommended.
- Prognosis is poor.

Growth hormone responsive dermatoses

See Chapter 12.

Acromegaly

Rare disease caused by overproduction of growth hormone in the mature dog and cat. In the cat, it usually presents as poorly controlled diabetes mellitus.

Cause and pathogenesis

Hypersecretion of growth hormone in the mature animal leads to overgrowth of connective tissue, bones and viscera Causes include the following:

- Progesterone-induced acromegaly through naturally occurring dioestrous in the bitch or exogenous administrations of progestagens – very common cause in the dog:
  - Unlike in the dog, progestagens do not stimulate excessive growth hormone secretion in the cat.
- Pituitary neoplasia – functional adenoma/adenocarcinoma of anterior pituitary gland – most common cause in the cat.
- Hypothalamic dysfunction – neoplasia – increased release of growth hormone releasing hormone.
- Ectopic growth hormone production – neoplastic lesions of lungs, ovaries, pancreas.

Clinical signs

- Dogs middle–old age; no breed or sex predilection.
- Cats male domestic short haired >10 years of age.
- Non-cutaneous signs:
  - Inspiratory stridor – due to excessive soft tissue in the oropharyngeal area (common dog, rare cat).
  - Increased size of extremities, paws and skull.
  - Organomegaly of heart liver, kidney and tongue (cat).
  - Polyuria, polydipsia, polyphagia, panting.
  - Prognathism, widening of interdental spaces.
  - Neurological signs may be present.
  - Renal and cardiac failure (common cat, rare dog).
  - Arthropathy common in the cat.
- Cutaneous signs:
  - Myxoedema, hypertrichosis
  - Hard claws

Differential diagnosis

- Hyperadrenocorticism
- Hypothyroidism
- Diabetes mellitus

Diagnosis

- History and clinical signs.
- Dog – haematology and biochemistry non-specific changes; hyperglycaemia and increase in SAP.
- Cat – more widespread changes including hyperglycaemia, hypercholesterolemia, mild increases in ALT and ALP (alkaline phosphatase). Associated renal failure may result in azotemia, isosthenuria, and proteinuria. A tentative diagnosis of acromegaly may be made in a cat with insulin-resistant diabetes (requiring >2 IU/kg insulin).
- Skin biopsy reveals an increase in collagen and mucin in dermis; myxoedema may be present.
- Diagnostic imaging with CT scan or MRI may help to identify a pituitary lesion.
- Basal growth hormone levels and insulin-like growth factor (IGF-1) are elevated.
- Dynamic function tests:
  - Plasma growth hormone levels remain unchanged in acromegalic dogs after intravenous glucose administration.

Treatment

- Progesterone-induced acromegaly therapy may be ovariohysterectomy or withdrawal of medication as appropriate.
- Pituitary/hypothalamic neoplasia:
  - Medical therapy with bromocriptine or octreotide unrewarding.
  - Neurosurgery – hypophysectomy.
  - Radiation treatment of pituitary.
- Prognosis dog is usually good as most cases are linked to excessive progestagen levels.
- Prognosis cat is guarded to poor with survival times of <4 years often <6 months. Most cats die from heart or renal failure.

Hyperoestrogenism in female dogs

Rare disease caused by excessive levels of oestrogen in female dogs.

Cause and pathogenesis

- Naturally occurring disease.
- Most commonly seen in intact females usually associated with ovarian cysts, less commonly with functional ovarian tumours (granulosa-theca cell in origin).
- In neutered females, it is caused by ectopic production of sex hormones. Iatrogenic.
- Administration of oestrogen for misalliance or as treatment for incontinence after spaying.

Clinical signs

- Cutaneous signs:
  - Bilaterally symmetrical alopecia initially affecting the perineum, inguinal and flank regions. In some cases, it is more generalised and can affect the whole of the trunk only sparing the head and limbs.
  - Alopecic skin is often hyperpigmented.
  - Remaining hair can be easily epilated.
  - Enlargement of nipples and vulva.
  - Comedones on ventrum and vulval skin.
  - Secondary pyoderma can be present.
- Non-cutaneous signs:
  - Oestrous cycle abnormalities, e.g. nymphomania
  - Endometritis or pyometra

Differential diagnosis

- Hypothyroidism
- Hyperadrenocorticism
- Hair cycle arrest alopecia
- Follicular dystrophies

Diagnosis

- History and clinical signs.
- Haematology and biochemistry are unremarkable except where oestrogen-induced bone marrow occurs, in which case non-regenerative anaemia, thrombocytopaenia and leukopaenia are seen. Haematology is obligatory in all cases to identify bone marrow suppression.
- Laboratory rule out of other endocrine diseases.
- Skin biopsy reveals signs of non-specific endocrine changes.
- Elevated blood oestrogen levels may be measured in some dogs; however, false-positive and false-negative results are common.
- Exploratory laparotomy to investigate ovaries and ovariohysterectomy together with an appropriate response to therapy.

Treatment

- Therapy for any concurrent infections together with supportive care if oestrogen-induced myelosuppression is present, i.e. fluid therapy and whole blood transfusion.
- In intact bitches, ovariohysterectomy is the therapy of choice. Radiographs of thorax are useful prior to surgery to check that there is no evidence of metastases in the case of neoplasia.
- Prognosis is good in that most dogs show an improvement in cutaneous disease in 3–6 months.

Oestrogen responsive alopecia

See Chapter 12.

Testosterone responsive alopecia

See Chapter 12.

Testicular neoplasia

Testicular neoplasia only leads to skin changes when tumours are functional and are producing hormones that can affect the skin. Clinical signs are associated with excessive production of sex hormones. Cryptorchid testes are 10 times more likely to become neoplastic than normal ones. The principal tumours that can affect the testicles are as follows:

- Sertoli cell tumours
- Interstitial cell tumours
- Seminomas

All three tumours occur with approximately equal incidence.

Sertoli cell tumour

Cause and pathogenesis

About a third of all Sertoli cell tumours are functional; most of these are found in cryptorchid testicles. Cutaneous and systemic signs are attributable to hyperoestrogenism. A hereditary syndrome of Sertoli cell tumour and feminisation has been recognised in miniature schnauzers.

Clinical signs

- Signs are seen most commonly in middle-aged–old dogs.
- Predisposed breeds include the Boxer, Shetland sheepdog (Figure 8.22), Weimaraner, Cairn terrier, Pekinese.
- Non-cutaneous signs:

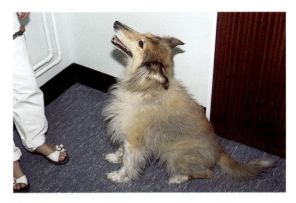

Figure 8.22 Generalised alopecia in rough collie with a Sertoli cell tumour.

- □ Palpable testicular tumour usually obvious in one testicle with concurrent atrophy of the other testicle.
- □ Feminisation – gynaecomastia, pendulous prepuce (Figure 8.23), attraction of other male dogs, galactorrhoea.
- □ Enlarged prostate and associated signs, e.g. faecal/urinary tenesmus.
- □ Oestrogen-induced bone marrow suppression.
- Cutaneous signs:
  - □ Alopecia starts on collar, rump and perineum (Figure 8.24) and progresses slowly; head and limbs are generally spared.
  - □ Hair coat is poor and hair can be easily epilated.

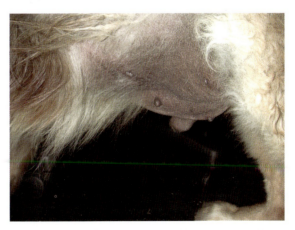

Figure 8.23 Sertoli cell tumour in a dog showing pendulous prepuce.

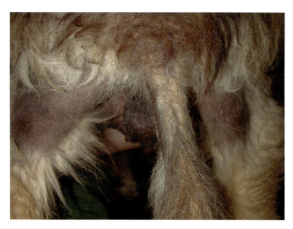

Figure 8.24 Sertoli cell tumour in a dog showing perineal hair loss.

- ☐ Linear erythematous preputial dermatosis common (Figure 8.25).
- ☐ Pruritus often associated with generalised seborrhoea.
- ☐ Secondary pyoderma and *Malassezia* infections are common.

Differential diagnosis

- Hypothyroidism
- Hyperadrenocorticism
- Hair follicle cycle arrest

Diagnosis

- History and clinical signs.
- Laboratory rule out for other diseases.

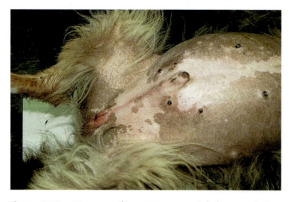

Figure 8.25 Linear erythematous preputial dermatosis in a dog with a Sertoli cell tumour.

- Haematology and biochemistry are unremarkable except where oestrogen-induced bone marrow occurs, in which case non-regenerative anaemia, thrombocytopaenia and leukopaenia are seen. Haematology is obligatory in all cases to identify bone marrow suppression.
- Sex hormones assays may be useful in some cases to assess oestrogen levels. However, false-negative results are common.
- Ultrasonography of testicles to identify a tumour is rarely needed as most are palpable. However, if clinical signs are present with obvious mass, ultrasound may be useful.
- Skin biopsy reveals signs of a non-specific endocrine pattern.
- Response to castration together with histopathology of neoplastic testicle after castration is important to confirm a retrospective diagnosis.

Treatment

- Bilateral castration is the treatment of choice in all cases.
- Assessment prior to surgery for therapy for any concurrent infections especially skin and prostate together with supportive care if oestrogen-induced myelosuppression is present, i.e. fluid therapy and whole blood transfusion.
- Prognosis is good in that most dogs show an improvement in cutaneous disease in 3–6 months.

Seminoma

Cause and pathogenesis

Seminomas are found in about 30% of all cases of testicular neoplasia. They are rarely functional so that most produce no dermatological signs.

Clinical signs

- Predisposed breeds include the Boxer, German shepherd dog.
- Oestrogen producing tumours have clinical signs that mimic Sertoli cell tumour.

- They are only locally invasive with a low rate of metastases.

Differential diagnosis

As Sertoli cell tumour.

Diagnosis

As Sertoli cell tumour.

Treatment

As Sertoli cell tumour.

Interstitial cell tumour

Cause and pathogenesis

Interstitial cell tumours are found in about 30% of all cases but are uncommonly functional, most produce no dermatological signs. Can be multiple tumours seen in some testicles. Malignancy and metastases are rare. Clinical signs when they occur are of hyperandrogenism.

Clinical signs

- No recognised breed predisposition.
- Non-cutaneous signs:
  - Prostatic disease including signs of faecal and urinary tenesmus
  - Perianal adenoma
  - Perineal hernia
  - Hypersexual behaviour including aggression towards other dogs
- Cutaneous signs:
  - Tail and perianal gland hyperplasia (Figure 8.26)
  - Macular melanosis
  - Greasy seborrhoea often with secondary pyoderma and Malassezia infection
  - Symmetrical trunk hair loss sparing of the extremities (Figure 8.27)

Differential diagnosis

As Sertoli cell tumour.

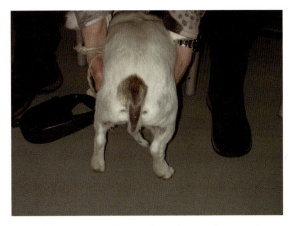

Figure 8.26 Tail gland hyperplasia due to a functional interstitial cell tumour.

Diagnosis

As Sertoli cell tumour, except that testosterone levels should be checked. These are inconsistently elevated and false negatives can occur.

Treatment

- Bilateral castration should be performed and testicles should be submitted for histopathology.
- Behavioural modification often needed for the first few months after surgery.
- Treatment of skin infection is important prior to surgery. Shampoo therapy may be useful post-operatively with sulphur, salicylic acid

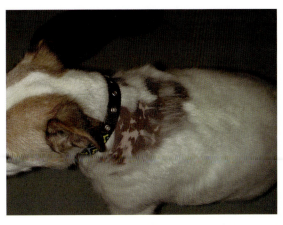

Figure 8.27 Alopecia on neck due to a functional interstitial cell tumour.

or tar shampoos to control the greasy seborrhoea whilst the skin and coat recover.
- Prognosis is good in that most dogs show an improvement in cutaneous disease in 3–6 months.

Castration responsive dermatoses

See Chapter 12.

Adrenal sex hormone imbalance

See Chapter 12.

Diabetes mellitus

Cause and pathogenesis

Diabetic dogs and cats have abnormal cell mediated immunity leaving them susceptible to infection and ectoparasite problems.

Clinical signs

- Recurrent bacterial pyoderma is common with *Staphylococcus* spp.
- Yeast infection can be seen with both *Malassezia* spp. and *Candida* spp.
- Diabetes mellitus can be an underlying cause for adult onset demodicosis in both dogs and cats.
- Generalised seborrhoea is common.
- Thin hypotonic skin often with alopecia (Figure 8.28).

Differential diagnosis

- Other causes of skin disease with polyuria and polydipsia especially
  - Hyperadrenocorticism – cat and dog
  - Hyperthyroidism – cat
  - Renal disease
- These diseases can occur concurrently with diabetes mellitus.

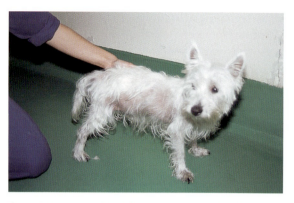

Figure 8.28 Generalised alopecia in a dog with diabetes mellitus.

Diagnosis

- History and clinical signs.
- Rule out of other differential with routine bloods and dynamic function tests where appropriate.
- Diabetic animals have hyperglycaemia and glucosuria.

Treatment

- Therapy of the diabetes is crucial to the management of the skin:
  - A full discussion of the management of diabetes mellitus is beyond the scope of this book; the reader is referred to more specialised endocrine texts for guidance. Dietary manipulation and insulin therapy are necessary in most cases.
- Symptomatic therapy of skin disease should be undertaken to control concurrent infections and ectoparasites.

Necrolytic migratory erythema (NME; hepatocutaneous disease)

Cause and pathogenesis

A very rare skin disease that is a cutaneous manifestation of an internal problem. This may be

Endocrine and metabolic skin disease 159

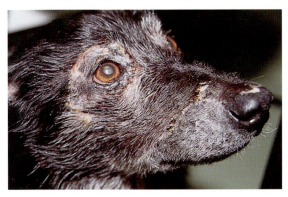

Figure 8.29 Ulceration and crusting on the face of a dog with NME.

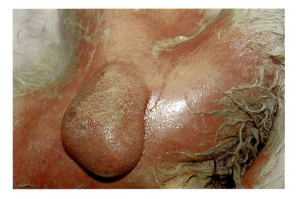

Figure 8.31 Severe ulceration of the external genitalia in a young dog with NME secondary to a pancreatic carcinoma.

chronic liver disease or else a glucagon secreting pancreatic tumour. It is thought that an increase in gluconeogenesis triggered by the hyperglucagonaemia or increased hepatic catabolism of amino acids produces low plasma amino acid concentration and epidermal depletion of protein leading to cutaneous lesions. It is an uncommon disease in the dog and a rare disease in the cat.

Clinical signs

- No sex predilection.
- Affects old animals. Predisposed breeds include Shetland sheepdog, West Highland white terrier, cocker spaniel and Scottish terrier.
- Cutaneous lesions:
  - Lesions are erythematous with scaling, crusting, erosions and ulcers.
  - Areas of trauma on hocks, elbows, ventrum, mucocutaneous junctions of face (Figures 8.29 and 8.30), distal limbs and external genitalia (Figure 8.31).
  - Footpads are usually hyperkeratotic and may be ulcerated and fissured (Figure 8.32).
  - Variable degrees of pruritus.
- Non-cutaneous signs:
  - Debilitating systemic disease leading to lethargy, inappetence and weight loss.
  - Polyuria and polydipsia may be present and should stimulate checks for diabetes if recognised.

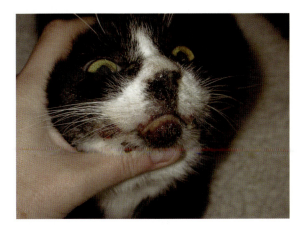

Figure 8.30 Ulceration of the face of cat with NME.

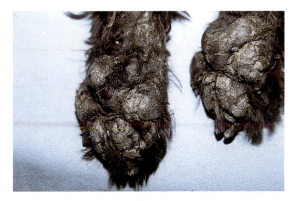

Figure 8.32 Footpad hyperkeratosis in a dog with NME.

Differential diagnosis

- Demodicosis
- Dermatophytosis
- Systemic lupus erythematosus
- Zinc deficiency
- Generic dog food dermatosis
- Pemphigus foliaceus
- Epitheliotropic lymphoma

Diagnosis

- History and clinical signs.
- Haematology reveals a normocytic, normochromic, non-regenerative anaemia.
- Biochemistry reveals a hyperglycaemia with increases in serum ALP and ALT, total bilirubin and bile acids. Hypoalbuminaemia and decreased blood urea nitrogen are commonly present. Plasma amino acids are reduced.
- Serum glucagon concentration is elevated if a glucagonoma is present.
- Ultrasound of liver where chronic liver disease is present typically presents with a 'honeycombed' pattern. Where pancreatic pathology is present, this too should be visible on ultrasound scans.
- Liver biopsy in cases of chronic liver disease reveals a vacuolar hepatopathy with parenchymal collapse, occasionally liver cirrhosis.
- Skin biopsy of early lesions reveals a very typical red, white and blue appearance. Blue is of the parakeratosis/hyperkeratosis of the stratum corneum. White is of the oedema of upper half of epidermis. Keratinocyte degeneration with hyperplastic basal cells gives the low red band to complete the colour triad.

Treatment

- Poor prognosis as most cases die or euthanised.
- Surgical intervention possible in some cases to remove the neoplastic tissue.
- Medical treatment:
  Topical therapy:
  - Symptomatic shampoos with gentle moisturising and soothing products.

  Systemic therapy:
  - Treatment of any secondary bacterial and yeast infection, based, where possible, on culture and sensitivity.
  - Symptomatic therapy of liver disease where it is identified together with correction of any underlying liver pathology where possible. Suitable drugs include the following:
    - Vitamin E 400 IU po bid
    - Ursodil 10 mg/kg po sid
    - S-adenosylmethionine (s-AME) denosyl 18–22 mg/kg po sid
  - Treatment of liver cirrhosis where identified on biopsy can be undertaken with colchicine 0.03 mg/kg po sid. This drug can cause gastrointestinal signs if used for long periods.
  - Amino acid supplementation can prolong survival time. Suitable products include the following:
    - 10% crystalline amino acid solution 25 ml/kg iv over 6–8 hours.
    - 3% amino acid and electrolyte solution 25 ml/kg iv over 6–8 hours.
    - Treatment may need to be repeated after 7–10 days; improvement is usually seen within 1–3 weeks.
  - Alternative amino acid supplements can be made by feeding 3–6 raw eggs daily together with zinc and amino acid therapy.
  - Anti-inflammatory doses of prednisolone at 1 mg/kg po sid may give some temporary relief but due to the underlying liver or pancreatic pathology, side effects such as diabetes or a deterioration of the animal's condition are possible.
- Prognosis is poor in all cases due to the severity of the underlying disease. Death is rarely from skin lesions or complications thereof.

Xanthoma

Cause and pathogenesis

Granulomatous lesions associated with abnormalities in lipid metabolism including the following:

- Hereditary hyperlipoproteinaemia
- Diabetes mellitus (naturally occurring and drug induced)
- Idiopathic disease

Clinical signs

- Cutaneous signs:
  - Lesions typically affect head, extremities and bony prominences.
  - Multiple white or yellow papules, nodules or plaques.
  - Surrounding skin appears erythematous.
  - Often painful and pruritic.
- Non-cutaneous signs:
  - Associated with concurrent diabetes or hyperlipoproteinaemia.

Differential diagnosis

- Eosinophilic granuloma complex
- Cutaneous neoplasia (lymphoma, mast cell tumour)
- Cutaneous horn
- Callus
- Calcinosis cutis

Diagnosis

- History and clinical signs.
- Skin biopsy reveals signs of multinucleate giant cells with foamy macrophages.
- Investigation of underlying fault in lipid metabolism, including biochemistry and glucose levels.

Treatment

- Medical treatment:
  - Therapy of underlying problem will result in spontaneous resolution of lesions, i.e. stabilisation of diabetes mellitus, high fibre/low fat diet in idiopathic cases.
- Surgical treatment:
  - Unsuccessful; only results in recurrence of lesions.

Selected references and further reading

Byrne, K.P. (1999) Metabolic epidermal necrosis-hepatocutaneous syndrome. *Vet Clin North Am Small Anim Pract*, 29, 1337–1355

Feldman, E.C. and Nelson, R.W. (1996) Hyperadrenocorticism (Cushing's syndrome). In: *Canine and Feline Endocrinology and Reproduction*. 2nd edn. pp. 187–265. WB Saunders, Philadelphia

Frank, L.A. (2004) Sex hormone dermatoses. In: Campbell, K.L. (ed) *Small Animal Dermatology Secrets*. pp. 280–288. Hanley and Belfus, Philadelphia

Medleau, L. and Hnilica, K. (2006) Alopecia. In: *Small Animal Dermatology: A Color Atlas and Therapeutic Guide*. 2nd edn. pp. 229–273. WB Saunders, Philadelphia

Paradis, M. (2004) Thyroid dysfunction. In: Campbell, K.L. (ed) *Small Animal Dermatology Secrets*. pp. 260–268. Hanley and Belfus, Philadelphia

Rosychuk, R.A. (1998) Cutaneous manifestations of endocrine disease in dogs. *Compend Small Anim*, 20, 287–302

Scott, D.W. et al. (2001) Endocrine and metabolic diseases. In: *Muller and Kirk's Small Animal Dermatology*. 6th edn. pp. 780–885. WB Saunders, Philadelphia

Schulman, R.L. (2004) Adrenal dysfunction. In: Campbell, K.L. (ed). *Small Animal Dermatology Secrets*. pp. 269–279. Hanley and Belfus, Philadelphia

Otitis externa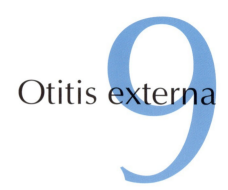

Otitis externa is defined as inflammation of the ear canal (Figure 9.1) and is a common disease in the dog but less common in the cat. To treat otitis successfully every effort should be made to identify the primary, predisposing and perpetuating factors for each case.

In many cases the primary trigger is low grade, meaning that when the perpetuating factor is tackled, e.g. bacterial infection, no recurrence is seen.

Where the condition constantly relapses, the primary trigger must be identified and treated.

Primary causes

Primary causes are present in every case of otitis externa. In uncomplicated disease where it is occurring on the first occasion they may not need to be investigated and treated (see Table 9.1), but where disease is recurrent or where a dog or cat presents with chronic disease, it is essential to investigate.

Predisposing factors

These factors by themselves will not cause otitis externa but will tend to make both dogs and cats more susceptible to disease. The main categories and diseases within each group are listed in Table 9.2.

Perpetuating factors

These factors are the pathogenic organisms that occur or pathological changes that progress when a potent primary trigger is not addressed and the ear is treated symptomatically; for example, *Pseudomonas* otitis externa is not a disease but a perpetuating microbe secondary to another disease. These categories are listed in Table 9.3.

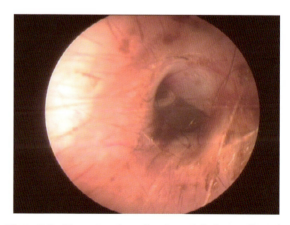

Figure 9.1 Normal eardrum showing soft fleshy pars flaccida and the opaque pars tensa below. The malleus can be seen behind the tensa.

Otitis externa

	Diseases within the category
Hypersensitivity	Atopy (Figure 9.2), food intolerance (Figure 9.3), contact hypersensitivity
Parasites	*Otodectes cynotis, Demodex* spp. (Figure 9.4) *Sarcoptes scabiei* (Figure 9.5), *Notoedres cati*, pediculosis, *Eutrombicula*, fleas (*Spilopsylla cuniculi*)
Fungal	Dermatophytes, *Sporothrix schenckii*
Endocrine disease	Hypothyroidism (dog) (Figure 9.6), hyperthyroidism (cat), hyperadrenocorticism
Immunological disease	Lupus erythematosus, pemphigus foliaceus (Figure 9.7), pemphigus erythematosus, erythema multiforme (Figure 9.8), cold agglutinin disease, vasculitis, bullous pemphigoid (Figure 9.9), drug eruption (Figure 9.10)
Foreign bodies	Plant material, hair, soil, sand, ear medication
Keratinisation disorders	Vitamin A responsive dermatoses, primary seborrhoea (Figure 9.11), sebaceous adenitis
Miscellaneous	Juvenile cellulitis (Figure 9.12), glandular disorders (idiopathic hyperplasia of glands), abnormalities of cerumen production (Figure 9.13)

Table 9.2 Predisposing factors in otitis externa.

Category	Diseases within the category
Anatomical configuration	Stenotic ear canals, e.g. shar-pei (Figure 9.14), hairy canals, e.g. poodles (Figure 9.15), pendulous pinnae, e.g. basset, hairy concave pinna, e.g. spaniel
Excessive moisture	'Swimmer's ear' especially gun dogs, water-based cleaners, water-based antibiotics
Treatment effects	Iatrogenic trauma, over zealous ear cleaning Irritant ear preparations, e.g. strong acids, Superinfection created by treatment effects on normal flora of ear, e.g. chronic antibiotic therapy
Obstructive ear disease – this category could be included in primary triggers; however, many animals tolerate growths in the ears until they obstruct	Polyps – derived from middle ear especially in cats and external ear canal both dogs and cats (Figures 9.16 and 9.17); neoplasia of external ear canal
Systemic disease	Any disease leading to immunosuppression especially in cats FIV, FeLV, FIP

Table 9.3 Perpetuating factors in otitis externa.

Category	Diseases within the category
Bacteria	Gram positive, e.g. *Staphylococcus* spp. (Figure 9.18), *Streptococcus* spp. Gram negative, e.g. *Proteus* spp., *Pseudomonas* spp. (Figure 9.19)
Yeast	*Malassezia* spp. (Figure 9.20) *Candida albicans*
Progressive pathological change – progressive changes will eventually become non-reversible	Hyperplasia, oedema, fibrosis (Figure 9.21), severe ceruminous gland hyperplasia, mineralisation of ear canals, failure of epithelial migration and formation of ceruminoliths (Figure 9.22)
Otitis media	Infection, excessive granulation tissue in tympanic bulla

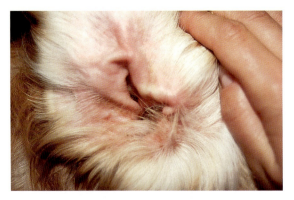

Figure 9.2 Otitis externa in a dog with atopy showing typical erythematous changes on medial aspect of ear pinnae.

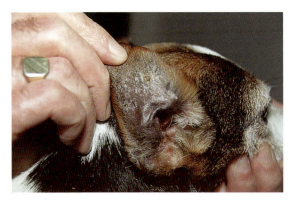

Figure 9.3 Chronic lichenification and hyperpigmentation in a dog with food allergy.

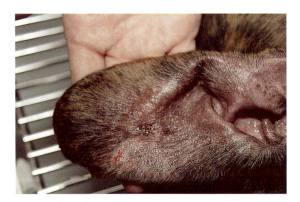

Figure 9.4 Boxer dog with demodicosis showing comedone formation on ear pinna.

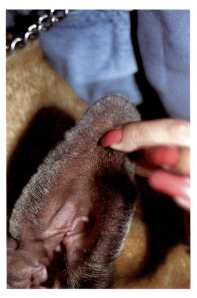

Figure 9.5 Scabies affecting the ear showing erythema of ear pinna and crusting and scaling around the periphery of the ear.

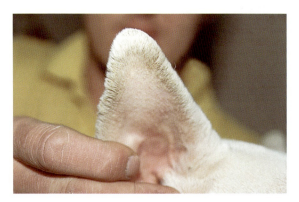

Figure 9.6 Hypothyroidism showing marked crusting around periphery of ear tip.

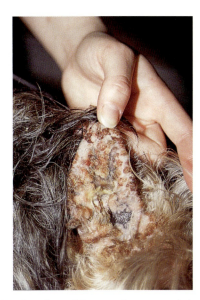

Figure 9.7 Pemphigus foliaceus affecting a Yorkshire terrier's ear showing primary pustules and papules.

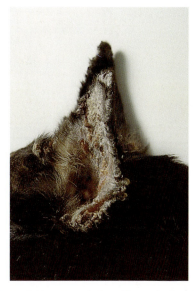

Figure 9.10 Otitis externa induced by topical medication.

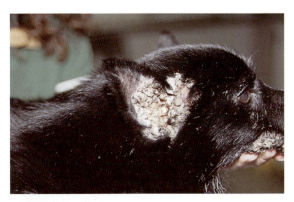

Figure 9.8 Erythema multiforme affecting the external ear canal.

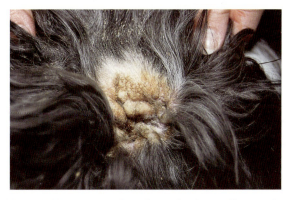

Figure 9.11 Primary idiopathic seborrhoea affecting the external ear canal of a cocker spaniel.

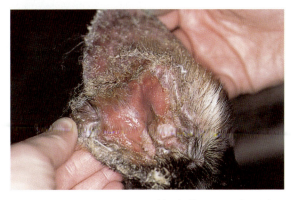

Figure 9.9 Otitis externa caused by bullous pemphigoid.

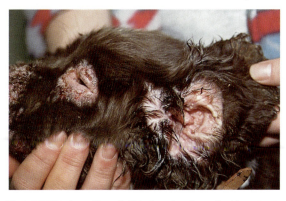

Figure 9.12 Juvenile cellulitis showing signs of otitis externa.

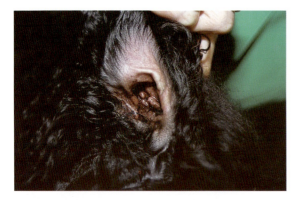

Figure 9.13 Ceruminous otitis externa.

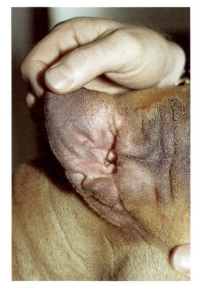

Figure 9.14 Stenotic ear canal in a shar-pei.

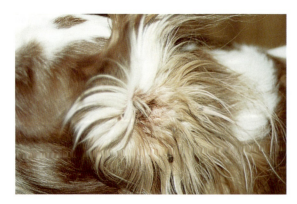

Figure 9.15 Hairy ears in a cavalier King Charles spaniel.

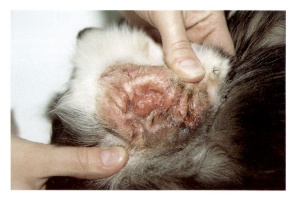

Figure 9.16 Polyp in external ear canal of Old English sheepdog.

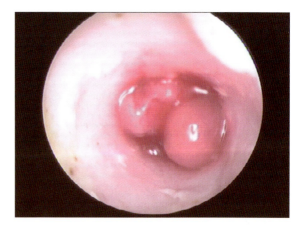

Figure 9.17 Oropharyngeal polyp in cat's ear.

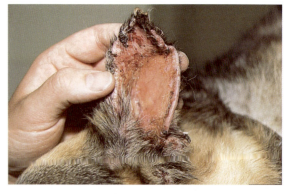

Figure 9.18 Staphylococcal infection superimposed on allergy.

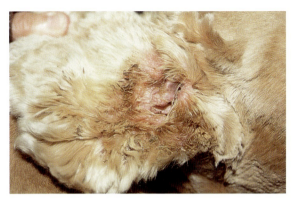

Figure 9.19 Pseudomonas otitis secondary to hypothyroidism.

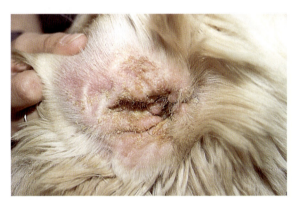

Figure 9.20 Malassezia otitis secondary to allergy.

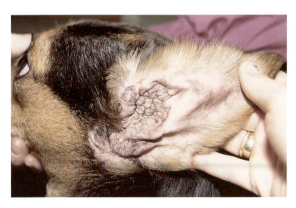

Figure 9.21 Chronic irreversible change in a dog with long-standing atopic dermatitis.

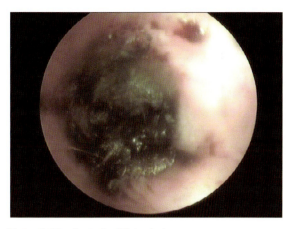

Figure 9.22 Ceruminolith in dog's ear.

Approach to otitis externa

- History, physical and dermatological examination will usually give clues as to the primary trigger for otitis externa, e.g. pruritus on other areas of body with hypersensitivity.
- Aural examination to check the ear pinnae, vertical, horizontal canal plus skin around external auditory meatus.
- Otoscopic examination – under sedation or general anaesthetic if necessary.
- Assessment of vertical and horizontal canals important plus integrity of tympanic membrane and the middle ear if the eardrum is ruptured (Figure 9.23).

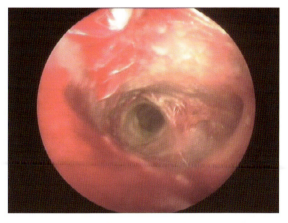

Figure 9.23 Ruptured tympanic membrane in a dog's ear; compare with Figure 9.1.

Table 9.4 Basic diagnostic tests in otitis externa.

Diagnostic test	Clinical findings
Cotton wool swab of discharge	
(a) Visual inspection	Moist brown exudate – *Staphylococcus, Malassezia* Purulent yellow/green exudate – Gram negative especially *Pseudomonas* Ceruminous brown black discharge – endocrine, keratinisation defects, anaerobic infection Dry coffee grounds – *Otodectes cynotis*
(b) Direct examination of earwax	Parasites – *O. cynotis, Demodex* spp.
(c) Examination of stained earwax (Diff-Quik or Gram stain)	Inflammatory cells – neutrophils degenerate in infectious disease, non-degenerate immune mediated disease Bacteria • Cocci –*Staphylococcus* spp ., *Streptococcus* spp. • Rods –*Proteus* spp.,*Pseudomonas* spp. Yeast • *Malassezia* spp.*Candida* spp. (rare)
Culture and sensitivity	Where cocci present and not responded to appropriate empirical therapy Where rods are present Where mixed infection is present
Skin scrape of pinna into potassium hydroxide or liquid paraffin	Parasites – *Demodex* spp. *Sarcoptes scabiei, Notoedres cati*, lice
Tape strip of pinna stained with Diff-Quik	Cellular infiltrate Neoplastic cells, e.g. lymphoma, Parakeratotic keratinocytes in keratinisation disorder, Infectious organisms – cocci, rods, yeasts as above
Biopsy of pinna or vertical ear canal	Elliptical biopsy taken with scalpel (not punch biopsy) to identify pemphigus, erythema multiforme, vasculitis, neoplasia

- Advanced diagnostic techniques – brain stem auditory evoked responses (BAER) assessment, MRI, radiography.

Diagnostic tests

See Chapter 3 on diagnostic tests for a more detailed description of specific tests.

As an absolute minimum database all cases should have cytology performed on ear discharge. This allows an informed decision to be made regarding the selection of cleaning fluids and antibiotic therapy. Culture of discharge is only really necessary when animals have failed to respond to rational therapy for Gram positive infection or where a mixed infection or Gram negative infection has been identified on cytology.

Basic diagnostic tests and possible clinical findings are described in Table 9.4.

More advanced diagnostic tests are often only possible in referral centres with the use of video-otoscopic imaging:

- Myringotomy may be necessary if an eardrum is intact but there is a suggestion that the eardrum is abnormal (Figure 9.24) or discharge (Figure 9.25) can be visualised behind the eardrum. This is best achieved by video-otoscopic visualisation with either a fine urinary catheter or by CO_2 laser. Fluid can be aspirated from the middle ear for cytology and culture. If the area appears 'dry' 2 ml of sterile

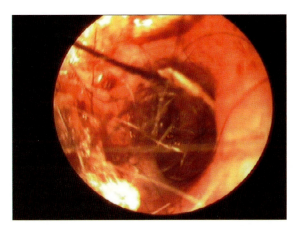

Figure 9.24 Abnormal eardrum; compare with Figure 9.1.

saline can be instilled through the myringotomy incision and then aspirated back for analysis.
- Pinch biopsy of the horizontal canal or of masses within the canal or middle ear can also be performed by video-otoscopic guidance with grasping tools.

Treatment

- Topical treatment:
  - Ear cleaners:
    - Indications: – Ear cleaners are essential in all cases of otitis. In many cases epithelial migration has been altered

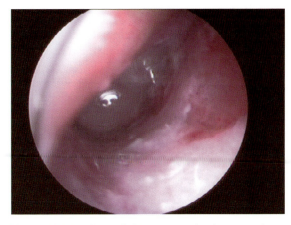

Figure 9.25 Eardrum is bulging outwards. There is evidence of fluid behind it.

so that wax will accumulate inside the canal of dogs leading to repeat infection and ceruminolith formation. Table 9.5 gives details of ear cleaning agents and their mode of action.
- Topical antibacterial products:
  - Indications: Antibiotics and antibacterial flushes should be based initially on cytology. Where Gram positive infection (cocci on cytology) is present, drugs can usually be prescribed empirically without cultures being necessary (Table 9.6). Where Gram negative infection (rods on cytology) is present, empirical therapy can be used based on drugs from Table 9.7 pending culture results.
- Topical glucocorticoids:
  - Indications: Topical glucocorticoids can be used to produce a variety of benefits in the ear (see Table 9.8). Hydrocortisone and prednisolone have minimal cutaneous absorption. More potent steroids such as dexamethasone and betamethasone have greater degrees of systemic absorption. Initial therapy may be undertaken with a potent steroid but topical drugs should be switched to the least potent topical drug as possible to avoid pituitary adrenal axis suppression. They should not be used on a daily basis over long periods.
- Topical anti-yeasts:
  - Indications: Anti-yeast drugs and flushes can be used on an empirical basis after cytology. Yeast infection can occur concurrently with both Gram positive and Gram negative infections. Suitable drugs are detailed in Table 9.9. In uncomplicated cases where only yeast is identified on cytology it is unusual to see the eardrum is damaged.
- Topical anti-parasitic agents:
  - Indications: Topical anti-parasitic drugs need to have activity against *Otodectes cynotis* and *Demodex* spp. Suitable drugs are listed in Table 9.10.

Table 9.5 Ear cleaners and their mode of action.

Agent	Agents with an unknown ototoxicity	Agents with recognised ototoxicity when the eardrum is ruptured	Agents with no recognised ototoxicity when the eardrum is ruptured[1]
Ceruminolytic agents		Dioctyl sodium/calcium sulphosuccinate Carbamate peroxide	
Lubricants	Glycerine	Triethanolamine polypeptide oleate condensate Propylene glycol	Squalene
Flushing agents		Povidone iodine >0.05% chlorhexidine	Water Sterile saline 0.05% chlorhexidine 2.5% acetic acid EDTA-tris
Drying agents	Lactic acid Malic acid Benzoic acid Salicylic acid Aluminium silicate/acetate	Isopropyl alcohol	2.5% acetic acid Boric acid

[1] No drug can ever be completely safe in the middle ear. No medication is licensed for use in the middle ear. Current recommendations are based on expert opinion and current veterinary literature.

Table 9.6 Useful topical drugs in Gram positive infections.

Topical drugs that should only be considered if the eardrum is intact	Topical drugs that may be considered if the eardrum is ruptured [1,2]
Ciprofloxacin Enrofloxacin Framycetin Fusidic acid Gentamicin Neomycin Polymyxin B Tobramycin	Ciprofloxacin Enrofloxacin Marbofloxacin

[1] See note above with Table 9.5.
[2] Injectable formulations of these antibiotics are preferable. Where possible licensed drugs should be used.

Table 9.7 Useful topical drugs in Gram negative infections.

Topical drugs that may only be used if the eardrum is intact	Topical drugs that may be used if the eardrum is ruptured[1,2]
Amikacin sulphate Ciprofloxacin Colistin Framycetin Gentamicin Neomycin Ofloxacin Silver sulphadiazine Polymyxin B sulphate Ticarcillin Tobramycin	Enrofloxacin 2.5% acetic acid EDTA-tris Marbofloxacin

[1] See note above with Table 9.5.
[2] Injectable formulations of these antibiotics are preferable. Where possible licensed drugs should be used.

Table 9.8 Uses of glucocorticoids in otitis externa.

Acute otitis	Chronic otitis
Reduction of erythema	As acute otitis
Reduction of oedema	Reduction of hyperplasia
Decreased inflammatory cell infiltrate	Reduction of ceruminous gland hyperplasia
Reduction in pain due to reduce nerve entrapment	Widening of lumen

- Systemic therapy:
  - Indications:
    - Antibiotics are rarely indicated in either otitis externa or media and it remains controversial whether adequate levels enter the aural tissue to produce benefit (for dose rate of systemic therapy, see Chapter 4).
    - Anti-yeast therapy appears to be more successful than that for bacterial infection (for suitable drugs and dose rates for yeast infection, see Chapter 5).

Table 9.9 Topical anti-yeast drugs for treatment of otitis externa.

Topical drugs that should only be considered if the eardrum is intact	Topical drugs that may be used if the eardrum is ruptured[1,2]
Ketoconazole Miconazole Nystatin Monosulfiram Thiabendazole Zinc undecylenate	Boric acid Clotrimazole

[1,2] See notes with Tables 9.5 and 9.6.

- Glucocorticoids may be used in acute allergy in the form of prednisolone at a dose of 1 mg/kg once daily by mouth for 2 weeks then tapering down to lowest possible alternate day dosage. In immune mediated disease, prednisolone is used at a dose of 2 mg/kg once daily for 2 weeks before

Table 9.10 Topical anti-parasitic drugs for use in otitis externa.

Topical drugs should only be used when the eardrum is intact[1]	Drugs with anti-demodex activity	Drugs with anti-otodectes activity	Systemic drugs with anti-mite activity available in spot on formulation or po (see Chapter 7)	Drugs with activity against demodex	Drugs with activity against otodectes
Amitraz[2]	✓[5]	✓[5]	Ivermectin	✓	✓
Fipronil[3]		✓[5,6]	Milbemycin	✓	✓
Ivermectin[4]	✓[5,6]	✓[5,6]	Moxidectin	✓	✓
Monosulfiram		✓[5,6]	Selamectin		✓
Pyrethrins		✓[5,6]			
Rotenone	✓[5]				
Thiabendazole	✓[6]	✓[5,6]			

[1] Where any of the listed drugs are not found in licensed otic products, their usage corresponds to an extra label usage.
[2] Amitraz may be diluted with 2 ml of 5% solution added to 20 ml of mineral oil and used topically. It is also available as a licensed spot on preparation.
[3] Fipronil spot on preparations have been used topically in ear canals.
[4] Ivermectin may be used diluted 1:9 with mineral oil and used topically.
[5] Applies to use in the dog.
[6] Applies to use in the cat.

switching to alternate day medication and then tapering to the lowest possible maintenance dose.
- Surgery:
  - Surgery should only be undertaken where irreversible pathological changes have occurred and the ear is no longer responsive to medical management.
  - This should not replace a thorough diagnostic work-up.

Selected references and further reading

Angus, J.C. (2004) Diseases of the ear. In: Campbell, K.L. (ed) *Small Animal Dermatology Secrets*. pp. 364–384. Hanley and Belfus, Philadelphia

Bensignor, E. (2003) An approach to otitis externa and media. In: Foster, A.P. and Foil, C.S. (eds) *BSAVA Manual of Small Animal Dermatology*. 2nd edn. pp. 104–112. BSAVA, Gloucester

Gotthelf, L. (ed) (2005) Diagnosis and treatment of otitis externa. In: *Small Animal Ear Disease*. 2nd edn. pp. 275–304. WB Saunders, Philadelphia

Harvey, R. et al. (2001) *Ear Disease of the Dog and Cat*. Iowa University State Press, Ames

Logas, D. (2000) Appropriate use of glucocorticoids in otitis externa. In: *Kirk's Current Veterinary Therapy XIII. Small Animal Practice*. pp. 585–586. WB Saunders, Philadelphia

Medleau, L. and Hnilica, K. (2006) Otitis externa. In: *Small Animal Dermatology: A Color Atlas and Therapeutic Guide*. 2nd edn. pp. 376–390. WB Saunders, Philadelphia

Morris, D.O. (2004) Medical therapy of otitis externa and otitis media. In: Matousek, J.L. (ed) *Veterinary Clinics of North America, Small Animal Practice, Ear Disease*. Vol. 34. pp. 541–556. WB Saunders, Philadelphia

Scott, D.W. et al. (2001) Otitis externa. *Muller and Kirk's Small Animal Dermatology*. 6th edn. pp. 1204–1232. WB Saunders, Philadelphia

White, P.D. (1999) Medical management of chronic otitis in the dog. *Compend Contin Educ*, **21**(8), 716–728

10 Allergic skin disease

Urticaria and angioedema

Cause and pathogenesis

- Immunological or non-immunological degranulation of mast cells of basophils.
- Immunological trigger type I, III hypersensitivity reaction.
- Non-immunological:
  - physical forces (pressure, sunlight, heat, exercise)
  - genetic abnormalities
  - drugs and chemicals including foods and food additives
  - venomous insects
  - plants

Uncommon disease in dogs and rare in cats.

Clinical signs

Urticaria:

- Localised or generalised weals (Figure 10.1).
- Pruritus and exudation variable.
- Hair tufts over areas of swelling.
- Generally benign, self-limiting disease but can occur in waves as old lesions resolve and new lesions appear.

Angioedema:

- Localised or generalised area of large oedematous swelling; usually involves the head (Figure 10.2).
- Pruritus and exudation variable.
- May be fatal if oedema involves pharynx, larynx or nasal mucosa leading to dyspnoea.
- Anaphylactic shock is rare.

Differential diagnosis

Urticaria:

- Folliculitis especially with hair tufting (bacteria, demodex, dermatophyte)
- Vasculitis
- Erythema multiforme
- Neoplasia especially lymphoma, mast cell tumours

Angioedema:

- Juvenile cellulitis
- Infectious cellulitis

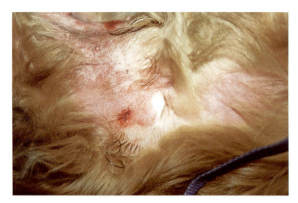

Figure 10.1 Urticarial weals in a dog with atopic dermatitis.

- Neoplasia especially lymphoma, mast cell tumour
- Myxoedema
- Lymphoedema

Diagnosis

- History and clinical signs. Identification of an underlying cause is not always possible but time spent taking an extensive history is particularly useful in cases of urticaria and angioedema.
- Diascopy of lesion (see Chapter 3). Urticaria lesions will blanch suggesting erythema is due to vasodilation not haemorrhage as in vasculitis.

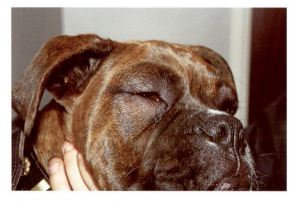

Figure 10.2 Angioedema in a Boxer due to a food intolerance.

- Skin biopsy reveals a variable, non-diagnostic pattern often superficial perivascular dermatitis.

Treatment

- Elimination and avoidance of trigger factors when they can be identified.
- Treatment of symptoms:
  - Angioedema:
    - Adrenalin 1:10,000 0.5–1.0 ml iv in severe reactions and 0.2–0.5 ml iv, sq in mild reactions as single treatments.
    - Dexamethasone sodium phosphate 1–2 mg/kg iv or prednisolone sodium succinate 100–500 mg/dog iv as single treatments.
  - Urticaria:
    - Glucocorticoids in the form of prednisolone as a single treatment of 2 mg/kg po, iv, im in acute disease followed by antihistamine therapy.
    - Antihistamines work best as maintenance therapy and in recurrent disease especially hydroxyzine or chlorpheniramine (see Table 10.1).

Canine atopy (atopic dermatitis)

This is defined as a genetic predisposition to develop allergic skin disease mediated through a type I hypersensitivity reaction to environmental allergens.

Cause and pathogenesis

- Atopy is thought to be genetically inherited disease. Parasites, viral infection, and vaccination are thought to augment the production of IgE specific for environmental allergens.
- The amount of allergen exposure appears to be critical in determining development of atopy.
- Route of allergen still remains controversial and may be percutaneous, inhaled or ingested.

Clinical signs

- Approximately 10% of all dogs are affected with atopy.
- Age of onset 6 months to 7 years, although more commonly 1–3 years of age.
- Eighty per cent of dogs start with seasonal disease during the summer months but many eventually become non-seasonal.
- Breed predilection is recognised, and the shar-pei, West Highland white terrier, Scottish terrier, English setter, Labrador retriever, Boxer, golden retriever are recognised as predisposed breeds.
- Cutaneous lesions:
  - Pruritus moderate – severe involving face (Figure 10.3), distal extremities (Figures 10.4 and 10.5), anterior elbows and ventrum (Figure 10.6).
  - Atopic otitis externa is seen in more than 50% of cases (Figure 10.7).
  - Conjunctivitis: approximately 50% affected.
  - Other signs include bacterial pyoderma, acute moist dermatitis, acral lick dermatitis (65–70%).
  - *Malassezia* infection seen in many as a secondary factor.
- Non-cutaneous signs are uncommon:
  - Respiratory disease especially rhinitis, asthma.
  - Gastrointestinal diseases intermittent diarrhoea, colitis.
  - Ocular signs less well established but possible links to cataract and keratoconjunctivitis sicca.
  - Urogenital disease in the form of abnormal cycling in bitches.

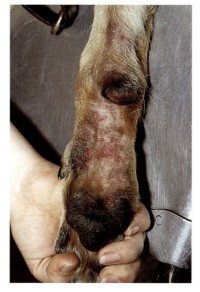

Figure 10.4 Erythema and lichenification of the flexural aspects of the carpus in an atopic German shepherd dog.

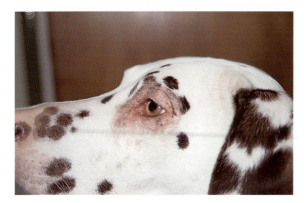

Figure 10.3 Periocular pruritus and pyoderma in an atopic Dalmatian.

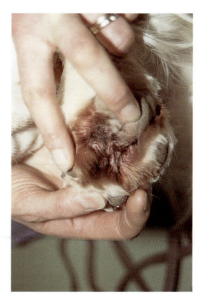

Figure 10.5 Interdigital pedal saliva staining in an atopic West Highland White terrier.

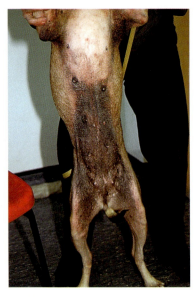

Figure 10.6 Chronic lichenification and hyperpigmentation in a long-standing atopic dog.

Differential diagnosis

- Flea-allergic dermatitis
- Food hypersensitivity/intolerance
- Scabies
- Contact dermatitis
- *Malassezia* dermatitis
- Bacterial folliculitis

Many of these diseases can occur concurrently in atopic dogs.

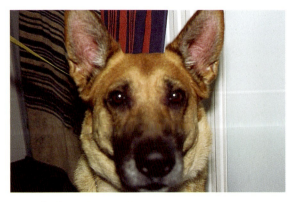

Figure 10.7 Erythema of the ear pinnae in an atopic German shepherd dog.

Diagnosis

- History and clinical signs.
- Diagnostic rule outs of other pruritic skin disease especially ectoparasites, bacterial and yeast infection. Atopy is a diagnosis of exclusion.
- Elimination food trial to rule out concurrent food 'allergy'.
- Skin biopsy may be useful as part of the investigation to rule out other diseases but cannot be used to make a diagnosis of atopy. Histopathology reveals signs of a non-specific superficial perivascular dermatitis.
- Specific allergy tests to investigate atopy may be undertaken once a diagnosis has been made to help in the management of the disease.
- Allergy testing:
  - Intradermal skin testing thought to be the 'gold standard' test for atopic dogs but needs to be performed by an experienced clinician. Most useful tests are performed using individualised allergens rather than mixes (Figure 10.8).
  - In vitro allergy tests also very useful in many cases but should be submitted to a laboratory with expertise in this area.

Treatment

Treatment of concurrent disease, e.g. bacterial and *Malassezia* infections, ectoparasite control

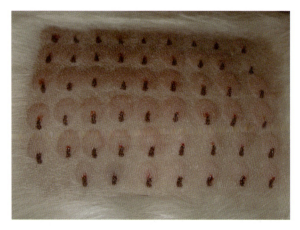

Figure 10.8 Intradermal allergy test in a dog.

and food regulation are important as part of the overall management of atopy

Environmental modification:

- Natural desensitisation is rare.
- Avoidance is not often possible but exposure to specific allergens can be decreased significantly through environmental changes, e.g. house dust mite, allergic dogs may be housed outside or bedding can be switched to avoid natural fibres especially feathers. Dogs should be kept out of bedrooms and bedding can be treated with sprays to decrease mite numbers or washed at high temperatures.

Topical therapy:

- Antipruritic agents may be useful in the form of creams, rinses, sprays and shampoos.
- Cooling solutions containing menthol, hamamelis extract, aloe vera and colloidal oat meal are available.
- Topical glucocorticoids may be used but long-term use of potent topical products should be avoided.

Systemic therapy:

- A range of systemic drugs can be used to control pruritus in atopic dogs. Table 10.1 details some of the potential medications and dose rates.
- Allergen-specific immunotherapy:
  - Useful in dogs where allergen avoidance is impossible and where topical and systemic treatment is unsuccessful; produces side effects or is prohibitively expensive. Dogs are injected with increasing amounts of allergen to induce immune 'tolerance'. Success rate 60–80%. Some dogs (60%) can be controlled with vaccines alone, others (80%) require concurrent medical therapy.

Contact hypersensitivity

Rare dermatitis manifested as an allergic maculopapular reaction affecting sparsely haired contact areas.

Cause and pathogenesis

Contact allergy – type IV hypersensitivity reaction; must be distinguished from contact irritants.

Approximately 1–5% of all canine dermatoses are caused by contact hypersensitivity. It is an uncommon disease in dogs and is rare in cats. Prolonged contact with the offending allergen is normally required (up to 2 years) to produce a reaction. It can be triggered by plants, e.g. poison ivy, poison oak; metals, e.g. cobalt, nickel; rubber, resins, carpet deodorisers, floor cleaners, plastic dishes, chews, toys, etc. Hypersensitivity reactions to topical drugs can also occur most commonly with neomycin.

Clinical signs

- No breed predilection has been recognised.
- Where only a single animal in a household is affected it tends to suggest a hypersensitivity reaction, where several animals are affected an irritant reaction is more likely.
- Lesions confined to hairless or sparsely haired areas (except where signs caused by creams, shampoos, etc.), e.g. ventral abdomen (Figure 10.9), thorax, neck, scrotum, perineum, ventral aspect of paws (not usually the pads). If the lips and muzzle are affected then the allergen is usually being chewed or is a feed bowl.
- Lesions show variable degrees of pruritus:
  - Acutely – erythema, macules, papules, alopecia, pustules variable.

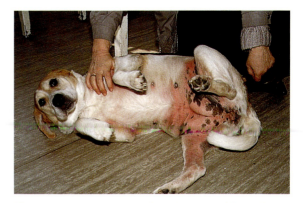

Figure 10.9 Erythema in axilla and groin in a dog with contact hypersensitivity.

Table 10.1 Anti-inflammatory medication shown to have benefits in canine atopy.

Drug	Dose rate	Comments
Antihistamines	Success rates range from 1 to 30%; different drugs may be for 7–10 day therapeutic trials to assess efficacy. They can be used in combination with other drugs	
Amitriptyline	1.0–2.0 mg/kg po bid	
Astemizole	1.0 mg/kg po bid/sid	
Cetirizine	0.5–1.0 mg/kg po sid	
Chlorpheniramine	0.2–3.0 mg/kg po tid/bid	May be used in atopy and urticaria
Clemastine	0.05–1.5 mg/kg po bid	
Clomipramine	1.0–3.0 mg/kg po sid	
Cyproheptadine	0.1–2.0 mg/kg po tid/bid	
Diphenhydramine	1.0–4.0 mg/kg po tid	
Doxepin	0.5–1.0 mg/kg pot id/bid	
Hydroxyzine	3.0–7.0 mg/kg po bid	May be used in atopy and urticaria
oratadine	0.5 mg/kg po sid	
Promethazine	1.0–2.5 mg/kg po bid	
Terfenadine	0.25–1.5 mg/kg po bid/sid	
Trimeprazine	0.5–5.0 mg/kg po tid/bid	
Non-steroidal anti-inflammatory drugs	Often not successful as sole form of therapy but drugs below can be used with glucocorticoids in a steroid sparing capacity	
Pentoxifylline	10–25 mg/kg po bid/tid	
Misoprostol	6.0 mg/kg po tid	
Chinese herbal medicines	Clinical trials have shown these drugs to have benefit in about 30% of cases; they can be used in conjunction with other drugs	
Essential fatty acids	Clinical trials have shown these drugs to be beneficial in 20–50% of pruritic dogs; benefits take 8–12 weeks; they have synergism with glucocorticoids and antihistamines	
Cyclosporine	5.0 mg/kg po sid	Successful in 60–75% of dogs; initial dose given for 4–6 weeks then tapered to lowest possible maintenance dose; should only be given to fit animals and should be regularly monitored by routine blood samples and where appropriate urine analysis
Glucocorticoids	Produce control in 75% of dogs; most suitable for animals with short pruritus season (<4 months); side effects can be seen with long-term use; they should not be used on a daily basis for long-term maintenance and always tapered to lowest possible dose rate	
Prednisolone	0.25–0.5 mg /kg po bid	Induction phase of 5–10 days to control pruritus
	0.5–1.0 mg/kg po eod	For maintenance tapering to lowest possible dose rate
Methyl prednisolone	0.2–0.4 mg/kg po bid	Induction phase of 5–10 days to control pruritus
	0.4–0.8 mg/kg po eod	For maintenance tapering to lowest possible dose rate

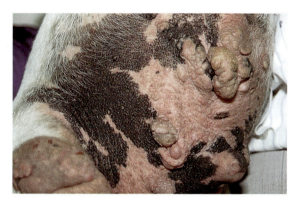

Figure 10.10 Lichenification and erythema in a chronic contact allergic dog.

- Chronically – alopecia, variable pigment changes (hypo- or hyperpigmentation), lichenification (Figure 10.10).
- Secondary infection with both bacterial pyoderma and *Malassezia* are common.

Differential diagnosis

- Irritant contact dermatitis
- Atopy
- Food hypersensitivity
- Scabies
- *Pelodera* dermatitis
- Hookworm dermatitis
- *Malassezia* dermatitis

Diagnosis

- History and clinical signs.
- Provocative exposure can be undertaken by confining the animal to hypoallergenic environment for 14 days, e.g. stainless steel cage. Careful re-exposure to potential allergens can then be undertaken to try and trigger reaction.
- Patch testing is technically difficult to achieve. This can be done by open or closed methods:
  - Closed patch test is undertaken when a test substance is applied to clipped skin on lateral thorax on gauze pad or in sterile stainless steel chamber, secured in place by a body bandage. Examination after 48 hours reveals signs of hypersensitive reaction.
  - Open patched test is performed when a test substance is rubbed into skin and then observed over a 5 day period.
- Skin biopsy is of little value and reveals a non-specific picture of superficial perivascular dermatitis.

Treatment

- Topical treatment with hypoallergenic baths to remove cutaneous allergens may be useful.
- Secondary infection with bacteria or yeast need to be treated.
- Allergen avoidance is important but requires identification of the offending allergen, which can be difficult. Where avoidance is impossible, a mechanical barrier may be useful with socks or a t-shirt.
- Pentoxifylline is useful in some cases in dogs at a dose of 10–25 mg/kg po tid.
- Glucocorticoids:
  - Short-term therapy is useful if the offending allergen is identified and removed from the animal's environment. Topical steroids may be used once or twice daily for 7–10 days or systemic prednisolone may be used at a dose of 1.0 mg/kg po sid (dogs) or 2.0 mg/kg po sid (cats) for the same period.
  - Chronic therapy may be necessary when the allergen cannot be identified or its removal from the animal's environment is not possible. Prednisolone or methyl prednisolone may be used under the same treatment protocol as for atopy.
- Prognosis is good if the offending allergen can be identified and removed from the animal's environment.

Canine food hypersensitivity (food intolerance/food allergy)

Non-seasonal pruritic skin disease associated with ingestion of components of the diet

Cause and pathogenesis

- Food allergy – type I reactions to food (III and IV may also occur); where true allergy occurs the reaction is usually triggered by glycoproteins.
- Food intolerance clinically indistinguishable from allergy but is a non-immunological reaction. Caused by food containing histamine or related substances, or histamine-releasing factors.
- Foods implicated in hypersensitivity include beef, dairy products, chicken, wheat, eggs, corn and soya. Additives and flavourings are rare causes of allergy in dogs.

Clinical signs

- Cause of approximately 1% of all canine skin disease.
- No age or sex predilection is reported although often seen in young dogs. Thirty per cent of affected dogs are <1 year old.
- No breed predilection is recognised.
- Cutaneous signs:
  - Pruritus and erythema can cause a papular eruption, but not a consistent finding.
  - Secondary lesions of self-inflicted trauma (Figure 10.11), often acute moist dermatitis.
  - Distribution of lesions variable, often distal limbs (Figure 10.12), axilla, groin, perineum, face and neck.

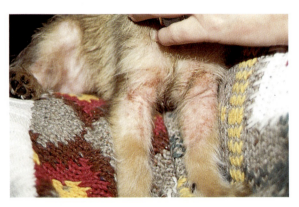

Figure 10.12 Self-inflicted trauma of elbow flexures in food-allergic puppy.

- Can mimic both atopy and flea-allergic dermatitis.
- Pruritus often poorly responsive to steroids and is non-seasonal.
- Lesions can be confined to the ears.
- May present with signs of acral lick dermatitis.
- Secondary bacterial and *Malassezia* infections can occur.
- Non-cutaneous signs:
  - Gastrointestinal signs seen in 30% of cases as increase in faecal frequency, tenesmus, colitis, vomiting, poor appetite.
  - Central nervous system signs are rare. Seizures have been reported, associated with dietary reactions.

Differential diagnosis

- Atopy
- Contact allergy
- Flea-allergic dermatitis
- Pediculosis
- Scabies
- Cheyletiellosis
- *Malassezia* dermatitis

Diagnosis

- History and clinical signs.
- Elimination diets:
  - Response to elimination diet is the best way to establish a diagnosis. The diet

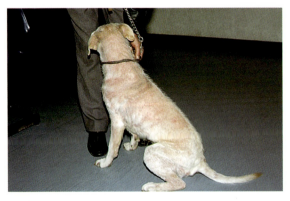

Figure 10.11 Generalised pruritus and erythema in a dog with food allergy.

should be fed for 10–13 weeks where possible; some improvement should be seen in 4 weeks. Provocative challenge should be undertaken if improvement is seen to establish a definitive diagnosis.
- Selection of diet is important and it should be individualised for each dog to include the following:
  - Novel protein and carbohydrate source.
  - Free of additives, colourants where possible.
  - Suitable proteins include fish, rabbit, venison, turkey, kangaroo, chicken, duck, soya.
  - Suitable carbohydrates include rice, potatoes, corn.
- Types of diet:
  - Home cooked are ideal but owner compliance is often poor and these are unbalanced for young dogs.
  - Commercial hypoallergenic diets are not a 'pure' diet but more convenient for busy owners and is nutritionally complete.
  - Hydrolysed diets are a new generation of commercial diets where the protein is hydrolysed to a size to render it non-allergenic, rendering the type of protein less critical.
■ Food allergy testing using both intradermal and serological tests is currently unreliable.
■ Skin biopsy is non-diagnostic and reveals a non-specific superficial perivascular dermatitis.

Treatment

■ Treatment of secondary infection is essential. Where other allergies are present concurrently, e.g. flea allergy or atopy, these also need to be managed.
■ Once a diagnosis has been made and offending allergens have been identified by provocative re-exposure, food allergen avoidance should be maintained. Provocative re-exposure can be achieved by adding new challenge food to the hypoallergenic diet every 7–10 days.
■ Selection of diet for long term can either be in the form of home-cooked diets with additional minerals, vitamins and essential fatty acid supplements or proprietary diets that do not contain any of the identified allergens.
■ Symptomatic anti-inflammatory therapy is rarely beneficial unless the diet is managed concurrently.
■ Prognosis is good, provided the offending allergens are identified and avoided on a long-term basis.

Feline atopy (atopic dermatitis)

An exaggerated or inappropriate response to environmental allergens.

Cause and pathogenesis

■ Thought to be an immediate hypersensitivity reaction to a heat labile antibody resembling IgE.
■ Route of allergen remains unclear; may be percutaneous absorption, inhaled or ingested.

Clinical signs

■ No breed or sex predilection is recognised although young cats appear to be predisposed.
■ Pruritus is a consistent finding.
■ Different cutaneous patterns can be seen:
  - Self-induced alopecia, usually ventral but also on caudal thighs, forelegs or lateral thorax (Figures 10.13 and 10.14).
  - Eosinophilic granuloma complex.
  - Miliary dermatitis.
  - Facial (Figure 10.15) and pedal pruritus (often secondary bacterial paronychia, Figure 10.16).
  - Pruritic ceruminous otitis externa.
■ Many cats have concurrent food hypersensitivity, flea-allergic dermatitis.

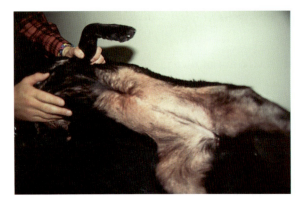

Figure 10.13 Ventral alopecia secondary to atopy.

- Respiratory signs of bronchitis and asthma may also be seen in some cats.

Differential diagnosis

- Flea-allergic dermatitis
- Food hypersensitivity
- Cheyletiella
- Ectopic otodectes
- Dermatophytosis
- Psychogenic alopecia

Diagnosis

- History and clinical signs.
- Laboratory rule outs for other diseases especially flea/food allergy.
- Intradermal skin testing useful as an aid to diagnosis but is difficult to undertake in the cat as reactions are more subtle than in the dog:
  - Reactions often occur and fade rapidly within 10 minutes.
  - Systemic fluorescein may improve the diagnostic accuracy of intradermal allergy testing in cats.
  - Must be read by an experienced investigator.
- Serology testing not adequately evaluated to date.
- Skin biopsy reveals a non-specific picture of superficial perivascular dermatitis and acts as a rule out rather than as a diagnosis.
- Bloods unremarkable; however, a peripheral eosinophilia usually present unless glucocorticoids have been prescribed.

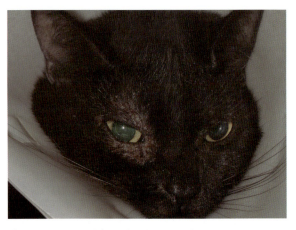

Figure 10.15 Facial pruritus in an atopic cat.

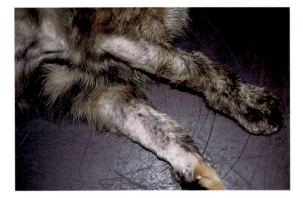

Figure 10.14 Pedal alopecia secondary to atopy.

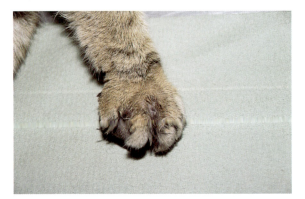

Figure 10.16 Bacterial paronychia secondary to atopy.

Treatment

Treatment of concurrent disease, e.g. bacterial and *Malassezia* infections, ectoparasite control and food regulation are important as part of the overall management of atopy.
Environmental modification:

- Natural desensitisation is rare.
- Avoidance is not often possible but exposure to specific allergens can be decreased significantly through environmental changes; for example, house dust mite cats may be moved to an outdoor cattery. Cats should be kept out of bedrooms and bedding can be treated with sprays to decrease mite numbers or washed at high temperatures.

Topical therapy:

- Topical antipruritic agents are rarely useful due to the problems with application in cats.
- Topical glucocorticoids may be used but long-term use of potent topical products should be avoided.

Systemic therapy:

- A range of systemic drugs can be used to control pruritus in atopic cats. Table 10.2 details some of the potential medications and dose rates.
- Allergen-specific immunotherapy:
  - Useful in cats where allergen avoidance is impossible and where topical and systemic treatments are unsuccessful, produce side effects or are prohibitively expensive. Cats are injected with increasing amounts of allergen to induce immune 'tolerance'. Suggested success rate is 50–70%.

Feline food hypersensitivity (food intolerance/food allergy)

Non-seasonal pruritic skin disease associated with ingestion of components of the diet.

Cause and pathogenesis

- Pathogenesis is poorly understood. A type I hypersensitivity (III and IV may also occur) to food is thought to be present. Where true allergy occurs the reaction is usually triggered by glycoproteins.
- Food intolerance clinically indistinguishable from allergy but is a non-immunological reaction. Caused by food containing histamine or related substances, or histamine-releasing factors.
- Foods implicated in hypersensitivity include beef, pork, dairy products especially milk, chicken, lamb, eggs and fish. Additives and flavourings are rare causes of allergy in cats.

Clinical signs

- No age or sex predilection is reported although often seen in cats 4–5 years of age.
- Siamese cats may be predisposed.
- Cutaneous signs very variable:
  - Pruritus often poorly responsive to steroids and is non-seasonal.
  - Facial pruritus (Figure 10.17), including pinnae and neck.
  - Ventral or flank alopecia (self-inflicted due to overgrooming).
  - Miliary dermatitis.
  - Eosinophilic granuloma complex (Figure 10.18).
  - Urticaria – less common.
  - Secondary bacterial and *Malassezia* infections can occur.
- Non-cutaneous signs:
  - Gastrointestinal signs include diarrhoea and vomiting.
  - Respiratory signs include sneezing.
- Twenty-five per cent of cases have other concurrent allergies.

Differential diagnosis

- Atopy
- Contact allergy

Table 10.2 Anti-inflammatory medication shown to have benefits in feline atopy.

Drug	Dose rate	Comments
Antihistamines	Success rates range from 40 to 70%; different drugs may be for 7–10 day therapeutic trials to assess efficacy; they can be used in combination with other drugs	
Amitriptyline	5.0–10.0 mg/cat po sid/bid	
Chlorpheniramine	2.0–4.0 mg/cat po sid/bid	May be used in atopy and urticaria
Clemastine	0.68 mg/cat po bid	
Cyproheptadine	2.0 mg/cat po bid	
Diphenhydramine	2.0–4.0 mg/cat po bid	
Hydroxyzine	5.0–10.0 mg/cat po tid/bid	May be used in atopy and urticaria
Essential fatty acids	Clinical trials have shown these drugs to be beneficial in 20–50% of pruritic dogs; benefits take 8–12 weeks; they have synergism with glucocorticoids and antihistamines	
Cyclosporine	5.0 mg/kg po sid	Successful in many cats but each animal needs careful assessment to ensure physically well and no concurrent viral/toxoplasma immunosuppression; initial dose given for 4–6 weeks then tapered to lowest possible maintenance dose; should be regularly monitored by routine blood samples and where appropriate urine analysis
Glucocorticoids	Produce control in most cases of feline atopy; most suitable for animals with short pruritus season (<4 months); side effects can be seen with long-term use; they should not be used on a daily basis for long-term maintenance and always tapered to lowest possible dose rate	
Prednisolone	2.0 mg/kg po sid	Induction phase of 2–8 weeks to control pruritus and lesions then taper
	2.0 mg/kg po eod	Maintenance therapy initially for 2–4 weeks then tapering to lowest possible dose rate
Methyl prednisolone acetate	20 mg/cat or 4.0 mg/kg sq or im every 2–3 months	Should not be used more than 3–4 times a year
Triamcinolone acetonide	5.0 mg/cat sq or im every 2–3 months	Should not be used more than 3–4 times a year

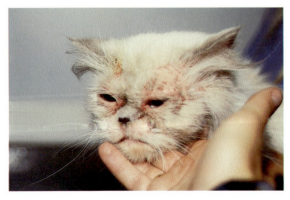

Figure 10.17 Facial pruritus secondary to food allergy.

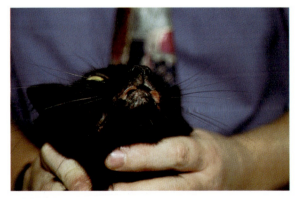

Figure 10.18 Indolent ulcer in a food-allergic cat.

- Flea-allergic dermatitis
- Pediculosis
- Cheyletiellosis
- Psychogenic alopecia
- Dermatophytosis
- Ectopic otodectes

Diagnosis

- History and clinical signs.
- Elimination diets:
  - Response to elimination diet is the best way to establish a diagnosis. The diet should be fed for 10–13 weeks where possible; some improvement should be seen in 4 weeks. Provocative challenge should be undertaken if improvement is seen to establish a definitive diagnosis.
  - Selection of diet is important and it should be individualised for each cat to include the following:
    - Novel protein source.
    - Free of additives, colourants where possible.
    - Suitable proteins include venison, kangaroo, turkey, duck, soya.
  - Types of diet:
    - Home cooked are ideal but owner compliance is often poor and these are unbalanced for cats and may need both taurine and calcium supplements.
    - Commercial hypoallergenic diets are not a 'pure' diet but more convenient for busy owners and is nutritionally complete.
    - Hydrolysed diets are a new generation of commercial diets where the protein is hydrolysed to a size to render it non-allergenic, rendering the type of protein less critical.
    - Cats often have multiple feeding stations and are best kept inside during the period of their food trial.
- Food allergy testing using both intradermal and serological tests is currently unreliable.
- Skin biopsy is non-diagnostic and reveals a non-specific superficial perivascular dermatitis.

Treatment

- Treatment of secondary infection is essential. Where other allergies are present concurrently, e.g. flea allergy or atopy, these also need to be managed.
- Once a diagnosis has been made and offending allergens have been identified by provocative re-exposure, food allergen avoidance should be maintained. Provocative re-exposure can be achieved by adding new challenge food to the hypoallergenic diet every 7–10 days.
- Selection of diet for long term can either be in the form of home-cooked diets with additional minerals, vitamins and essential fatty acid supplements or proprietary diets that do not contain any of the identified allergens.
- Symptomatic anti-inflammatory therapy is rarely beneficial unless the diet is managed concurrently.
- Prognosis is good, provided the offending allergens are identified and avoided on a long-term basis.

Flea-allergic dermatitis

See Chapter 7.

Mosquito bite hypersensitivity

See Chapter 7.

Eosinophilic furunculosis of the face

Acute sterile furunculosis of nose and muzzle.

Cause and pathogenesis

The exact pathomechanism is unknown. It is thought to be hypersensitivity reaction to venomous insect or arthropod. Exposure to fleas or wasps is seen in many cases. It is an uncommon to rare disease that has only been recognised in dogs.

Clinical signs

- Young dog usually medium to large outdoor dogs.
- No breed or sex predilection.
- Acute onset of lesions, which develop within hours and progress rapidly.
- Lesions appear as nodules, papules, ulceration, haemorrhage and crust.
- Painful lesions with only minimal pruritus.
- Sites usually affected are the bridge of the nose (Figure 10.19), also muzzle and periocular skin.
- In rare cases, the ventral abdomen chest and ear pinnae are involved.
- Lesions often sterile; secondary infection is uncommon in acute cases.

Differential diagnosis

- Nasal pyoderma – Staphylococcal infection
- Dermatophytosis – *Trichophyton mentagrophytes*
- Burns
- Drug eruption
- Autoimmune skin disease – pemphigus foliaceus, discoid lupus erythematosus

Diagnosis

- History and clinical signs.
- Diagnostic rule outs for other differentials, e.g. fungal culture.
- Cytology reveals in the acute stages an eosinophil-rich infiltrate with no evidence of infectious organisms.
- Skin biopsy reveals signs of an eosinophilic perifolliculitis, folliculitis and furunculosis. Also a mixed inflammatory infiltrate with dermal haemorrhage and collagen degeneration.

Treatment

- Good prognosis.
- Antibiotics based on culture and sensitivity where infection is present for 3–4 weeks.
- Systemic glucocorticoids in the form of prednisolone 1–2 mg/kg po sid until a response is seen (usually 7–10 days) then tapered to 1–2 mg/kg po sid every other day for a further 7–10 days. After this drugs can usually be stopped.
- Prognosis is good. Many dogs will improve without glucocorticoids. However, therapy speeds the rate of resolution and makes the dog more comfortable.

Selected references and further reading

Bloom, P. (2004) Symptomatic management of pruritus. In: Campbell, K.L. (ed) *Small Animal Dermatology Secrets*. pp. 43–56. Hanley and Belfus, Philadelphia

Bruner, S.R. (2004) Dietary hypersensitivity. In: Campbell, K.L. (ed) *Small Animal Dermatology Secrets*. pp. 196–201. Hanley and Belfus, Philadelphia

Chesney, C.J. (2002) Food hypersensitivity in the dog a quantitative study. *J Small Anim Pract*, **43**, 203–207

Guaguere, E. et al. (2004) Cyclosporin A: a new drug in the field of veterinary dermatology. *Vet Derm*, **15**, 61–74

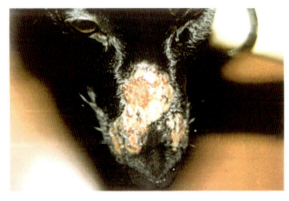

Figure 10.19 Erythema with crusting and exudation in a dog with eosinophilic furunculosis of the face.

Medleau, L. and Hnilica, K. (2006) Hypersensitivity disorders. In: *Small Animal Dermatology: A Color Atlas and Therapeutic Guide.* 2nd edn. pp. 159–188. WB Saunders, Philadelphia

Olivry, T. (ed) (2001) The ACVD task force on atopic dermatitis (XXIII). *Vet Immunol Immunopathol*, 81, 143–385.

Prelaud, P. (2004) Atopy. In: Campbell, K.L. (ed) *Small Animal Dermatology Secrets.* pp. 188–196. Hanley and Belfus, Philadelphia

Roudebush, P. (2000) Hypoallergenic diets for dogs. In: Bonagura, J.D. (ed) *Kirk's Current Veterinary Therapy XIII Small Animal Practice.* pp. 530–535. WB Saunders, Philadelphia

Scott, D.W. et al. (2001) Skin immune system and allergic skin disease. *Muller and Kirk's Small Animal Dermatology.* 6th edn. pp. 543–666. WB Saunders, Philadelphia

Immune mediated skin disease

Pemphigus complex

Very rare vesiculobullous pustular diseases of the skin and mucous membranes.
In the dog and cat five different forms are recognised:

- Pemphigus vulgaris
- Pemphigus erythematosus
- Pemphigus foliaceus
- Panepidermal pustular pemphigus
- Paraneoplastic pemphigus

Pemphigus can be associated with drugs (including food substances), chronic disease and immune system related tumours.

Pemphigus vulgaris

Cause and pathogenesis

Autoantibodies are thought to react with cadherins (cell to cell adhesion molecules), which is found in the suprabasilar epidermal layers and may extend into the basal cell membrane. Antibody binding leads to loss of intercellular cohesion and acantholysis at the suprabasilar level. It is the most severe form of pemphigus due to the depth of the target antigen in the skin and its additional location in mucosa. It is rare amongst both dogs and cats.

Clinical signs

- No age, breed or sex predilection.
- Cutaneous signs:
    - Vesicles, bullae, erosions, ulcers found in oral cavity (90%, Figure 11.1) and mucocutaneous junctions (Figure 11.2).
    - Oral lesions lead to salivation and halitosis.
    - Occasionally lesions seen in groin, axilla and flanks.
    - Ulcerative paronychia and onychomadesis.
    - Nikolsky sign may be present.
- Non-cutaneous signs:
    - Anorexia, pyrexia

Differential diagnosis

- Bullous pemphigoid
- Systemic lupus erythematosus
- Cat flu – especially calici virus

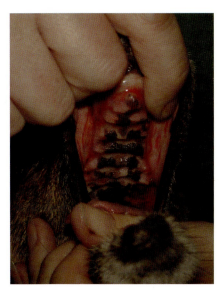

Figure 11.1 Ulceration of the mouth in a dog with pemphigus vulgaris.

- Toxic epidermal necrolysis
- Drug eruption
- Erythema multiforme
- Epitheliotropic lymphoma

Diagnosis

- History and clinical signs.
- Diagnostic rule outs of other differentials.
- Bacterial culture usually sterile.

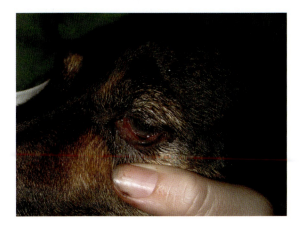

Figure 11.2 Ulceration of the mucocutaneous junctions in a dog with pemphigus vulgaris.

- Skin biopsy of primary lesion reveals suprabasilar acantholysis 'tombstones' of basement membrane, also perivascular interstitial or lichenoid inflammation.
- Immunofluorescence or immunohistochemistry of skin biopsy specimens to detect intercellular antibody deposition. False negative and positive results can occur; positive results should also have compatible histopathology.

Treatment

- Very poor prognosis – without treatment this disease is fatal.
- Difficult to achieve and maintain animals in remission.
- Symptomatic therapy with gentle keratolytic shampoos such as sulphur may be useful.
- Antibacterial and anti-yeast therapy should be prescribed where appropriate and may need to be continued until the disease is under control.
- Immunosuppressive therapy is necessary; see Tables 11.1–11.3 for drugs, monitoring and side effects in dogs and cats.
- In view of the severity of pemphigus vulgaris several different immunosuppressive drugs may need to be used together. Glucocorticoids are usually used with a non-steroidal immunosuppressive drug.
- Prognosis is poor in most cases and animals need long-term therapy and monitoring.

Pemphigus foliaceus

Cause and pathogenesis

Autoantibodies react with 150 kD glycoprotein (desmoglein I) from cadherin group of adhesion molecules. The binding of the antibody leads to loss of intercellular cohesion and acantholysis at the intragranular or subcorneal level.

Clinical signs

- The most common form of pemphigus complex disease in the dog and cat.

Table 11.1 Therapy for autoimmune disease in dogs.

Drug	Induction dose	Maintenance dose
Glucocorticoids		
Prednisolone	1–3 mg/kg po sid /bid	0.5–2 mg/kg po every 48 hours
Methylprednisolone	0.8–2.4 mg/kg po sid/bid	0.4–0.8 mg/kg po every 48 hours
Triamcinolone	0.1–0.3 mg/kg po sid/bid	0.1–0.2 mg/kg po every 48 hours
Dexamethasone	0.1–0.2 mg/kg po sid/bid	0.05–0.1 mg/kg po every 48–72 hours
Methylprednisolone sodium succinate (pulse therapy)	1 mg/kg iv over 3–4 hours once daily for 2–3 consecutive days	Alternate day oral glucocorticoids
Dexamethasone	1 mg/kg iv once or twice daily on two occasions 24 hours apart	Alternate day oral glucocorticoids
Tetracycline/niacinamide	Dogs >10 kg 500 mg of each drug po qid Dogs <10 kg 250 mg of each drug po qid	Dogs >10 kg 500 mg of each drug po sid/bid Dogs <10 kg 250 mg of each drug po sid/bid
Doxycycline/niacinamide	Niacinamide as above doxycycline 5–10 mg/kg bid	Niacinamide as above; doxycycline taper to lowest effective dose rate
Cyclosporine	5.0–12.5 mg/kg po sid/bid until clinical remission	Taper to lowest possible dose rate; aim for 2.5–5.0 mg/kg po sid or every 48 hours
Vitamin E	400 IU po bid	400 IU po bid
Azathioprine	1.5–2.5 mg/kg po sid or every 48 hours	1.5–2.5 mg/kg po every 48–72 hours
Chlorambucil	0.1–0.2 mg/kg po sid	0.1–0.2 mg/kg po every 48 hours
Mycophenolate mofetil	22–39 mg/kg divided tid until clinical remission	Taper to lowest effective dose rate
Gold sodium thiomalate	1 mg/kg im weekly until clinical remission	Taper to monthly administration

Table 11.2 Therapy of autoimmune disease in cats.

Drug	Induction dose	Maintenance dose
Glucocorticoids		
Prednisolone	2–2.5 mg/kg po sid /bid	2.5–5 mg/kg po every 2–7 days
Triamcinolone	0.3–1 mg/kg po sid/bid	0.6–1 mg/kg po every 2–7 days
Dexamethasone	0.1–0.2 mg/kg po sid/bid	0.05–0.1 mg/kg po every 48–72 hours
Methylprednisolone sodium succinate (pulse therapy)	1 mg/kg iv over 3–4 hours once daily for 2–3 consecutive days	Alternate day oral glucocorticoids
Dexamethasone	1 mg/kg iv once or twice daily on two occasions 24 hours apart	Alternate day oral glucocorticoids
Chlorambucil	0.1–0.2 mg/kg po sid	0.1–0.2 mg/kg po every 48 hours

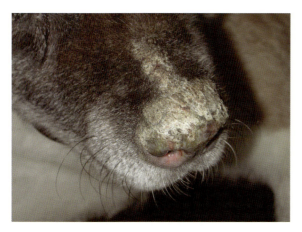

Figure 11.3 Pemphigus foliaceus in an Akita.

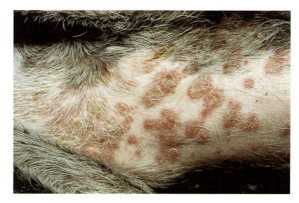

Figure 11.5 Primary pustules and macules on the ventral abdomen of a dog with pemphigus foliaceus.

Dogs:

- No age or sex predilection.
- Predisposed breeds – Akita (Figure 11.3), chow, Doberman pinscher, dachshund, bearded collie.
- Cutaneous signs:
  - Initial signs usually face (Figure 11.4), waxing and waning course often.
  - Mucocutaneous and oral signs rare.
  - Primary lesions macules and pustules progressing to severe crusting (Figure 11.5).
  - Footpad and nasal hyperkeratosis seen in 90% of cases (Figure 11.6).
  - Nose often depigmented chronically.
  - Claw abnormalities can occur but rare.
  - Nikolsky sign may be present.
- Non-cutaneous signs:
  - Anorexia, pyrexia

Cats:

- No age, sex or breed predilection.
- Cutaneous signs:
  - Most commonly sterile paronychia, with a thick caseous discharge (Figure 11.7).
  - Primary lesions macules and pustules progressing to severe crusting (Figure 11.8).
  - Involvement of nipples and footpads common (Figure 11.9).

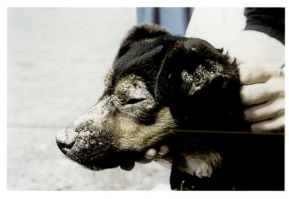

Figure 11.4 Crusting on the nose and ears in a dog with pemphigus foliaceus.

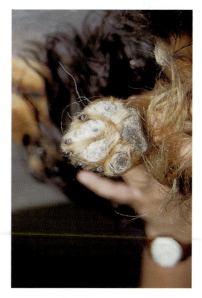

Figure 11.6 Footpad hyperkeratosis in a dog with pemphigus foliaceus.

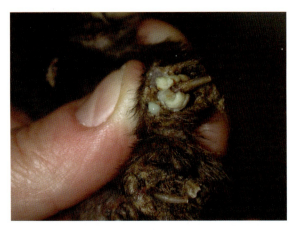

Figure 11.7 Sterile paronychial in a cat with pemphigus foliaceus.

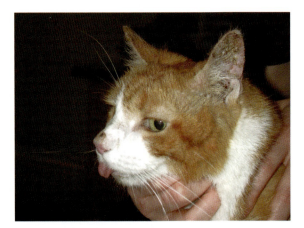

Figure 11.8 Lesions on the face of a cat with pemphigus foliaceus.

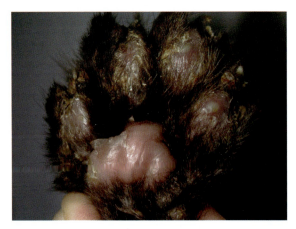

Figure 11.9 Hyperkeratosis and pustular lesions of footpads of a cat with pemphigus foliaceus.

- ☐ Nose often depigmented chronically.
- ☐ Claw and oral signs rare.
- ☐ Nikolsky sign may be present.
- Non-cutaneous signs:
  - ☐ Anorexic, depression, pyrexia

Differential diagnosis

- Bacterial impetigo-folliculitis
- Dermatophytosis
- Demodicosis
- Lupus erythematosus
- Subcorneal pustular dermatosis

Diagnosis

- History and clinical signs.
- Cytology of primary lesions or nail bed exudate reveals acanthocytes, non-degenerate neutrophils and/or eosinophils, no bacteria in uncomplicated cases.
- Antinuclear antibodies are negative but false positives can be seen.
- Skin biopsy reveals intragranular/subcorneal acantholysis with cleft and pustule formation (granular cells 'cling-ons'). Variable numbers of eosinophils.
- Immunofluorescence or immunohistochemistry of skin biopsy specimens to detect intercellular antibody deposition. False negative and positive results can occur; positive results should also have compatible histopathology.
- Bacteriology only isolates infection when it is there as a secondary problem.

Treatment

- Symptomatic therapy with gentle keratolytic shampoos such as sulphur may be useful.
- Antibacterial and anti-yeast therapy should be prescribed where appropriate and may need to be continued until the disease is under control.
- Immunosuppressive therapy is necessary; see Tables 11.1–11.3 for drugs, monitoring and side effects in dogs and cats. In dogs the author's preferred combination of therapy is azathioprine with prednisolone. In cats the

Table 11.3 Side effects and monitoring drug therapy in autoimmune skin disease.

Drug	Side effects	Monitoring
Glucocorticoids	Polyuria, polydipsia, weight gain, behavioural changes, panting, increased risk of infection, poor hair coat, scaly coat, muscle atrophy gastrointestinal ulceration, pancreatitis, steroid hepatopathy, diabetes mellitus	Twice yearly blood counts, chemistry profile, urine analysis and urine cultures
Tetracycline/niacinamide	Vomiting diarrhoea, anorexia, increased liver enzyme levels	Not required
Doxycycline/niacinamide	As above	As above
Cyclosporine	Anorexia, vomiting and diarrhoea, weight loss, nephrotoxicity, gingival hyperplasia, papillomatosis, hirsutism	Twice yearly blood counts, chemistry profile, urine analysis and urine cultures
Vitamin E	Rarely reported	Not required
Azathioprine	Myelosuppression, diarrhoea, increased susceptibility to infection, vomiting, hepatotoxicity, pancreatitis	Blood counts with platelet count and chemistry profile every 2–3 weeks for the first 3 months then every 3 months going to every 6 months once case is in remission
Chlorambucil	Myelosuppression, diarrhoea, increased susceptibility to infection, vomiting	As azathioprine
Mycophenolate mofetil	Myelosuppression, diarrhoea, increased susceptibility to infection, vomiting	As azathioprine
Gold sodium thiomalate	Skin rashes, oral ulceration, proteinuria, myelosuppression	As azathioprine but urine analysis should be included

author's preferred drug is prednisolone or dexamethasone.
- Prognosis is moderate to good in most cases. Animals usually need long-term therapy and monitoring except where lesions are drug induced, where therapy can be tapered and withdrawn.

Pemphigus erythematosus

Cause and pathogenesis

Benign form of pemphigus foliaceus and may possibly be a crossover between pemphigus and lupus erythematosus. It is rare in both dogs and cats.

Sunlight may play a part in pathogenesis.

Clinical signs

- No age or sex predilection.
- Predisposed dog breeds include the Shetland sheepdog, collie, German shepherd dog.
- No feline breed predisposition.
- Affects face and ears – pustules, leading to crusts, scale and erosions (Figure 11.10).
- Nikolsky signs may be present.
- Nose often depigmented chronically, uncommonly footpads affected.
- No oral signs.

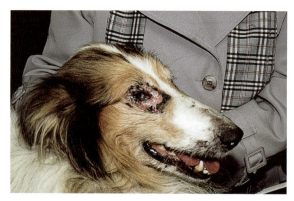

Figure 11.10 Ulceration and crusting of the periocular skin in a rough collie with pemphigus erythematosus.

Differential diagnosis

As pemphigus foliaceus.

Diagnosis

- History and clinical signs.
- Cytology of primary lesions or nail bed exudate reveals acanthocytes, non-degenerate neutrophils and/or eosinophils, no bacteria in uncomplicated cases.
- Antinuclear antibodies are often positive but only useful if other diagnostic signs are compatible with pemphigus erythematosus.
- Skin biopsy reveals subcorneal pustules that contain acanthocytes, neutrophils and variable numbers of eosinophils. Also lichenoid infiltrate with mixed mononuclear cells, plasma cells and polymorphs.
- Immunofluorescence or immunohistochemistry of skin biopsy specimens to detect intercellular and dermal–epidermal junction antibody deposition. False negative and positive results can occur; positive results should also have compatible histopathology.
- Bacteriology only isolates infection when it is there as a secondary problem.

Treatment

- Symptomatic therapy with gentle keratolytic shampoos such as sulphur may be useful.
- Antibacterial and anti-yeast therapy should be prescribed where appropriate and may need to be continued until the disease is under control.
- Sunlight exposure should be reduced and sun blocks should be used if animals spend time outdoors during the warmest times of the day (10.00 a.m. to 4.00 p.m.).

Mild cases:

- In mild disease good levels of control can be achieved with topical therapy (table 11.4).

Moderate to severe cases:

- In more severe cases systemic medication is required. Due to the localised nature of the problem the author will generally use the non-steroidal drugs such as niacinamide, tetracycline and vitamin E before using more potent medication; see Tables 11.1–11.3
- Prognosis is good in most cases as lesions remain benign and localised. Animals that need systemic immunosuppressive therapy require long-term monitoring. Where lesions are sunlight induced, more intensive therapy is required during the summer months and can often be withdrawn during the winter.

Table 11.4 Topical therapy in autoimmune skin disease.

Drug	Use
Glucocorticoid	Initial therapy should be with a potent steroid, e.g. betamethasone twice daily for 4–6 weeks to achieve remission, then the frequency and the potency of the cream should be reduced to the lowest possible levels
Tacrolimus 0.1%	Initial therapy bid or tid for 4–6 weeks to achieve remission, then the frequency can be reduced to lowest maintenance levels
Cyclosporine 1–2%	As tacrolimus

Panepidermal pustular pemphigus

A rare form of pemphigus that may be a variant of pemphigus foliaceus, erythematosus and vulgaris. Histopathologically, pustules are found at all levels of the epidermis and follicular epithelium.

Lesions are found predominantly on the face but can generalise and take the form of fragile pustules that rupture to form a thick crust.

Paraneoplastic pemphigus

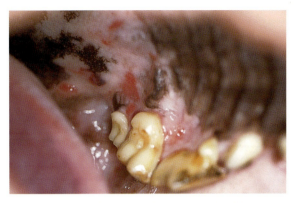

Figure 11.11 Oral vesicles in a dog with bullous pemphigoid.

A very rare form of pemphigus that is associated with neoplastic disease. Autoantibody binding leads to acantholysis as well as necrosis and vacuolation of basal layer keratinocytes.

Lesions can mimic erythema multiforme, pemphigus vulgaris and bullous pemphigoid.

Associated neoplasms include malignant lymphoma, leukaemia, thymoma and sarcoma.

Bullous pemphigoid

Rare vesiculobullous ulcerative canine skin disease of skin, oral mucosa or both.

Cause and pathogenesis

- Autoantibodies are directed against antigen associated with epidermal basal cell hemidesmosomes and lamina lucida of the basement membrane. Antibody attack disrupts dermo–epidermal cohesion leading to dermo–epidermal separation and vesicle formation.
- Two forms of the disease:
  - Spontaneous occurring bullous pemphigoid.
  - Drug-induced bullous pemphigoid especially due to sulphonamides.

Clinical signs

- Very rare disease.
- No age or sex predilection.

- Predisposed breeds include collies and Doberman pinschers.
- Cutaneous signs:
  - Eighty per cent of cases have oral lesions (Figure 11.11).
  - Other mucous membranes of anus, vulva, prepuce and conjunctiva also involved.
  - Vesicles and bullae are rarely seen but occur at mucocutaneous junctions (Figure 11.12), skin especially axilla and groin. Usually secondary ulcerative lesions are present.

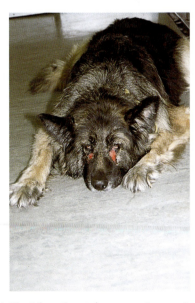

Figure 11.12 Ulceration at the mucocutaneous junctions in a German shepherd dog with bullous pemphigoid.

- Ulcerative paronychia, onychomadesis, footpad ulceration also seen.
- True Nikolsky sign not present.
- Pruritus, pain variable.
- Secondary pyoderma common:
  - Non-cutaneous signs.
  - Anorexia and pyrexia.

Differential diagnosis

- Pemphigus vulgaris
- Systemic lupus erythematosus
- Erythema multiforme
- Toxic epidermal necrolysis
- Drug eruption
- Epitheliotropic lymphoma

Diagnosis

- History and clinical signs.
- Cytology is not useful due to the depth of the damage in the skin; acanthocytes are not present.
- Skin or mucosal biopsy of primary lesion if present reveals subepidermal clefting and vesicles with a mild perivascular to lichenoid mononuclear and neutrophilic inflammation.
- Immunofluorescence or immunohistochemistry of skin biopsy specimens to detect immunoglobulin along the dermal–epidermal junction. False negative and positive results can occur; positive results should also have compatible histopathology.
- Bacteriology only isolates infection when it is there as a secondary problem.

Treatment

- Symptomatic therapy with gentle keratolytic shampoos such as sulphur may be useful.
- Antibacterial and anti-yeast therapy should be prescribed where appropriate and may need to be continued until the disease is under control.
- Spontaneous occurring bullous pemphigoid:
  - Immunosuppressive therapy is necessary; see Tables 11.1–11.3 below for drugs, monitoring and side effects in dogs and cats.
  - In view of the severity of bullous pemphigoid, several different immunosuppressive drugs may need to be used together. Glucocorticoids are usually used with a non-steroidal immunosuppressive drug.
  - Prognosis is moderate to poor in most cases and animals need long-term therapy and monitoring.
- Drug-induced bullous pemphigoid especially
  - home-cooked exclusion diet and supportive fluid therapy for 2 weeks before starting immunosuppressive treatment;
  - many dogs only require supportive therapy;
  - prognosis is good providing the drug is withdrawn.

Systemic lupus erythematosus (SLE)

Rare multisystemic autoimmune disease.

Cause and pathogenesis

Multifactorial disease; a variety of factors contribute to its pathogenesis including genetic susceptibility, immunological factors, drugs, viral infection, hormonal and ultraviolet light components; these are all thought to be important. Over reactive B cells produce antibodies against a variety of body tissues leading to immune complex formation and a type III hypersensitivity reaction. Skin lesions thought to be caused by autoantibodies to antigens on epidermal basal cells inducing antibody-dependent cytotoxicity.

Clinical signs

Dogs:

- No age or sex predilection.
- Predisposed dog breeds include collies, Shetland sheepdogs, and German shepherd dogs.
- Clinical signs are non-specific and wax and wane.

Table 11.5 Major and minor clinical signs seen in SLE.

Major signs	Minor signs
Joint disease – non-infectious usually non-erosive	Pyrexia – steroid responsive
Skin disease – variable, most commonly symmetrical, diffuse scale with scarring alopecia, lesions usually involve face, ears and distal limbs (Figures 11.13 and 11.14)	Central nervous system signs – seizures
Anaemia – Coomb's positive	Pleuritis – without evidence of infection
Thrombocytopaenia	
Glomerulonephritis with proteinuria	
Neutropaenia	
Polymyositis	

- Skin lesions are frequently seen in SLE and most commonly are those described under major signs in Table 11.5. Lesions though can mimic many other different diseases including
    - cutaneous or mucocutaneous vesiculobullous disorders,
    - footpad ulcers and hyperkeratosis,
    - refractory secondary bacterial pyoderma,
    - panniculitis.

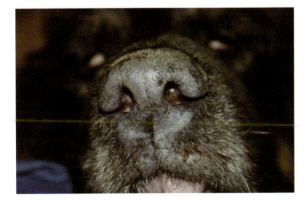

Figure 11.13 Inflammation of the planum nasale in a dog with SLE.

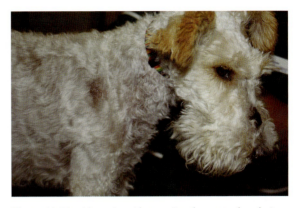

Figure 11.14 Alopecia with associated crust and scale in a dog with SLE.

- Multisystemic disease signs are seen in the approximate order of incidence within each column of Table 11.5.

Cats:

- No age or sex predilection.
- Predisposed breeds include Siamese, Persian, Himalayan cats.
- Cutaneous lesions seen in about 20% of cases include the following:
    - Generalised scaling disease
    - Exfoliative erythroderma
    - Paronychia
    - Erythematous, scaling and crusting alopecia involving the face, pinnae and paws
- Systemic signs that may be present include the following:
    - Weight loss
    - Glomerulonephritis
    - Haemolytic anaemia
    - Pyrexia
    - Polyarthritis
    - Neurological abnormalities
    - Myopathy
    - Oral ulceration (Figure 11.15)

Differential diagnosis

Almost any skin disease with multiple organ involvement including

- drug eruption,
- leishmaniasis,

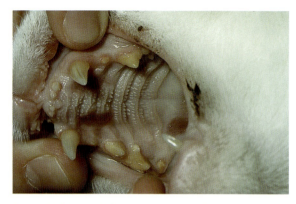

Figure 11.15 Oral ulceration in a cat with systematic lupus. (Source: Picture courtesy of J. Henfrey.)

- infection – bacterial, viral or fungal disease,
- neoplasia.

Diagnosis

- Systemic lupus is diagnosed by two major diagnostic signs or two minor and one major diagnostic sign with supporting serological evidence.
- Haematology may show any one or combination of anaemia (that may be Coombs positive), thrombocytopaenia, leukopaenia, leukocytosis.
- Urine analysis reveals proteinuria.
- Arthrocentesis in cases of polyarthritis reveals sterile purulent inflammation (positive Rheumatoid factor is a variable finding).
- Serology reveals a positive antinuclear antibody test (ANA) in 90% of cases. Useful supportive test but not diagnostic as false positives can occur with many other chronic diseases.
- Positive lupus erythematosus (LE) test is further diagnostic evidence but again by itself is not diagnostic.
- Cutaneous LE diagnosed by clinical signs and histopathology. Skin biopsy can be non diagnostic; however, changes of focal thickening of basement membrane zone, subepidermal vacuolation, hydropic or interface dermatitis or a leukocytoclastic vasculitis are highly suggestive of SLE.
- Immunofluorescence or immunohistochemistry of skin biopsy specimens can be used to detect immunoglobulin or complement at the basement membrane zone. False negative and positive results can occur; positive results should also have other compatible clinical findings.

Treatment

- Symptomatic therapy with gentle keratolytic shampoos such as sulphur may be useful.
- Antibacterial and anti-yeast therapy should be prescribed where appropriate and may need to be continued until the disease is under control.
- Success of treatment depends on the organ systems affected. When concurrent anaemia, thrombocytopaenia and neutropaenia are present, then the prognosis is more guarded.
- Topical therapy may be useful on localised nasal lesions (see Table 11.5).
- Systemic immunosuppressive therapy is used in the form of glucocorticoids (see Table 11.1). Non-steroidal immunosuppressive therapy may be used in combination with glucocorticoids, provided side effects of medication, e.g. myelosuppression, are not detrimental in therapy. All medication must be carefully monitored (see Table 11.3).

Discoid lupus erythematosus (DLE)

Uncommon cutaneous autoimmune disease with no evidence of systemic involvement seen in both dogs and cats.

Cause and pathogenesis

- Type III hypersensitivity is caused by autoantibodies to antigens on epithelial basal cells.
- Fifty per cent of cases are aggravated by ultraviolet light. Lesions therefore often start or are more severe in the summer/warm climates.

Immune mediated skin disease

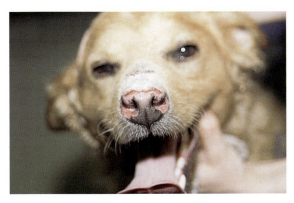

Figure 11.16 Ulceration and loss of normal architecture of nose in a collie with DLE.

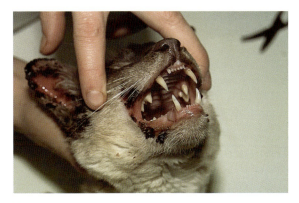

Figure 11.17 Facial lesions in DLE.

Clinical signs

Dogs:

- No age or sex predilection.
- Predisposed breeds include the Shetland sheepdog, German shepherd dog, collies and German short-haired pointers.
- Lesions usually occur on the nose. Acute signs reveal depigmentation and loss of normal architecture (Figure 11.16). Chronically these are replaced by erosions, ulcers and crusting.
- Less commonly periocular, pinnal, distal limbs, genitalia, lips and oral cavity affected.
- Footpad hyperkeratosis and oral ulcers are rare.
- Deep ulcers can cause haemorrhage.

Cats:

- No sex, age or breed predisposition.
- Lesions are confined usually to the face and ear pinnae (Figure 11.17), nasal signs less common.
- Initial signs are of erythema, alopecia and crusting, which will progress to ulceration.
- Paronychia can be seen (Figure 11.18).
- Pruritus variable.

Differential diagnosis

- Nasal pyoderma
- Dermatophytosis
- Dermatomyositis
- Pemphigus erythematosus/foliaceus
- Epitheliotropic lymphoma
- Drug reaction
- Uveodermatologic syndrome

Diagnosis

- History and clinical signs.
- Laboratory tests in the form of routine haematology and biochemistry are usually unremarkable. ANA commonly negative.
- Skin biopsy reveals signs of hydropic or lichenoid interface dermatitis with focal thickening of basement membrane zone. Pigment incontinence is a common finding with apoptotic keratinocytes.

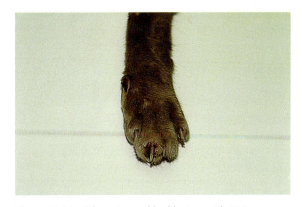

Figure 11.18 Ulcerative nail bed lesions with DLE.

- Immunofluorescence or immunohistochemistry of skin biopsy specimens can be used to detect patchy deposits of immunoglobulin or complement at the basement membrane zone. False negative and positive results can occur; positive results should also have other compatible clinical findings.

Treatment

- Prognosis good due to the localised nature of the disease.
- Sun avoidance should be undertaken from 8.00 a.m. to 5.00 p.m. Where possible, the animals should be taken out of the sun, or where practical topical sunscreens can be used.
- Symptomatic therapy with gentle keratolytic shampoos such as sulphur may be useful.
- Antibacterial and anti-yeast therapy should be prescribed where appropriate and may need to be continued until the disease is under control.
- Topical therapy is the treatment of choice (see Table 11.5) in mild to moderate cases.
- Systemic immunosuppressive therapy may also be used. In mild cases, non-steroidal immunosuppressive therapy with drugs such as vitamin E or doxycycline and niacinamide may be used before using glucocorticoids (Tables 11.1 and 11.2). All medication must be carefully monitored (see Table 11.3).

Vesicular cutaneous lupus erythematosus

Vesicular variant of cutaneous LE.

Cause and pathogenesis

Uncommon disease only recoded in dogs. Precise cause unknown but thought to be triggered by exposure to ultraviolet radiation. The disease was previously described as ulcerative dermatosis of Shetland sheepdogs and rough collies.

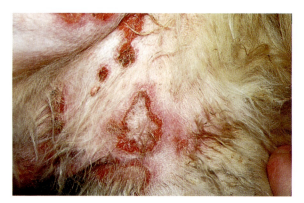

Figure 11.19 Serpiginous ulcers in the groin of a Sheltie with vesicular cutaneous LE.

Clinical signs

- Predisposed breeds include Shetland sheepdog and rough collie.
- Disease commonly occurs in adult dogs with no previous history of skin disease.
- Lesions show a marked seasonal incidence with most starting in the summer months. Many go into spontaneous remission in the winter.
- Vesiculobullous lesions are initially found in the groin and axilla. These are fragile and rapidly develop into crateriform and serpiginous ulcers (Figure 11.19).
- Eyelids, pinnae, mouth, external genitalia, anus and footpads occasionally involved.
- Lesions tend not to be pruritic but are painful.
- Affected dogs can develop secondary infection, which can lead to more severe generalised disease.
- Cyclical disease, which can make maintenance difficult.

Differential diagnosis

- Bullous pemphigoid
- Erythema multiforme
- SLE
- Pemphigus vulgaris
- Drug eruptions
- Epitheliotropic lymphoma

Diagnosis

- History and clinical signs especially in predisposed breed.
- Diagnostic rule outs of other differentials.
- Skin biopsy reveals signs of a lymphocytic interface dermatitis and folliculitis with vesiculation at dermo–epidermal junction.
- Immunofluorescence or immunohistochemistry of skin biopsy specimens can be used to detect deposits of immunoglobulin along the dermo–epidermal junction. False negative and positive results can occur; positive results should also have other compatible clinical findings.
- ANA tests are usually negative using conventional laboratory techniques.

Treatment

- Sun avoidance should be undertaken from 8.00 a.m. to 5.00 p.m. Where possible the animals should be taken out of the sun, or where practical topical sunscreens can be used.
- Antibacterial and anti-yeast therapy should be prescribed where appropriate and may need to be continued until the disease is under control.
- Topical therapy may be used to supplement systemic medication but is rarely enough by itself (see Table 11.5).
- Systemic immunosuppressive therapy is needed in most cases. The authors initial combination of choice would be glucocorticoids with azathioprine (see Tables 11.1 and 11.3 for drug regimes, monitoring and side effects in dogs). Prednisolone is initially used at a full immunosuppressive dose rate and tapered down to the lowest maintenance dose once clinical remission has been achieved (2–8 weeks). It is not uncommon to have to use several different immunosuppressive drugs together.
- In mild cases, non-steroidal immunosuppressive therapy with drugs such as vitamin E or doxycycline and niacinamide may be used before using glucocorticoids (Tables 11.1 and 11.2) or may be added in as secondary drugs where glucocorticoids are needed at high doses and/or produce unacceptable side effects.
- Prognosis is moderate in most cases; all animals need long-term therapy and monitoring.

Cold agglutinin disease (CAD)

Cause and pathogenesis

CAD is a type II hypersensitivity reaction associated with cold reacting autoantibodies to erythrocytes. Cryoglobulins and cryofibrinogens precipitate from serum and plasma, respectively, by cooling leading to vascular damage and clinical lesions. Autoantibodies are most active at temperatures from 0 to 4°C. Formation of antibodies may be idiopathic or associated with lead poisoning in dogs plus respiratory disease in cats. Rare disease of dogs and cats.

Clinical signs

- No age, sex or breed predilection.
- Lesions are typically seen on the extremities especially tips of ears, tail, nose and footpads.
- Initial lesions are painful and are erythematous with acrocyanosis and ulceration progressing to necrosis (Figures 11.20 and 11.21). Lesions have typical appearance of a punched-out ulcer.

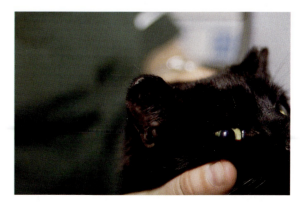

Figure 11.20 Ear tip slough in CAD.

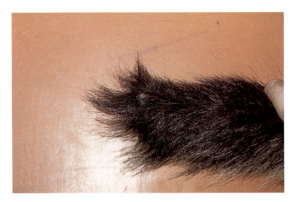

Figure 11.21 Necrosis of tip of tail due to CAD.

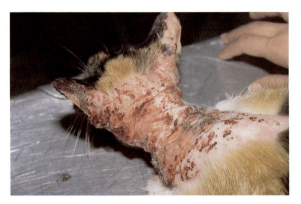

Figure 11.22 EM caused by carbimazole in a hyperthyroid cat.

- Seasonal disease seen in cold conditions in the winter as signs are only associated with exposure to cold.

Differential diagnosis

- Vasculitis
- SLE
- Frostbite
- Dermatomyositis
- Drug eruption

Diagnosis

- History and clinical signs.
- Diagnostic rule outs of other diseases.
- Typically autoagglutination is seen of blood in heparin or EDTA on slide at room temperature from affected animals. The reaction is accentuated by cooling to 0°C and reversed on warming to 37°C.
- Typically a Coomb's test at 4°C is positive.
- Skin biopsy reveals signs of necrosis and ulceration. In some cases vasculitis with thrombosis and necrosis of blood vessels is seen.

Treatment

- Where underlying triggers are recognised these must be corrected.
- Further exposure to cold should be avoided.

- Immunosuppressive therapy with systemic drugs is usually necessary to treat the vascular damage (see Tables 11.1 and 11.2).

Erythema multiforme (EM) and toxic epidermal necrolysis (TEN)

Cause and pathogenesis

The precise aetiology of these two diseases is unknown. They are thought to represent a cell mediated hypersensitivity reaction, which can be triggered by a variety of antigens including the following:

- Infections (bacteria, viruses)
- Drugs (Figure 11.22)
- Neoplasia
- Connective tissue disorders
- Idiopathic

Antigens lead to alteration in keratinocytes structure making them targets for an aberrant immune attack. It is not clear if EM and TEN represent separate diseases or TEN is a more severe form of EM.

Clinical signs

Erythema multiforme:

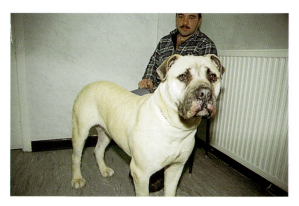

Figure 11.23 Ulceration around the mouth in a dog with EM due to potentiated sulphonamides.

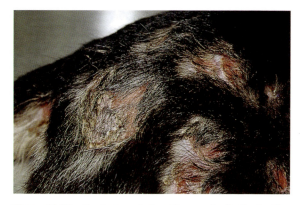

Figure 11.25 Erosions and ulceration on the flank of a dog with TEN.

- Cutaneous lesions:
    - Lesions have an acute onset and are multifocal to diffuse.
    - They affect mucocutaneous junctions (Figure 11.23), pinnae, axilla and groin.
    - Lesions can be variable in their presentation:
        - Erythematous annular 'bullseyes' (Figure 11.24).
        - Urticarial papules and plaques that spread peripherally.
        - Vesicles and bullae.
        - Scaling, crusting and alopecia less common.
- Non-cutaneous lesions:
    - Depression, anorexia, pyrexia

Toxic epidermal necrolysis:

- Cutaneous lesions:
    - Lesions can be found on any area of the body but especially mouth, mucocutaneous junctions and feet.
    - Lesions tend to be painful.
    - Present as vesicles, bullae, erosions, ulceration and necrosis (Figure 11.25).
- Non-cutaneous lesions:
    - Depression, anorexia, pyrexia often leading to collapse and death (Figure 11.26).

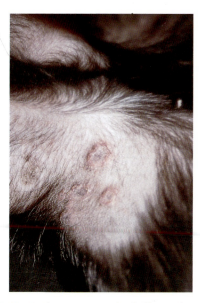

Figure 11.24 Erythematous annular 'bullseyes' lesions of EM on the flank of a dog.

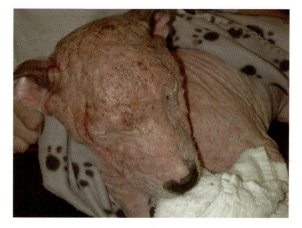

Figure 11.26 TEN in a young dog.

Differential diagnosis

- Thermal or chemical burn
- Pustular demodicosis
- Deep infection (bacterial or fungal)
- Urticaria
- Vasculitis
- Drug eruption
- Other autoimmune vesicular and pustular diseases

Diagnosis

- History and clinical signs.
- Laboratory rule out of other conditions.
- Skin biopsy reveals a variable picture depending on the type of lesion. In EM histopathological changes are confined to the epidermis where typically apoptosis is present. Epithelial cells of outer root sheath and hair follicle may be similarly affected. In TEN full thickness necrosis of the epidermis can be seen.

Treatment

- Where possible an underlying cause needs to be identified and treated.
- All drugs suspected of causing a reaction should be withdrawn. Substances in food have also been implicated as causes, so the author will generally put all animals on a home-cooked low-allergy diet.
- Symptomatic and supportive treatment should be given with whirlpool baths, fluid therapy and supportive nutrition.
- Treatment of secondary bacterial infection should be undertaken where necessary, but care should be taken not to use any drugs related to those previously administered.
- Mild cases of EM can spontaneously resolve with only supportive care.
- In severe cases of EM or TEN systemic therapy is needed using either glucocorticoids or immunoglobulin therapy (see Table 11.6).
- Prognosis is good to fair for EM but poor for TEN.

Table 11.6 Drug therapy for EM and TEN.

Drug	Protocol
Prednisolone	1–2 mg/kg (dog) or 2–4 mg/kg (cat) po sid for 7–14 days; therapy can be tapered once improvement is seen, aiming to withdraw it
Human intravenous immunoglobulin	5–6% solution in 0.9% saline; 0.5–1.0 g/kg given over 4–6 hours by slow iv infusion once or twice over 24 hours

Vasculitis

Cause and pathogenesis

- Type III hypersensitivity reaction leads to formation of immune complexes and subsequent blood vessel damage.
- A variety of causes have been implicated including the following:
  - Infection – bacterial, rickettsial, viral, fungal
  - Malignancy
  - Hypersensitivity to foods
  - Vaccination especially rabies vaccination
  - Connective tissue disease, e.g. rheumatoid arthritis
  - Metabolic disease, e.g. diabetes mellitus, uraemia
  - Drugs
  - Idiopathic

It is an uncommon disease in dogs and rare in cats.

Clinical signs

- No age or sex predisposition.
- Predisposed breeds include Rottweilers and dachshunds.
- Cutaneous lesions:

Immune mediated skin disease

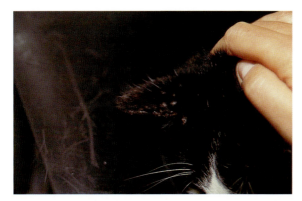

Figure 11.27 Punched-out ulcers on the ear of a cat with vasculitis.

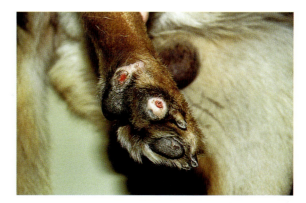

Figure 11.29 Punched-out ulcers on the footpads of a dog with vasculitis.

- ☐ Extremities usually affected especially ear pinnae (Figures 11.27 and 11.28) oral mucosa, footpads (Figures 11.29 and 11.30), tail and scrotum.
- ☐ Typical lesions are purpura, haemorrhagic bullae with punched-out ulcers.
- ☐ Pain variable.
- ☐ In cases of vasculitis caused by rabies vaccination, areas of alopecia develop at the site of the vaccination 1–5 months after administration. This is often followed by multifocal lesions caused by generalised ischaemic dermatopathy.
- ■ Non-cutaneous lesions:
  - ☐ Anorexia, lethargy, pyrexia.
  - ☐ Oedema of extremities.
  - ☐ Polyarthropathy, myopathy.

Differential diagnosis

- ■ SLE
- ■ CAD
- ■ Frostbite
- ■ EM/TEN
- ■ Bullous pemphigoid
- ■ Pemphigus vulgaris
- ■ Dermatomyositis

Diagnosis

- ■ History and clinical signs.
- ■ Diagnostic rule outs of other differentials.
- ■ Skin biopsy reveals signs of a neutrophilic, eosinophilic or lymphocytic vasculitis. In cases of rabies-induced vasculitis ischaemic dermatopathy with moderate follicular

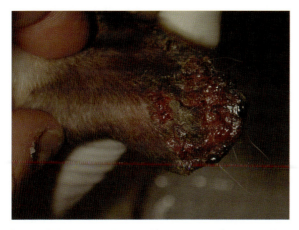

Figure 11.28 Vasculitis of the ear pinna due to a drug eruption.

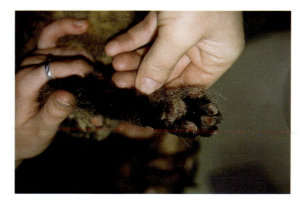

Figure 11.30 Ulceration of footpads due to vasculitis.

Table 11.7 Drugs for treatment of vasculitis.

Drug	Dosage regime
Prednisolone	1–2 mg/kg po (dogs) or 2–4 mg/kg po (cats) every 12 hours until lesions resolve (may take 2–4 weeks); then taper over next 8–10 weeks to the lowest possible alternate day dosage
Dexamethasone	0.05 mg/kg po every 12 hours until lesions resolve (2–4 weeks); then taper over next 8–10 weeks to the lowest possible alternate day dosage
Dapsone	(Dogs only) 1 mg/kg po qid until lesions resolve, which takes 2–4 weeks; once remission is achieved the drug is cut to twice, then once, then alternate day dosing aiming to withdraw
Sulphasalazine	10–20 mg/kg (up to 3 g daily) po qid until remission is achieved (2–4 weeks); once remission is achieved the dose rate is cut to twice, then once, then alternate days aiming to withdraw the drug
Tetracycline/ niacinamide	See dose rates in Table 10.3; drugs are given qid to achieve remission (2–4 weeks), then tapered to at least daily medication
Pentoxifylline	(Dogs only) 10–15 mg/kg po qid ± vitamin E 400 IU po bid
Other anti-inflammatory drugs	Drugs such as azathioprine, cyclophosphamide, chlorambucil and cyclosporine may be used for disease; see Table 11.1

atrophy, hyalinisation of collagen, cell poor interface dermatitis and mural folliculitis can be seen.

Treatment

- Identification and treatment of underlying cause where possible.
- Therapy can be undertaken with a variety of different drugs in both the dog and cat (see Table 11.7).
- In many cases after 4–6 months therapy can be discontinued. The prognosis of this disease depends on the underlying cause that precipitates the immune reaction.

Cutaneous drug reactions

Uncommon cutaneous or mucocutaneous reaction to a drug.

Cause and pathogenesis

Route of administration is variable. Drugs may be administered orally, topically or injected. Reactions can occur after the first, second or several treatments with the drug. It is an uncommon disease in both dogs and cats.

Type of reactions:

- Predictable – dose dependent, related to pharmalogical action of the drug.
- Unpredictable – idiosyncratic reaction or drug intolerance.

Groups of drugs leading to reactions:

- Antibiotics, especially potentiated sulphonamides
- Non-steroidal anti-inflammatory drugs
- Anthelmintics
- Vaccines

Clinical signs

- Many different cutaneous patterns can be associated with drug reactions, these include
  - papules and plaques,
  - urticaria, angioedema (Figure 11.31),
  - scaling and exfoliation,
  - EM,

Immune mediated skin disease

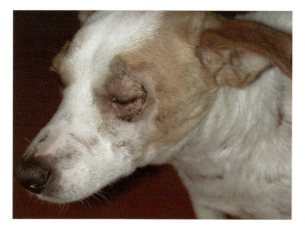

Figure 11.31 Periocular urticaria in a dog due to an allergic reaction to an anaesthetic agent.

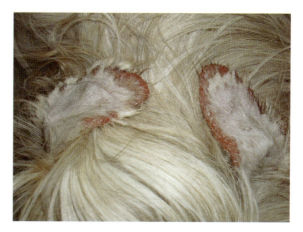

Figure 11.33 Vasculitis of ear tip due to an ampicillin reaction.

- TEN,
- vesicles and bullae, e.g. bullous pemphigoid (Figure 11.32),
- pustular disease, e.g. pemphigus foliaceus,
- vasculitis (Figure 11.33).
- Drug reactions can mimic almost any disease and can be localised, multifocal or diffuse.
- Onset of reaction is usually within 2 weeks of the drugs administration.
- Non-cutaneous signs can include
  - pyrexia and depression,
  - lameness – polyarthropathy,
  - ocular disease – keratoconjunctivitis sicca.

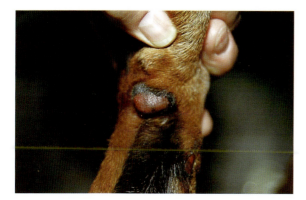

Figure 11.32 Drug eruption in a Doberman due to potentiated sulphonamides; histologically this appeared as bullous pemphigoid like.

- Resolution 10–14 days after withdrawal of drug.

Differential diagnosis

- Almost any other disease.

Diagnosis

- History is especially important in drug eruptions.
- Diagnostic rule outs of other differentials.
- Haematology and biochemistry may show a variety but inconsistent range of changes.
- Biopsy reveals many different patterns. No one specific pattern is diagnostic. However, necrotic keratinocytes often seen throughout the epidermis in drug eruptions.

Treatment

- Discontinuation of offending drug leads to resolution of clinical signs within 2–3 weeks.
- Symptomatic and supportive treatment for clinical signs are important, e.g. fluid therapy, whirlpool baths, etc.
- Avoid chemically related drugs at any stage in the future.

- Drug therapy may be undertaken in severe cases with either glucocorticoids in the form of prednisolone or human intravenous immunoglobulin (see Table 11.6).

Canine Linear IgA Dermatosis

Cause and pathogenesis

Immunological disease leading to subcorneal pustules with IgA deposited at basement membrane zone. The precise cause of the clinical lesions is unknown.

Clinical signs

- No sex or age predisposition.
- Only recognised in dachshunds.
- Multifocal to generalised pustules usually on the trunk.
- Secondary lesions appear as annular areas of alopecia, epidermal collarettes with some hyperpigmentation, scaling and crusting.
- Pruritus is generally mild.

Differential diagnosis

- Bacterial folliculitis
- Dermatophytosis
- Demodicosis
- Sterile pustular disease, e.g. pemphigus foliaceus, subcorneal pustular dermatosis

Diagnosis

- History and clinical signs especially in predisposed breeds.
- Diagnostic rule outs of other diseases.
- Cytology of pustules reveals evidence of non-degenerate neutrophils, rare acanthocytes and no evidence of bacterial infection.
- Culture in uncomplicated cases is usually sterile.
- Skin biopsy reveals signs of intraepidermal pustules with numerous non-degenerate neutrophils and occasional acanthocytes.
- Immunofluorescence or immunohistochemical testing reveals evidence of IgA deposited at basement membrane zone.

Treatment

- Symptomatic therapy with mild anti-seborrhoeic shampoo, e.g. sulphur;
- prednisolone 2.2–4.4 mg/kg po sid until remission achieved then alternate days for maintenance; or
- dapsone 1 mg/kg po tid until remission then as required.

Amyloidosis

Rare cutaneous manifestation of abnormal extracellular deposition of one of the family of unrelated amyloid proteins.

Cause and pathogenesis

Amyloid can accumulate in both internal organs and the skin produced due to a variety of different pathogenic mechanisms including chronic inflammatory disease especially renal disease and neoplasia.

Clinical signs

- Cutaneous signs:
  - Solitary or grouped dermal or subcutaneous nodules and plaques; any site but especially the ears.
  - Tongue, gingiva, footpads and pressure points can be affected with whitish oozing plaques and papules.
  - Cutaneous haemorrhage has been reported in some cases of amyloidosis when the skin is affected.
- Non-cutaneous signs:
  - Clinical signs depend on the organ systemically involved. Amyloid may be deposited in kidneys, spleen and liver.

Differential diagnosis

- Neoplasia
- Infectious nodular granulomas
- Sterile nodular granulomas

Diagnosis

- History, especially of chronic internal disease, plus clinical signs.
- Diagnostic rule outs of other diseases.
- Skin biopsy reveals deposition of eosinophilic amorphous substance that is congophilic and bifringent when polarised.

Treatment

- Solitary nodules without internal disease best resolved by surgical incision.
- Where associated with systemic disease or where multiple nodules are identified, treatment is rarely successful and the prognosis is guarded.

Alopecia areata

Cause and pathogenesis

Thought to be immunological attack mediated by both humoral and cell mediated mechanisms on antigens in the wall of the hair follicle leading to non-inflammatory hair loss. It is a rare disease in both the dog and cat.

Clinical signs

- No sex or breed predilection.
- Most commonly occurs in adult animals.
- Focal or multifocal patches of asymptomatic non-inflammatory alopecia especially on head (muzzle, periocular areas, ears, chin and forehead) neck, trunk.
- Facial lesions can be bilaterally symmetrical.
- Skin in chronic areas of alopecia can become hyperpigmented.
- Leukotrichia can also be seen.

Differential diagnosis

- Injection site reaction
- Demodicosis
- Dermatophytosis
- Superficial folliculitis
- Traction alopecia

Diagnosis

- History and clinical signs.
- Diagnostic rule outs of other differentials.
- Trichography reveals signs of typical 'exclamation point' hairs, which have a tapered end and are dysplastic.
- Skin biopsy: typically early lesions reveals signs of peribulbar and intrabulbar lymphocytes, histiocytes and plasma cells – 'swarm of bees'. Chronic lesions show signs of follicular atrophy and predominantly catagen and telogen follicles, later lesions; hair follicles are completely destroyed. Changes are not seen on all biopsies so that multiple biopsies are usually needed to find characteristic histopathological findings.

Treatment

- No specific treatment has been described.
- Many cases will recover spontaneously in 6 months to 2 years.
- Topical therapy can be undertaken with glucocorticoids, cyclosporine or tacrolimus used daily on affected areas until hair growth restarts.
- Systemic glucocorticoids with immunosuppressive doses of glucocorticoids (see Table 11.1) may be used but have a variable success rate.
- Prognosis for a complete hair regrowth is moderate. Hair loss is essentially cosmetic and does not affect the dog's general health.

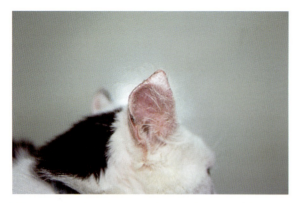

Figure 11.34 Polychondritis showing deformity of the ear pinna.

Relapsing polychondritis

Rare immune mediated disease caused by inflammation and destruction of both articular and non-articular cartilaginous structures.

Cause and pathogenesis

- Precise aetiology unknown; thought to be an immune mediated attack on type II collagen.
- Rare disease only reported in cats. All reported cases have been either FeLV or FIV positive

Clinical signs

- No age, sex or breed predisposition.
- Lesions affect the ear pinnae.
- Acutely painful, swollen, erythematous/violaceous pinnae becoming curled and deformed (Figure 11.34).
- Systemic signs variable; cats may be quiet, pyrexic and anorexic.

Differential diagnosis

- Trauma
- Aural haematoma
- Actinic damage
- Neoplasia – squamous cell carcinoma
- Hyperadrenocorticism

Diagnosis

- History and clinical signs.
- Diagnostic rule outs of other disease.
- Skin biopsy of ear pinna reveals signs of lymphoplasmacytic inflammation with cartilage necrosis.

Treatment

- Permanent deformity of the pinna occurs whether the cat is treated or not.
- Immunosuppressive therapy with either prednisolone (see Table 11.2) or dapsone (1 mg/kg sid po) may be effective.

Sterile nodular panniculitis

Cause and pathogenesis

- An inflammatory disease of subcutaneous fat, which is found in both the dog and cat. It is a rare disease in both species.
- Lesions can occur as
  - solitary lesions, which can be associated with trauma, foreign bodies or idiopathic;
  - multiple lesions associated with immune mediated disease such as SLE, pancreatic dysfunction or idiopathic.

Clinical signs

- Cutaneous signs:
  - Solitary lesions:
    - Deep-seated cutaneous nodule often ulcerated with an oily/yellow often haemorrhagic discharge (Figure 11.35). They are a few millimetres to centimetres in diameter and may be found on the flanks, neck, abdomen (Figure 11.36).

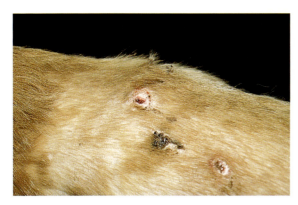

Figure 11.35 Deep-seated nodules producing a haemorrhagic fluid on the dorsum of a dog with idiopathic sterile panniculitis.

- Multiple lesions:
  - As solitary lesions, but usually occur in crops on dorsum and flanks.
- Non-cutaneous signs:
  - Inappetence, depression, lethargy.
  - Abdominal pain, vomiting seen with pancreatic involvement.

Differential diagnosis

- Infectious panniculitis of bacterial, mycobacterial, actinomycotic, fungal origin
- Foreign body/injection reaction
- Sterile pyogranulomatous disease
- Neoplasia
- Vitamin E deficiency (steatitis in cats)

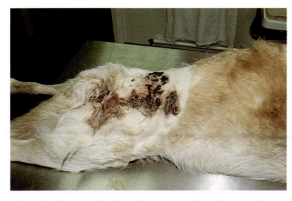

Figure 11.36 Sterile idiopathic panniculitis showing the typical distribution pattern.

Diagnosis

- History and clinical signs.
- Cytology of direct smear and fine needle aspirate reveals signs of neutrophils and foamy macrophages (which contain lipid). In uncomplicated cases no micro-organisms are present.
- Skin biopsy in the form of an excisional biopsy of a nodule is the best way to establish a diagnosis. Special stains are usually necessary to rule out infective organisms. Histopathology reveals signs of a suppurative, granulomatous to pyogranulomatous fibrosing septal of diffuse panniculitis.
- Microbial cultures if taken carefully are negative for aerobic, anaerobic, mycobacterial and fungal culture.
- Blood samples are necessary if underlying disease such as systemic lupus or pancreatic neoplasia is thought to be present.

Treatment

- Solitary lesions – surgical excision.
- Multiple lesions (see Table 11.8).
- Prognosis is moderately good, provided that there is no underlying disease present.

Proliferative arteritis of the nasal philtrum

Cause and pathogenesis

Proliferative arteritis is a rare but distinctive skin disease affecting the nasal philtrum in dogs.

Clinical signs

- No sex predisposition.
- Affected animals were 3–6 years of age.
- St Bernards, Newfoundlands as well as other large dogs may be predisposed.

Table 11.8 Drugs useful for the therapy of sterile nodular panniculitis.

Drug	Dosage	Details
Tetracycline/niacinamide	Dogs >10 kg 500 mg of each drug tid Dogs <10 kg 250 mg of each drug tid	Daily tid dosage up to 3 months to resolve lesions, then bid for 4–6 weeks then sid for maintenance
Doxycycline/niacinamide	Niacinamide as above Doxycycline 10 mg/kg bid	Niacinamide as above Doxycycline bid until response, then tapered to lowest possible maintenance dose
Cyclosporine	5 mg/kg po sid	Given daily until remission 6–8 weeks; then give eod for 4 weeks, then every 72 hours for 4 weeks then withdrawn if possible
Prednisolone	2 mg/kg (dog) or 4 mg/kg (cat) po sid or methyl prednisolone 1.6 mg/kg (dog) po sid	Dosage is given daily until remission 2–8 weeks, then tapered slowly to lowest dose rate with a view to withdrawal
Vitamin E	400 IU twice daily	May not control disease but can be sued as a steroid sparing medication

- Lesions present as well-demarcated linear ulcers affecting the nasal philtrum (Figure 11.37).
- Ulcers variable in size from 3–5 cm in length to 2–15 mm in width.
- Dogs develop signs of arterial haemorrhage from the ulcers.

Differential diagnosis

- Vasculitis
- Frostbite

Diagnosis

- History and clinical signs.
- Skin biopsy using a small punch biopsy from the periphery of the lesion. Histopathology reveals large V-shaped ulcers with subepidermal fibrosis and pigmentary incontinence. Exocytosis of inflammatory cells into the epidermis. Deep dermal arteries beneath the ulcer show subendothelial intimal proliferation of spindle cells, which leads to thickening and stenosis of vessels.

Treatment

- Topical therapy:
  - Tacrolimus may be useful if the animal will tolerate application.
- Systemic medication:
  - Glucocorticoids at anti-inflammatory dose rates of 1–2 mg/kg po sid for 14 days, then cut to alternate days and taper as required.

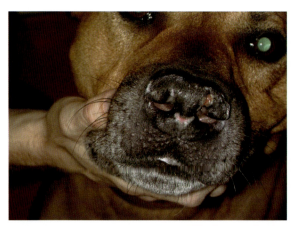

Figure 11.37 Proliferative arteritis of the planum nasale in a Rhodesian ridgeback.

- Pentoxifylline given at a dose of 10–25 mg/kg po bid/tid may act as a peripheral dilator and may also decrease production of fibrous tissue. May take 4 weeks to see full benefit.

Selected references and further reading

Hall, J. (2004) Erythema multiforme and toxic epidermal necrolysis. In: Campbell, K.L. (ed) *Small Animal Dermatology Secrets*. pp. 243–250. Hanley and Belfus, Philadelphia

Jackson, H.A. and Olivry, T. (2004) Ulcerative dermatosis of the Shetland sheepdog and rough collies: Clinical management and prognosis. *Vet Dermatol*, **15**, 37–41

Marsella, R. (2000) Canine pemphigus complex, diagnosis and therapy. *Compend Contin Educ Pract Vet*, **22**, 680–689

Medleau, L. and Hnilica, K. (2006) Autoimmune and immune-mediated skin disorders. In: *Small Animal Dermatology: A Color Atlas and Therapeutic Guide*. 2nd edn. pp. 189–228. WB Saunders, Philadelphia

Morris, D.O. (2004) Vasculitis and vasculopathy. In: Campbell, K.L. (ed) *Small Animal Dermatology Secrets*. pp. 254–260. Hanley and Belfus, Philadelphia

Nichols, P.R. et al. (2001) A retrospective study of canine and feline vasculitis. *Vet Dermatol*, **12**, 255–264

Rosenkrantz, W.S. (2004) Pemphigus: Current therapy. *Vet Dermatol*, **15**, 90–98

Scott, D.W. et al. (2001) Immune mediated diseases. *Muller and Kirk's Small Animal Dermatology*. 6th edn. pp. 667–779. WB Saunders, Philadelphia

Torres, S. (2004) Immune mediated skin disease. In: Campbell, K.L. (ed) *Small Animal Dermatology Secrets*. pp. 231–243. Hanley and Belfus, Philadelphia

White, S.D. (2000) Nonsteroidal immunosuppressive therapy, Bonagura (ed) In: *Kirk's Current Veterinary Therapy XIII Small Animal Practice*. pp. 536–538. WB Saunders, Philadelphia

12 Alopecia

Alopecia in the dog and cat will be discussed under four main headings detailed below:

(1) Follicular dystrophy
   (a) Congenital
      - Non-colour linked:
         □ Tardive onset
         □ Congenital hypotrichosis
         □ Pili torti
      - Colour linked:
         □ Colour dilute alopecia
         □ Black hair follicular dystrophy
   (b) Acquired
      - Anagen defluxion
(2) Hair cycle abnormalities
   (a) Alopecia associated with systemic disease, e.g. hyperadrenocorticism.
   (b) Alopecia of unknown cause, but where cycle arrest occurs this is a large group that includes the following:
      □ Post-clipping alopecia
      □ Alopecia X/growth hormone responsive dermatosis/adrenal sex hormone responsive dermatosis/congenital adrenal hyperplasia/castration responsive dermatosis
      □ Pattern baldness
      □ Idiopathic cyclic flank alopecia
      □ Telogen defluvium
      □ Idiopathic bald thigh syndrome of greyhounds
      □ Feline-acquired symmetrical alopecia
      □ Pancreatic paraneoplastic alopecia
      □ Feline preauricular and pinnal alopecia
      □ Hyperadrenocorticism
(1) Traumatic alopecia
   (a) Loss of normal hair
   (b) Loss of abnormal hair
(2) Scarring alopecia
   (a) Primary scarring
   (b) Secondary scarring

Follicular dystrophy

Abnormal hairs or follicles are formed due to abnormal development or growth of the hair.

This does not necessarily cause an alopecia although often does. It can be congenital or acquired.

Congenital follicular dystrophy

Non-colour linked follicular dystrophy

Hair loss is caused by abnormal hair follicle development or else structural abnormalities. Hair loss is not colour linked and shows no seasonal pattern.

Tardive onset
Affects a variety of different breeds and progresses slowly from puppyhood.

Clinical signs
- Doberman pinscher:
  - Black or red dogs affected.
  - Hair loss is often seen first at 1–4 years of age. Alopecia starts on the flanks and will spread caudodorsally (Figures 12.1 and 12.2).
  - Secondary bacterial infection is common.
- Siberian husky, malamute:
  - Hair loss is seen on trunks at 3–4 months of age.
  - Coat turned reddish.
  - Areas clipped for biopsies do not regrow.
- Irish water spaniel, Portuguese water dog:
  - Hair loss on the ventral neck and tail is normal for water dogs.
  - Irish water spaniel dystrophic alopecia affects neck, flanks, trunk and thigh:
    - In males hair loss starts in middle age and is non-seasonal and progressive.

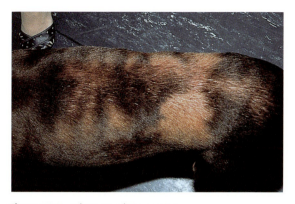

Figure 12.2 Close-up of Figure 12.1.

  - In females hair loss starts 6–8 weeks after first/second season and will regrow 3–4 weeks later.
  - Portuguese water dog dystrophic alopecia affects the flanks, caudodorsal trunk and periocularly (Figure 12.3).
    - Hair loss waxes and wanes but will grow back in many dogs. New hair is of poor quality and at each cycle less hair grows back leading to permanent alopecia.

Differential diagnosis
- Dermatophytosis
- Demodicosis
- Endocrine alopecia
- Superficial bacterial folliculitis

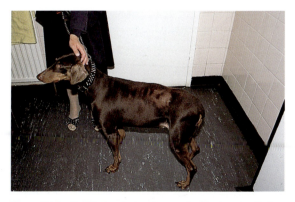

Figure 12.1 Follicular dystrophy on the flanks of a Doberman.

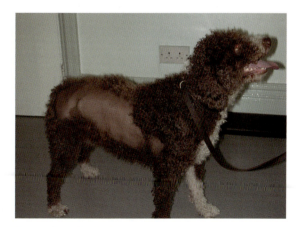

Figure 12.3 Follicular dysplasia in a Portuguese water spaniel.

Diagnosis
- History and clinical signs.
- Trichography of plucked hairs mounted in liquid paraffin reveals defects in cuticle, and hair cortices and medulla contain numerous large melanin clumps.
- Skin biopsy reveals the presence of dilated hair follicles filled with keratin, hair shaft fragments and melanin. Abnormal clumps of melanin are also apparent in follicular and epidermal basal cell layer and hair matrix cells.

Treatment
None.

Congenital hypotrichosis
Cause and pathogenesis
Dogs and cats with congenital hypotrichosis are born without hair. They do not have a follicular dystrophy but an ectodermal defect.

Clinical signs
- Most dogs and cats with congenital hypotrichosis are born with complete hair coat or with only partial loss of hair, which progresses through dystrophic change to almost whole body alopecia within 4 months. In some cases whiskers, claws and papillae on the tongue can be affected.
- Predisposed dog breeds: poodles (toy and miniature), whippets, beagle, Rottweiler, Yorkshire terrier, American cocker spaniel, Belgian shepherd dog, Labrador retriever. Chinese crested dog is a hairless breed where alopecia is caused through follicular dystrophy (Figures 12.4 and 12.5).
- Predisposed cat breeds include Birman, Burmese, Devon Rex and Siamese.

Differential diagnosis
- Demodicosis
- Nutritional deficiencies
- Dermatophytosis
- Pili torti

Diagnosis
- History and clinical signs.
- Diagnostic rule outs of other differential.

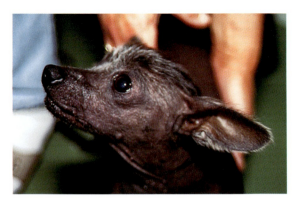

Figure 12.4 Chinese crested dog; naturally hairless breed due to follicular dystrophy.

- Skin biopsy reveals a variety of changes ranging from the presence of dystrophic hair follicles to complete lack of follicles often with similar changes in the adnexal glands.

Treatment
None.

Pili torti
Cause and pathogenesis
Rare disease caused by curvature of the hair follicle leading to a flattening and rotation of the hair shaft.

Clinical signs
- No breed or sex predilection.
- Young kittens are affected.
- Generalised hair loss occurs by 10 days of age.

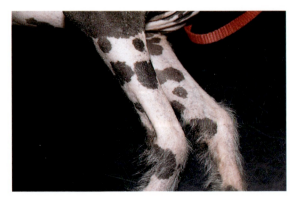

Figure 12.5 Alopecia of legs of Chinese crested dog showing comedones.

- Periocular and pedal dermatitis is commonly seen as well as paronychia.

Differential diagnosis
As congenital hypotrichosis.

Diagnosis
- History and clinical signs.
- Trichography of plucked hairs mounted in liquid paraffin reveals that all secondary hairs are flattened and rotated.
- Skin biopsy is not diagnostic. It reveals signs of hyperkeratosis and cystic dilatation of follicles.

Treatment
None.

Colour linked follicular dystrophy

Colour dilution alopecia (colour mutant alopecia)
Associated with blue (dilute black) or fawn (dilute brown) coat colours.

Cause and pathogenesis
Genetic factors appear to be important. Dystrophic change is associated with dilute-coloured hair, which has defective hair pigmentation in the form of large pigment granules, which leads to the formation of abnormal hair. In some cases lethal pigment changes cause hair loss due to shaft fractures.

Clinical signs
- Predisposed breeds include Doberman, dachshund, Great Dane, Yorkshire terrier (Figure 12.6), whippet, greyhound, miniature pinscher, Saluki, chow chow, Boston terrier, Shetland sheepdog, Chihuahua, poodles and Irish setter.
- Tardive condition as dog's hair coat appears normal at birth but hair loss becomes noticeable from 6 months of age.
- Lesions start dorsally as hypotrichosis, usually with bacterial folliculitis (Figure 12.7) and can become generalised.
- Non-colour dilute areas remain unaffected.

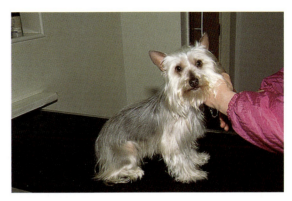

Figure 12.6 Blue colour dilute Yorkshire terrier.

Differential diagnosis
- Dermatophytosis
- Demodicosis
- Superficial bacterial folliculitis
- Endocrine skin disease especially hypothyroidism

Diagnosis
- History and clinical signs especially coat colour.
- Diagnostic rule outs of other differentials.
- Trichography of plucked hairs mounted in mineral oil reveals cortices and medullas contain numerous large pigment granules of irregular shape and size. Hair shafts are often fractured.
- Skin biopsy of colour dilute areas reveals dilated cystic keratin-filled follicles. Abnormal clumps of melanin are present in hair and

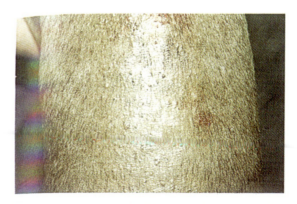

Figure 12.7 Dorsum of blue Doberman showing comedone formation, diffuse alopecia and folliculitis.

peribulbar melanophages, and epidermal and follicular basal cells with associated pigment incontinence.

Treatment
- No specific therapy is available other than symptomatic treatment to make the dog feel comfortable and prevent infection.
- Symptomatic treatment of secondary infection with appropriate antibiotics.
- Avoid harsh shampoos and excessive grooming as this increases hair loss due to shaft fracture, but gentle shampoo therapy with mild antiseborrhoeic and/or antibacterial product is useful.
- Prognosis is good in that this is only a cosmetic problem albeit a lifetime condition.

Black/dark hair follicular dystrophy
Cause and pathogenesis
A familial disease that is only seen in bicoloured or tricoloured puppies; only the black/dark hair affected. A defect in hair growth is thought to be associated with disorder of pigment transfer.

Clinical signs
- Predisposed breeds include the bearded collie, basset hounds, Saluki, beagle, dachshund, pointer, also bi- and tricoloured crossbreeds.
- Dogs appear to have a normal hair coat at birth; however, progressive loss of weaken black hairs occurs due to shaft fracture from 4 weeks of age.
- Alopecia areas can give appearance of complete alopecia or short stubble (Figures 12.8–12.10).

Differential diagnosis
- Demodicosis
- Dermatophytosis
- Superficial bacterial folliculitis
- Endocrine alopecia

Diagnosis
- History and clinical signs especially the coat colour.
- Trichography of plucked hairs mounted in mineral oil reveals cortices, and medullas

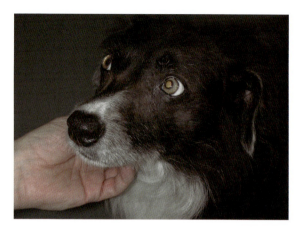

Figure 12.8 Black-haired follicular dystrophy in a collie.

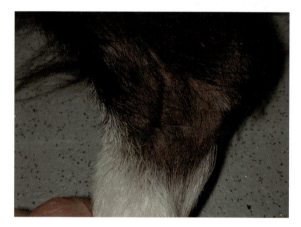

Figure 12.9 Black-haired follicular dystrophy affecting the legs in a collie.

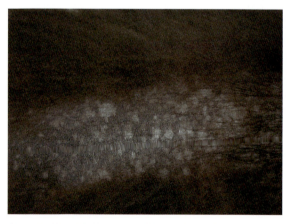

Figure 12.10 Black-haired follicular dystrophy affecting the dorsum in a collie.

contain numerous large melanin clumps. Hair cuticles have defective shafts, which are often fractured.
- Skin biopsy of black-haired areas reveals dilated cystic keratin-filled follicles. Abnormal clumps of melanin are present in epidermal and follicular basal cells and hair matrix cells. Samples from non–black-haired areas are completely normal.

Treatment
As colour dilution alopecia.

Acquired follicular dystrophy

Anagen defluvium

Cause and pathogenesis
Anagen growth phase is temporarily halted leading to abnormalities of the hair. The hair is usually lost within days of insult as the resulting dystrophic change is incompatible with normal hair growth. An uncommon disease in dogs and cats; it can be caused by a range of factors including

- antimitotic drugs, e.g. cancer, chemotherapy,
- infectious disease,
- endocrine disease,
- metabolic disease.

Clinical signs
- Hair loss starts acutely within days of the insult to the skin.
- Diffuse and widespread hair loss over most of the body (Figure 12.11), often sparing the head.
- Shed hair appears to be relatively normal.
- No primary lesions are present.

Differential diagnosis
- Endocrine alopecia
- Superficial folliculitis
- Demodicosis
- Dermatophytosis

Diagnosis
- History of previous insult to hair cycle and clinical signs.

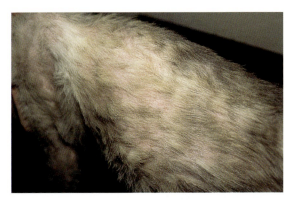

Figure 12.11 Anagen defluxion causing diffuse hair loss in a cat on chemotherapy.

- Trichography of plucked hairs in mineral oil reveals no sign of trauma to the tips, no shaft abnormalities, and bulbs are exclusively in anagen.
- Skin biopsy is often normal and is only useful before hair is lost completely. In the acute stages, abnormal hair matrix cells with dysplastic hair shafts may be seen.

Treatment
- None is necessary, provided the inciting factor is identified and removed.
- Prognosis is good and normal hair should grow back once the insult to the skin has resolved.

Hair cycle abnormalities

Hair cycle abnormalities result in alopecia when the anagen phase of the hair cycle is shortened or the telogen phase of the hair cycle is lengthened. In some cases, hair may be miniaturised due to changes in cycle length. Suspended animation can occur as hair cycle halts in telogen.

No further growth appears and hairs are retained for long periods in some cases or may be lost due to normal wear and tear.

Causes
- Alopecia associated with systemic disease, e.g. hyperadrenocorticism (see Chapter 8).

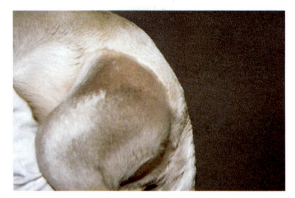

Figure 12.12 Post-clipping alopecia in a Labrador. All endocrine tests were normal in this dog. Hair grew back after approximately 12 months.

- Alopecia of unknown cause, but where cycle arrest occurs this is a large group that includes the following:
    - Post-clipping alopecia
    - Alopecia X/growth hormone responsive dermatosis/adrenal sex hormone responsive dermatosis/congenital adrenal hyperplasia/castration responsive dermatosis
    - Pattern baldness
    - Idiopathic cyclic flank alopecia
    - Telogen defluvium
    - Idiopathic bald thigh syndrome of greyhounds
    - Feline-acquired symmetrical alopecia
    - Pancreatic paraneoplastic alopecia
    - Feline preauricular and pinnal alopecia

Post-clipping alopecia

Cause and pathogenesis
- Hair fails to grow in areas that have been clipped either due to a presurgical clip (Figure 12.12) or part of the normal grooming process.
- Uncommon disease only found in dogs.
- Any breed can be affected but the chow chow and Siberian husky appear to be predisposed.
- Cycle arrest occurs at the time of clipping; hair will normally start to regrow after 3–4 months.

Clinical signs
- Unclipped areas of hair appear to be normal.
- Clipped areas appear alopecic due to the presence of short stubble; the coat, where present, is normal.

Differential diagnosis
- Endocrine diseases
- Telogen defluvium
- Follicular dystrophy
- Demodicosis
- Dermatophytosis

Diagnosis
- History and clinical signs.
- Diagnostic rule outs of other differentials.
- Skin biopsy may fail to reveal signs of abnormality. In some cases hairs appear to be in catagen arrest.

Treatment
- Hair will eventually regrow as hair cycle restarts, but can take up to 24 months in the plush-coated breeds.
- Hair growth stimulants have no proven benefit in therapy.
- Prognosis is good.

Alopecia X

Growth hormone responsive dermatosis/adrenal sex hormone responsive dermatosis/congenital adrenal hyperplasia/castration responsive dermatosis.

This disease represents a category of hair cycle arrest alopecia that is poorly understood. Various treatment modalities have been used to restart the hair cycle.

Cause and pathogenesis
Cycle arrest occurs in all cases so that hairs stay in telogen in suspended animation. Several theories exist for the pathogenesis including abnormal adrenal sex hormone imbalance and a growth hormone deficiency. Most recent work suggests that hair loss may be due to a local follicular receptor dysregulation. Uncommon disease only recognised in dogs.

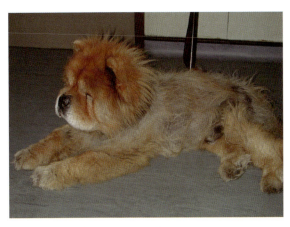

Figure 12.13 Alopecia X in a chow chow.

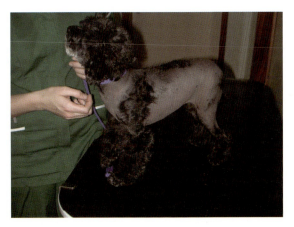

Figure 12.15 Progressive hair loss in a miniature poodle with Alopecia X.

Clinical signs
- Reported in young dogs usually aged 2–5 years.
- Predisposed breeds include the chow chow (Figure 12.13), Samoyed, keeshond, Pomeranian (Figure 12.14), Alaskan malamute, Siberian husky and miniature poodle.
- Hair coat becomes faded; truncal alopecia often starts in perineum and inguinal areas. Hair loss is progressive leading to complete alopecia of neck, tail, caudodorsal areas, perineum and caudal thighs (Figure 12.15).
- Head and neck tend to be spared but coat is made of secondary hairs, which have the appearance of 'puppy coat' (Figure 12.16).
- Alopecic skin may become hyperpigmented and thinned.
- Secondary seborrhoea and pyoderma can be present.

Differential diagnosis
- Endocrine alopecia
- Telogen defluxion

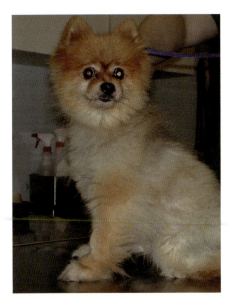

Figure 12.14 Alopecia X in a Pomeranian.

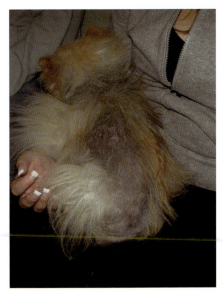

Figure 12.16 Alopecia X in a Pomeranian showing loss of dorsal hairs.

- Demodicosis
- Dermatophytosis

Diagnosis
- History and clinical signs especially in a predisposed breed.
- Diagnostic rule outs of other causes of alopecia.
- Skin biopsy reveals non-specific endocrine-type changes
- ACTH stimulation test (sex hormone assay profile – SHAP) may be performed by measuring cortisol and selected sex hormones before and after stimulation. Interpretation of results can be difficult due to false positive and negative results and lack of breed data for normal parameters.

Treatment
- Observation without undertaking therapy is appropriate in many cases due to the fact that hair loss is purely cosmetic and dogs are otherwise well.
- Neutering of intact male and female dogs may help with hair regrowth, but this is not a consistent finding.
- Medical therapy has been shown to be capable of producing some improvement but not a consistent finding:
    - Melatonin 3–12 mg/dog po sid–qid until maximum hair growth occurs. Levels can then be tapered every 2 months using 3–6 mg daily, then alternate days, every third day, then twice weekly. Side effects are rare.
    - Trilostane has been shown to be beneficial in some dogs. Various protocols have been suggested, including dogs <2.5 kg, 20 mg po sid, dogs 2.5–5.0 kg, 30 mg po sid, dogs 5.0–10.0 kg, 60 mg po sid, which produced hair regrowth within 4–8 weeks with most dogs. In difficult cases, the doses may be doubled but should be tapered to the lowest possible twice weekly dosage where possible once full hair regrowth has been achieved. Dogs should be monitored for adrenal insufficiency in the same way as those with hyperadrenocorticism (see Chapter 8).
    - Methyl testosterone 1 mg/kg up to 30 mg every other day for up to 3 months. Maintenance levels may be given 1–2 times weekly. Side effects of therapy include liver cholestasis and aggression. Due to potential hepatotoxicity, liver function should be monitored periodically.
    - Cimetidine at a dose of 5–10 mg/kg po qid. Side effects are rare but if they occur take the form of gastrointestinal signs.
    - Prednisolone 1 mg/kg po sid for 7 days then tapered to an alternate day regime of 0.5 mg/kg po sid.
    - Diethyl stilboestrol 0.1–1.0 mg by mouth every other day or daily for 3 weeks. Side effects of oestrogen therapy include severe bone marrow depression.
    - Porcine growth hormone has been used at a dose of 0.15 IU/kg sq twice weekly for a total of 6 weeks. Periodic retreatment may be necessary. Side effects include induction of diabetes so that blood glucose should be carefully monitored during therapy.
    - Leuprolide acetate 100 mg/kg im every 4–8 weeks until hair regrowth is seen.
    - Goserelin 60 mg/kg sq for 3 weeks until signs of hair regrowth become apparent.
- Not all dogs show a complete response to medical therapy. Some never grow back hair; other regain hair only to lose it again.

Pattern baldness

Cause and pathogenesis
An idiopathic hair cycle arrest that leads to alopecia. It is thought to be associated with miniaturisation of hairs. Uncommon disease; only recognised in dogs.

Clinical signs
In all cases, thinning of the hair progresses to complete alopecia of the affected area. Hair loss is usually symmetrical and hair in non-alopecic areas does not tend to epilate easily. Three syndromes are commonly recognised.

- Male dachshunds:
    - Alopecia of the pinnae, which usually starts at 6–9 months of age (Figure 12.17).

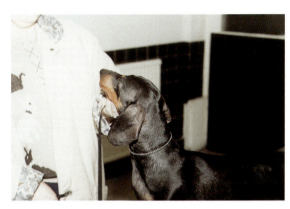

Figure 12.17 Pattern baldness in a dachshund showing striking pinnal alopecia.

- American water spaniels and Portuguese water dogs:
    - Alopecia of ventral neck, caudomedial thighs and tail from 6 months of age.
- Female dachshund, Chihuahua, whippet, greyhound:
    - Alopecia of the post-auricular area, ventrum and caudomedial thighs. Starts in early adulthood.

Differential diagnosis
- Endocrine alopecia
- Dermatophytosis
- Demodicosis
- Superficial folliculitis

Diagnosis
- History and clinical signs especially in predisposed breeds.
- Diagnostic rule outs of other diseases.
- Skin biopsy reveals signs of miniaturisation of the hair follicles.

Treatment
- No specific therapy has been shown to be useful.
- Hair may grow back spontaneously.
- Anecdotal reports success that melatonin at a dose of 3–12 mg/dog po sid–qid for 3–6 months may be useful.
- Prognosis is good, this is only a cosmetic disease and animals are never systemically unwell.

Idiopathic cyclic flank alopecia (seasonal flank alopecia, canine recurrent flank alopecia)

Cause and pathogenesis
Hair cycle arrest occurs at particular times of the year leading to alopecia on the flanks. The hair regrowth can be triggered in some breeds by changing photo period leading to the assumption that the pineal gland may be important in combination with prolactin production in stimulating hair growth. No specific hormonal abnormalities have been identified in animals. It is an uncommon condition in dogs and not recorded in cats.

Clinical signs
- Predisposed breeds include the Boxer, Airedale and bulldog, although signs can occur in any breed.
- In the Northern hemisphere hair loss occurs between November and March. It will normally regrow 3–8 months later.
- Dogs can lose and then regrow hair annually, biannually or not at all.
- Hair is lost from the thoracolumbar region and typically is bilaterally symmetrical (Figure 12.18), although asymmetrical hair loss can occur.
- Unlike endocrine hair loss the borders of alopecia tend to be well-demarcated and are often geometric in shape (Figure 12.19).
- Skin is usually hyperpigmented but not inflamed, and there is no pruritus.
- Dogs show no signs of systemic ill health.

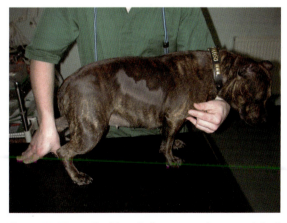

Figure 12.18 Staffordshire bull terrier with seasonal flank alopecia.

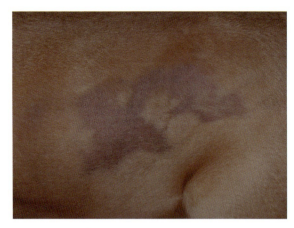

Figure 12.19 Close-up of alopecic patch on a mastiff with seasonal flank alopecia.

Differential diagnosis
- Endocrine disease, e.g. hypothyroidism, hyperadrenocorticism
- Superficial folliculitis
- Demodicosis
- Dermatophytosis
- Alopecia areata

Diagnosis
- Clinical signs and history, especially when dogs have a history of hair loss the previous year.
- Diagnostic rule outs of other differentials.
- Skin biopsy reveals signs of dysplastic, atrophic and dilated keratin-filled follicles that project down into the dermis like a 'witches foot'.

Treatment
- Observation without therapy may be appropriate in many cases as hair will often grow back without therapy.
- Medical therapy with either oral melatonin or melatonin implants:
  - Sustained release melatonin (1–4) 12 mg implants/dog sc once only.
  - Melatonin 3–12 mg/dog po sid qid for 3–4 months.
- Prognosis is variable as some dogs will grow back a normal hair coat; some never grow back hair and others have incomplete growth often with changes in quality and colour.

Telogen defluvium

Cause and pathogenesis
An abrupt stressful medical or surgical intervention, e.g. pyrexia, systemic illness, pregnancy, major surgery leads to cessation of the anagen phase of cycle. Hairs become synchronised in catagen, then move through to telogen to be lost 1–3 months after the initial insult.

Clinical signs
- Presents with sudden and widespread hair loss that progresses rapidly over a period of a few days (Figure 12.20). Hairs can be easily epilated.
- Hair loss is generalised but tends to spare the head.
- Skin is non-inflamed and there is no evidence of pruritus.

Differential diagnosis
- Endocrine disease, e.g. hypothyroidism, hyperadrenocorticism
- Superficial folliculitis
- Demodicosis
- Dermatophytosis
- Alopecia areata

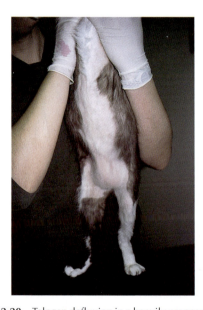

Figure 12.20 Telogen defluxion in a heavily pregnant queen.

Diagnosis
- Clinical signs and history especially when dogs have a history of systemic ill health 1–3 months prior to hair loss.
- Diagnostic rule outs of other differentials.
- Skin biopsy reveals no specific signs of abnormality. Often only changes that are present are that most of the hairs in sections are in telogen. Skin appears normal.

Treatment
- The underlying cause should be identified and treated where possible.
- Hair will grow back spontaneously once the underlying trigger is corrected.

Idiopathic bald thigh syndrome in the greyhound

Cause and pathogenesis
Alopecia of unknown origin reported to affect the thigh of greyhounds.

Clinical signs
- Alopecia is first noticed during late puberty or late adulthood and will progress as the animal becomes older.
- Hair loss is seen initially on the lateral and caudal aspects of the thighs (Figure 12.21), often extending onto the ventral abdomen.
- Underlying skin is not inflamed and the condition is non-pruritic.
- Animals appear to be systemically well.

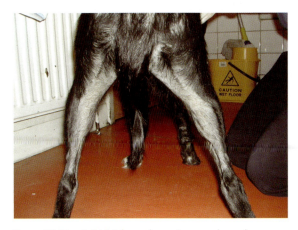

Figure 12.21 Bald thigh syndrome in a greyhound.

Differential diagnosis
- Endocrine disease, e.g. hypothyroidism, hyperadrenocorticism
- Superficial folliculitis
- Demodicosis
- Dermatophytosis
- Alopecia areata

Diagnosis
- Clinical signs and history in greyhounds.
- Diagnostic rule outs of other differentials.
- Skin biopsy reveals non-specific changes consistent with an endocrine type of pattern.

Treatment
- No specific therapy has been shown to be effective.
- Prognosis is good. Hair loss may be permanent but this is only a cosmetic disease.

Feline-acquired symmetrical alopecia

A very rare bilaterally symmetrical alopecia of unknown origin. Originally called feline endocrine alopecia, no true hormonal cause has been identified for this disease.

Cause and pathogenesis
- Thyroid function tests in these cats are normal. However, they may have a decreased thyroid reserve based on the fact many respond to thyroid supplementation with liothyronine.
- Response to thyroxine may be non-specific due to psychological factors rather than a deficiency state.

Clinical signs
- No breed or sex predilection recognised. Cats range in age from 2–12 years.
- Bilaterally symmetrical non-inflammatory alopecia.
- Hair can be easily epilated
- Affected sites are the anogenital area, proximal tail, caudomedial thighs and ventral abdominal skin. Relative sparing of face and feet.
- Non-pruritic.

Differential diagnosis

- Traumatic alopecia
- Ectoparasites (fleas, cheyletiella, otodectes, lice, demodex)
- Allergy (atopy, food)
- Psychogenic alopecia
- Dermatophytosis
- Non-pruritic alopecia
- Hypothyroidism (very rare)
- Hyperadrenocorticism (very rare)
- Telogen defluxion
- Anagen defluxion

Diagnosis

- History and clinical signs.
- Diagnostic rule out of other differentials.
- Routine blood samples including thyroid and adrenal function tests are normal.
- Trichography reveals no sign of trauma to the hair so that the distal hair tips are intact and pointed; the bulb are telogenised.
- Use of Elizabethan collar to establish if the hair loss is spontaneous or traumatic. If the cats are licking out their hair the coat will grow back with the use of a collar.
- Skin biopsy reveals a non-specific pattern other than the presence of telogenised hairs.

Treatment

Therapy should only be considered once a diagnosis has been made. Empirical therapy for alopecia is not appropriate.

Drugs that have been used include the following:

- Liothyronine 20 µg/cat orally twice daily may be increased to 50 µg/cat for 12 weeks.
  - *Side effects* – cardiac arrhythmia's.
- Androgen/oestrogen therapy – intramuscular injections of testosterone 12.5 mg total testosterone/cat with oestradiol 0.5 mg/cat. Injections of both are given on two occasions 6 weeks apart. Oestradiol is unlicensed for use in the cat.
  - *Side effects* – oestrous in females, urine spraying and aggressiveness in males. Hepatobiliary, renal and cardiac disease in cases of overdosage.
- Progestagens – megestrol acetate orally 2.5–5.0 mg/cat once every other day until hair regrows, then a maintenance dose of 2.5–5.0 mg/cat every 1–2 weeks, or intramuscular injection of medroxyprogesterone acetate 50–175 mg/cat two injections 6 weeks apart.
  - *Side effects* – adrenal suppression, diabetes mellitus, mammary gland fibroadenomatous hyperplasia, which can progress to neoplasia.

Pancreatic paraneoplastic alopecia

See Chapter 21.

Feline preauricular and pinnal alopecia

Cause and pathogenesis

Preauricular alopecia in cats is common and a normal finding. Pinnal alopecia is of unknown aetiology and is characterised by periodic alopecia of the ears.

Clinical signs

- Preauricular alopecia:
  - Presents generally in short-coated breeds as sparsely haired skin on the head between the ears and eyes (Figure 12.22).
  - No sex or breed predisposition.
  - No skin lesions are present.
- Pinnal alopecia:
  - Presents as non-pruritic alopecia (Figure 12.23).

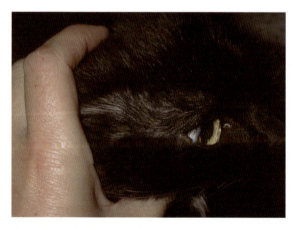

Figure 12.22 Feline preauricular alopecia.

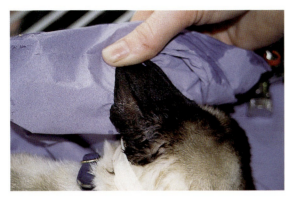

Figure 12.23 Patchy alopecia on the ear of a Siamese.

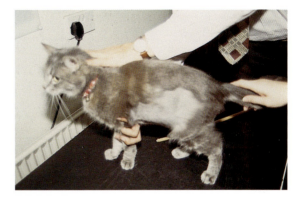

Figure 12.24 Flank alopecia secondary to flea allergy.

- No sex predilection but Siamese appear to be predisposed.
- Alopecia typically bilateral; may be patchy or more extensive.
- Hair will spontaneously regrow after several months.

Differential diagnosis
- Dermatophytosis
- Demodicosis
- Superficial pyoderma

Diagnosis
- History and clinical signs.
- Diagnostic rule outs of other differentials.

Treatment
- Preauricular alopecia:
  - No therapy needed as this is a normal finding.
- Pinnal alopecia:
  - No therapy necessary as hair will regrow after several months.

Traumatic alopecia

Pruritic/psychogenic alopecia

Hair is plucked out in association with underlying pruritic dermatoses or due to psychological factors (see Chapter 16). Traumatic hair loss tends to be much more important in cats than in dogs.

Cause and pathogenesis

Cats are often secret groomers and due to their fastidious nature overgrooming can produce areas of alopecia, as hair is either nibbled short or pulled out. The animal's hair coat remains normal. Any cause of overgrooming in dogs or cats can lead to traumatic hair loss including

- ectoparasites (fleas (Figure 12.24), cheyletiella, otodectes, lice, demodex),
- allergy (atopy (Figure 12.25), food),
- psychogenic alopecia,
- dermatophytosis,
- hyperthyroidism,

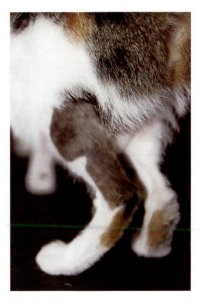

Figure 12.25 Alopecia on lower legs in a cat with atopy.

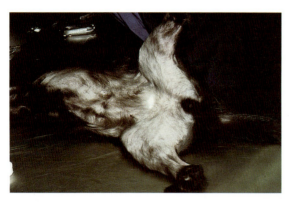

Figure 12.26 Ventral alopecia secondary to flea allergy.

- paraneoplastic pruritus,
- localised pain, e.g. abdominal or orthopaedic pain,
- seborrhoeic dermatitis.

Clinical signs

Alopecia can be complete if the hair is pulled out, or partial if the hairs have been barbered off to give the impression of extensive hair loss.

Patterns of alopecia are variable. In the dog, specific patterns of hair loss can give a clue to the underlying aetiology; for example, caudal dorsal traumatic hair loss is often associated with flea allergy. In cats, patterns of alopecia are not specific to any one disease. Feline patterns that are recognised include

- bilaterally symmetrical flank alopecia,
- ventral abdominal alopecia (Figure 12.26),
- alopecia of caudomedial thighs,
- alopecia of lower extremities,
- diffuse generalised hair loss.

These patterns can occur concurrently and also in combination with components of the eosinophilic granuloma complex in cats. Primary lesions are not usually present in cats. Traumatic hair loss in the dog is often accompanied by a papular eruption.

Differential diagnosis

- Hyperadrenocorticism
- Hypothyroidism
- Telogen defluxion
- Paraneoplastic alopecia
- Feline-acquired symmetrical alopecia

Diagnosis

- History and clinical signs.
- Diagnostic rule out for non-traumatic alopecia.
- Trichography.
- Loss of normal hairs reveals that both anagen and telogen hairs are represented. Hair shafts appear normal but hair tips are barbered suggesting overgrooming.

Treatment

Identification of underlying cause of pruritus/overgrooming essential where normal hair is lost.

Traction alopecia

Cause and pathogenesis

Hair loss is seen on the top of the head of dogs that have rubber bands or bows to tie up their hair. If these are applied tightly for prolonged periods hair loss can occur. It is an uncommon condition, only recognised in the dog.

Clinical signs

- Initial lesion is an erythematous plaque, which progresses to hair loss.
- Well-circumscribed areas of hair loss associated with area where hair was tied up, usually on the top of the head.

Differential diagnosis

- Dermatophytosis
- Demodicosis
- Alopecia areata

Diagnosis

- History and clinical signs.
- Skin biopsy reveals signs of mononuclear cell infiltrate with oedema, vasodilation and a fibrosing or scarring alopecia.

Treatment

- Proper use or else avoidance of bows.
- Resection of alopecia if permanent hair loss is seen.

Scarring alopecia

Cause and pathogenesis

Scarring alopecia occurs as a result of destruction or distortion of hair follicles so that hair is lost but does not grow back. This type of alopecia can occur in both the dog or cat but generally is more common in the dog.

(1) Primary
   Inflammatory reactions directed against hair follicles or organisms in lumen:
   - Bacterial folliculitis
   - Dermatophytic folliculitis (Figure 12.27)
   - Demodex folliculitis
   - Direct destruction of follicles, e.g. severe burns
(2) Secondary
   Hair follicles damaged as a bystander:
   - Infarcted hairs, e.g. vasculitis (Figure 12.28)
   - Perifollicular damage above hair bulb, e.g. sebaceous adenitis

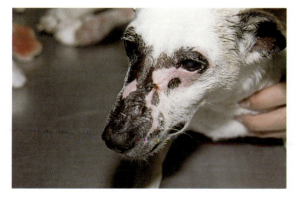

Figure 12.27 Scarring alopecia post *Trichophyton mentagrophytes* infection of the facial areas in a Jack Russell terrier.

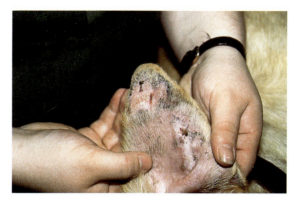

Figure 12.28 Scarring alopecia on the ear of a dog with dermatomyositis.

- Severe generalised cutaneous damage, e.g. burns

Selected references and further reading

Cerundolo, R. et al. (2000) An analysis of factors underlying hypotrichosis and alopecia in Irish water spaniels in the United Kingdom. *Vet Dermatol*, **11**, 107–122

Cerundolo, R. et al. (2004) Treatment of canine alopecia X with Trilostane. *Vet Dermatol*, **15**, 285–293

Diaz, S.F. et al. (2004) An analysis of canine hair regrowth after clipping for a surgical procedure. *Vet Dermatol*, **15**, 25–30

Frank, L.A. et al. (2004) Adrenal steroid hormone concentrations in dogs with hair cycle arrest alopecia (Alopecia X) before and after treatment with melatonin and mitotane. *Vet Dermatol*, **15**, 278–284

Medleau, L. and Hnilica, K. (2006) Hereditary, congenital and acquired alopecia. In: *Small Animal Dermatology: A Color Atlas and Therapeutic Guide*. 2nd edn. pp. 229–273. WB Saunders, Philadelphia

Morris, D.O. (2004) Disorders of hair and hair growth. In: Campbell, K.L. (ed) *Small Animal Dermatology Secrets*. pp. 99–105. Hanley and Belfus, Philadelphia

Paradis, M. (2000) Melatonin therapy in canine alopecia. In: Bonagura, E.D. (ed) *Kirk's Current Veterinary Therapy XIII Small Animal Practice*. pp. 546–549. WB Saunders, Philadelphia

Roperto, F. et al. (1995) Colour dilution alopecia (CDA) in ten Yorkshire terriers. *Vet Dermatol*, **6**, 171–178

Schoning, P.R. and Cowan, L.A. (2000) Bald thigh syndrome of Greyhound dogs: gross and microscopic findings. *Vet Dermatol*, **11**, 49–51

Scott, D.W. et al. (2001) *Acquired Alopecia Muller and Kirk's Small Animal Dermatology*. 6th edn. pp. 887–912. WB Saunders, Philadelphia

Nutritional skin disease

Dogs are by nature omnivorous and do not have the precise dietary requirements of the cat. Nutritional skin disease can occur through inadequate or unbalanced nutrition in either the dog or cat. Cats have a protein requirement of 25–30%, which is much higher than dogs, which is 18–20%. Cats unlike dogs require taurine in their diets. Deficiency of taurine leads to retinal degeneration and blindness. Cats cannot convert the fatty acid linoleic acid to arachidonic acid and must therefore consume preformed arachidonic acid, which is found in animal tissue. Cats cannot convert B carotene in plants to vitamin A and so must therefore consume preformed vitamin A also found in animal tissue. Cats cannot convert the amino acid tryptophan to the B vitamin niacin leading them to have a high requirement for niacin in their diets. Cats also have a high requirement for vitamin B6 (pyridoxine).

Protein Deficiency

Cause and pathogenesis

Normal hair growth requires 25–30% of the animal's total daily protein intake:

- Deficiency is usually seen when inappropriately low-protein diets are fed. This can occur when kittens or cats are fed on dog food, which has inadequate protein for cats.
- Low-protein prescription diets fed inappropriately for renal/hepatic disease.
- Systemic illness occurs, causing protein loss; diseases that may lead to this include protein-losing nephropathy, gastroenteropathy, hepatopathy, chronic blood loss.

Clinical signs

- Cutaneous signs will often precede weight loss.
- Generalised scaling and loss of hair pigment.
- Poor hair growth and the hair is thinner, dry, brittle (Figure 13.1).
- Patchy alopecia can be seen but more commonly the coat is diffusely thinned.

Differential diagnosis

Endocrine disease

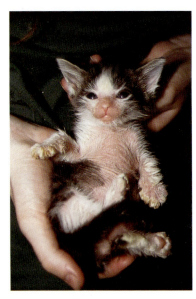

Figure 13.1 Generalised hair loss and seborrhoea oleosa in a protein-deficient kitten.

Diagnosis

- History and clinical signs.
- Investigation of dietary deficiency or search for source of protein loss.

Treatment

- Poor-quality diets should be replaced with ones with improved protein levels in diet.
- Correction of underlying diseases should be undertaken where possible.
- Specific dietary supplementation can be given with the use of prescription diets.

Fatty Acid Deficiency

Cause and pathogenesis

Essential fatty acids should constitute at least 2% of the caloric intake of the diet. Cats but not dogs require preformed linoleic acid and arachidonic acid, both are omega 6 fatty acids.

This is a rare disease in both the dog and cat. When it occurs, it is caused through the following:

- Inadequate diet especially poorly formulated or preserved foods, especially seen in young kittens; cats fed a vegetarian diet.
- Internal disease.
- Gastrointestinal disease especially inflammatory or neoplastic lesions leading to malabsorption and/or maldigestion.
- Chronic renal or hepatic disease.

Clinical signs

- Cutaneous signs:
  - Generalised scaling, loss of lustre of hair coat.
  - Chronic changes include a poor hair coat with seborrhoea oleosa plus often a ceruminous otitis.
  - Secondary infection with bacteria or yeast is common.
  - 'Hot spot' areas of acute moist dermatitis can be seen.
  - Miliary dermatitis in cats.
  - Impaired wound healing.
- Non-cutaneous signs:
  - Abnormal reproductive function.

Differential diagnosis

- Primary seborrhoea
- Other causes of secondary seborrhoea

Diagnosis

- History and clinical signs.
- Diagnostic rule outs of other differentials.
- Skin biopsy reveals signs of orthokeratotic hyperkeratosis with no underlying epidermal hyperplasia.
- Routine haematology, biochemistry, FeLV, FIP, FIV may be useful to identify any underlying disease.

Treatment

- Feeding a balanced diet is preferable to adding in fatty acid supplements.
- If supplements are given these should be balanced containing both omega 6 and omega 3 fatty acids. If these are unavailable,
    - natural sources of linoleic acid include soya or corn oil;
    - natural sources of arachidonic acid include poultry fat or lard.
- Identification of underlying disease and therapy of this is useful.

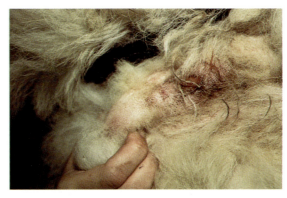

Figure 13.2 Pansteatitis affecting the groin.

Pansteatitis

Cause and pathogenesis

- Rare disease, caused by an excessive consumption of unsaturated fatty acids with inadequate dietary intake of antioxidants. Diets are usually high in oily fish especially tuna, sardines.
- The accumulation of reactive peroxides (end products of rancidification) in adipose tissue produces yellow discolouration of body fat. So-called 'yellow fat disease'. Rare disease; only recognised in cats.

Clinical signs

- Young and obese cats appear to be predisposed.
- Generalised signs:
    - Cats appear to be depressive, febrile and anorexic.
    - They appear unable to jump up or move freely.
    - Ascites is an uncommon finding but raises the suspicion of FIP as a major differential diagnosis.
- Cutaneous signs:
    - Cutaneous pain is present when cats are handled caused by the inflammation of subcutaneous fat. Usually generalised inflammation occurs of all fat deposits.
    - Nodular subcutaneous deposits of fat or fibrous tissue can be seen, especially in the groin and on the ventral abdomen (Figure 13.2).
    - Overlying skin usually appears normal unless traumatised by the cat.

Differential diagnosis

- Infectious causes of nodular skin disease including the following:
    - Bacterial infections such as
        - Bacterial pseudomycetoma
        - Mycobacteria
        - *Yersinia pestis* (plague)
        - Actinomycosis
        - Actinobacillosis
        - Nocardiosis
- Dermatophytic pseudomycetoma
- Fungal mycetoma
- Sterile causes of nodular skin disease
- Neoplasia
- Foreign body

Diagnosis

- Clinical signs and history, especially if a high-fat diet has been fed.
- Skin biopsy reveals that fat is characteristically brown/yellow/orange with lobular/septal panniculitis ± fat necrosis and

mineralisation. Due to the fact that many differentials are infectious special stains should be put on histopathology samples to rule out infectious causes.

Treatment

- Dietary changes are essential to feed a balanced cat food. Appetite stimulants/force feeding may be needed to encourage the cat to eat the new diet:
  - Cyproheptadine (2 mg po bid) or diazepam (1 mg po bid) can both be used as appetite stimulants in cats.
- Vitamin E supplementation (alpha tocopherol) 20–50 mg/kg body weight by mouth once daily. Should be given for 1 month beyond clinical cure.
- Glucocorticoids may be given as a short course at anti-inflammatory doses, which is
  - prednisolone 1–2 mg/kg once daily by mouth for 7 days, then every other day for 10 days.

Vitamin A deficiency

Cause and pathogenesis

Rare disease caused through inadequate levels of vitamin A in the diet. It is most commonly seen in cats fed a vegetarian diet. Cats cannot convert B carotene in plants to vitamin A and need preformed vitamin A from meat. Vitamin A is required for normal skin formation and ocular function.

Clinical signs

- Cutaneous signs:
  - Poor coat, alopecia, generalised scale
  - Marked follicular hyperkeratosis
- Generalised signs:
  - Retinal degeneration, photophobia,
  - Weakness of hind legs
  - Reproductive failure

Diagnosis

- History and clinical signs.
- Skin biopsy reveals signs of epidermal hyperplasia and follicular hyperkeratosis.

Treatment

- Single injection of vitamin A aqueous solution 6,000 IU/kg body weight is adequate for serious deficiency.
- Change of diet to a high-meat-based diet is often sufficient. Toxicity can occur through excess supplementation.

Vitamin A responsive disease

See Chapter 17.

Hypervitaminosis A

Cause and pathogenesis

A rare disease seen in cats that are fed a diet rich in vitamin A. This may be due to oversupplementation especially with cod-liver oil or diets containing large quantities of liver. This disease is very rare in dogs, but has been reported.

Clinical signs

- Cumulative disease that tends to be seen in elderly cats >8 years of age. Signs in dogs are similar to cats.
- Generalised signs:
  - Anorexia, weight loss.
  - Peri-articular exostoses especially forelimb and neck, leading to stiffness and eventual cervical spondylitis
- Cutaneous signs:
  - Hyperaesthesia.
  - Spondylitis leads to neck pain so that cats are reluctant to groom leading to poor-quality unkempt coat and generalised seborrhoea (Figure 13.3).

Nutritional skin disease

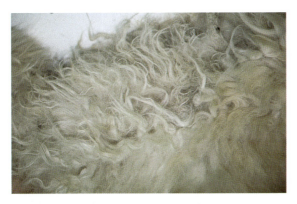

Figure 13.3 Unkempt coat in a cat with hypervitaminosis A. Cat is unable to groom due to cervical spondylitis.

Differential diagnosis

- Cutaneous lesions:
  - Seborrhoea related to chronic systemic disease
  - Hyperthyroidism

Diagnosis

- History and clinical signs
- Radiographic signs of bony changes

Treatment

- Institution of a balanced diet.
- This can be difficult, as cats can become obsessive about liver-based food.
- Force feeding and appetite stimulants may be necessary (see treatment for pansteatitis).
- Prognosis very guarded; often changes are irreversible.

Vitamin B deficiencies

Rare disease caused through deficiency of biotin, riboflavin, niacin (see Table 13.1).

Zinc responsive dermatosis

Cause and pathogenesis

Three deficiency syndromes are recognised:

- Syndrome I – huskies, Alaskan malamutes.
- Contributory factors:
  - Genetic defect leading to reduced zinc absorption from bowel in malamutes.
  - Diets high in calcium or cereal or soya protein prevent zinc absorption.
  - Chronic bowel problems – malabsorption.
- Syndrome II – rapidly growing puppies especially Great Danes, Dobermans, Labradors.

Contributory factors:

- Large breeds.
- High levels of calcium supplementation of diet.

Table 13.1 Vitamin B deficiencies: causes and clinical signs.

Vitamin B deficiency	Causes	Clinical signs	Treatment
Biotin	Diets high in uncooked eggs, chronic antibiotic therapy	Periocular alopecia, crusting on face, neck, body Lethargy, diarrhoea	Therapy is the same in all cases Balanced commercial dog foods Brewers yeast B complex injection
Riboflavin	Diets without meat or dairy products	Periocular and ventral seborrhoea, cheilosis	
Niacin	Diets low in protein/high in corn	Pellagra – dermatitis, neuritis, glossitis Ulceration of mucous membranes	

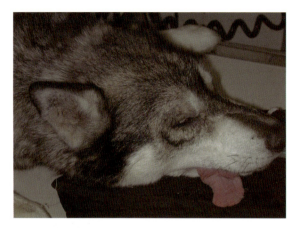

Figure 13.4 Periocular and aural erythema in a zinc-deficient husky.

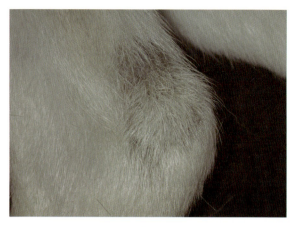

Figure 13.6 Crusting over elbows in a zinc-deficient husky.

- High cereal levels of diet.
■ Syndrome III – English bull terriers, lethal acrodermatitis (see Chapter 14).

Clinical signs

■ Syndrome I:
  □ Cutaneous signs:
    • Erythema, crusting, scaling around mouth, chin, eyes, ears and genitalia (Figures 13.4 and 13.5).
    • Generalised seborrhoea.
    • Thick crusting over the pressure points of elbows and stifles (Figure 13.6).
    • Secondary bacterial and yeast infections common.
    • Hyperkeratosis of footpads.
    • Mild to moderate pruritus.
  □ Non-cutaneous signs:
    • Depression, anorexia.
    • Lymphadenomegaly and pitting oedema of extremities.
    • Severely affected puppies may have stunted growth.
■ Syndrome II:
  □ Cutaneous signs:
    • Crusting of pressure points (Figure 13.7).
    • Nasal and footpad hyperkeratosis often with secondary fissuring.

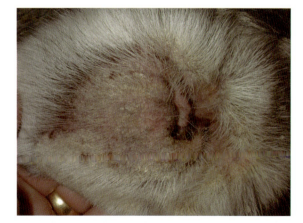

Figure 13.5 Close-up of the dog in Figure 13.4.

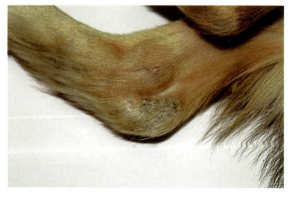

Figure 13.7 Zinc responsive disease in a collie showing crusting on pressure points. Lesions were caused by an unbalanced high-cereal diet.

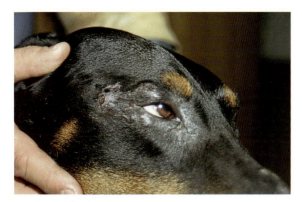

Figure 13.8 Periocular crusting and scaling in a Doberman with zinc responsive dermatosis caused through high calcium supplementation feeding with cereal-based diet.

- Crusting and scaling around eyes and mouth (Figure 13.8).
- Mild to moderate pruritus.

Differential diagnosis

- Other cause of nasal/footpad hyperkeratosis
- Primary and secondary seborrhoea

Diagnosis

- History and clinical signs especially in predisposed breeds.
- Skin biopsy reveals diffuse epidermal and follicular parakeratosis and superficial perivascular dermatitis. Evidence of secondary infection is common.
- Measurement of zinc in serum or hair is difficult and unreliable.
- Response to zinc therapy.

Treatment

- In both syndromes I and II correction of the diet and treatment of any underlying disease where possible, e.g. malabsorption, are essential.
- Any secondary bacterial and yeast infection should be treated with appropriate medical therapy for a minimum of 3–4 weeks.
- Oral essential fatty acid supplementation may allow the zinc supplementation levels to be reduced or withdrawn.
- Intact females should be neutered as oestrous can lead to a deterioration in their skin.
- Topical treatment:
  - Water soaks plus mild antiseborrhoeic shampoos and application of ointments may be useful.
- Zinc supplementation:
  - Syndrome I – essential and life long:
    - Zinc sulphate 10 mg/kg/daily with food.
    - Severe cases intravenous injection of 10–15 mg/kg weekly for 4 weeks then maintenance as required.
    - Zinc methionine 1–7 mg/kg daily.
    - Dogs should be removed from breeding programmes.
    - Side effects of zinc therapy include depression, anorexia, vomiting and diarrhoea.
  - Syndrome II:
    - Zinc supplementation is adequate as a short course to speed resolution.
- Prognosis is good for most dogs although some breeds need lifetime therapy.

Selected references and further reading

Medleau, L. and Hnilica, K. (2006) Keratinisation and seborrhoeic disorders. In: *Small Animal Dermatology: A Color Atlas and Therapeutic Guide*. 2nd edn. pp 295–326. WB Saunders, Philadelphia

Rosychuk, R.A. (2004) Zinc related dermatoses. In: Campbell, K.L. (ed) *Small Animal Dermatology Secrets*. pp. 304–311. Hanley and Belfus, Philadelphia

Roudebush, P. and Wedekind, K.J. (2002) Zinc responsive dermatosis in dogs. *Vet Dermatol*, **13**, 63

Scott, D.W. et al. (2001) *Nutritional Skin Disease Muller and Kirk's Small Animal Dermatology*. 6th edn. pp. 1112–1123. WB Saunders, Philadelphia

Congenital and hereditary skin diseases

Disorders of epithelial formation

Primary seborrhoea

Cause and pathogenesis

Canine:

Predisposed breeds include cocker spaniel, English springer spaniel, West Highland white terrier, basset hound, Irish setter. It is thought to be primary cellular defect in the dog. In cocker spaniels the epidermis, hair follicle infundibulum and sebaceous gland have all shown to be hyperproliferative.

Feline:

A very rare disease in the cat. In most cats seborrhoea is secondary to an underlying disease. Every effort should be made to identify this before a diagnosis of primary seborrhoea is made.

Often clinical signs can be quite mild due to the fastidious grooming behaviour of the cat.

Clinical signs

Canine:

- No sex predilection. It is seen in young dogs.
- Predisposed breeds include those listed below. Clinical signs differ between breeds. The initial signs are of mild scaling progresses to the following:
    - Irish setter and Doberman produce signs of dry generalised seborrhoea.
    - Cocker spaniel, West Highland white terrier, cavalier King Charles spaniel, basset and shar-pei produce signs of greasy malodorous skin, scaly and crusty pruritic patches (Figures 14.1 and 14.2).
- Ceruminous otitis externa is common. Dogs commonly have marked intertrigo.
- Secondary staphylococcal and Malassezia pachydermatis infection common.

Feline:

- No sex predilection. Age of onset is variable. Severe cases are seen in young kittens by 2–3 days of age. Mild cases become apparent by 6 weeks of age.
- Predisposed breeds include the Persian:
    - In Persian cats it has been identified as an autosomal recessive mode of inheritance.
    - Cats present with signs of generalised seborrhoea oleosa (Figure 14.3), which is malodorous.

Congenital and hereditary skin diseases 239

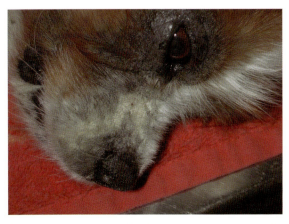

Figure 14.1 Idiopathic seborrhoea on the face of a cavalier King Charles spaniel.

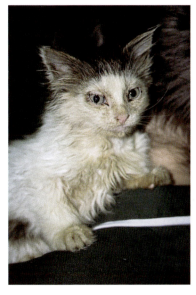

Figure 14.3 Generalised primary seborrhoea in a young kitten.

- Waxy debris accumulates in the face folds and ears (Figure 14.4).

Differential diagnosis

- Ichthyosis
- Sebaceous adenitis
- Vitamin A responsive dermatosis
- Causes of secondary seborrhoea:
  - ectoparasites, e.g. fleas, cheyletiella,
  - endocrine, e.g. hypothyroidism (dogs), hyperthyroidism (cats)
  - dermatophytosis
  - thymoma (cats)
  - allergy with secondary Malassezia overgrowth

Diagnosis

- History and clinical signs especially in young animals.
- Diagnostic rule outs of other secondary causes of seborrhoea.
- Skin biopsy reveals non-specific signs of follicular keratosis and a hyperplastic superficial perivascular dermatitis with orthokeratotic

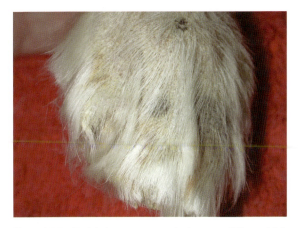

Figure 14.2 Pedal changes present in the case of Figure 14.1.

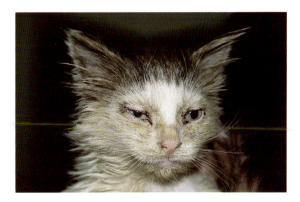

Figure 14.4 Close-up of facial area in Figure 14.3.

or parakeratotic hyperkeratosis. Secondary infection with yeast and bacteria is common.

Treatment

- Owners need to be made aware of the need for long-term therapy.
- Good nutritional support is important with a well-balanced, high-quality diet.
- Symptomatic treatment can include the following.
- Topical therapy:
  - Antiseborrhoeic shampoos:
    - Shampoo therapy for dogs is easily undertaken; however, many cats will tolerate regular shampoo therapy if they are started at a young age.
    - Animal's coat should be kept well groomed, clipping often helps.
    - Shampoo used once or twice weekly initially, then as required for maintenance. Shampoo therapy may be tailored to the type of seborrhoea:
      - Dry seborrhoea – sulphur, salicylic acid.
      - Dry seborrhoea with secondary infection – acetic acid, ethyl lactate, chlorhexidine, miconazole, sulphur, salicylic acid.
      - Greasy seborrhoea – benzoyl peroxide, selenium sulphide, tar. (Tar shampoos should not be used in cats.)
    - Shampoos for greasy seborrhoea are rarely needed for long-term maintenance.
- Topical rinses:
  - Suitable products contain essential fatty acids, moisturisers and humectants.
- Essential fatty acids:
  - Omega 3, omega 6 fatty acids supplements successful in some cases.
- Retinoids.
  - Retinoids are reported to be useful in dogs. Suitable drugs include isotretinoin 1.0–3.0 mg/kg po bid, etretinate 1.0 mg/kg po bid or acitretin 0.5–1 mg/kg po sid.
  - There are few reports of use of retinoids in cats.
  - Retinoids are potent teratogens and should be dispensed with care, especially to female owners of childbearing age.
  - Monitoring of the canine patient should include routine haematology, biochemistry, especially liver function, triglycerides and cholesterol.
- Glucocorticoids:
  - Glucocorticoids should be used as a last resort when other problems are controlled.
  - Prednisolone 1.0–2.0 mg/kg to reduce greasiness for a maximum of 2 weeks then the lowest possible dose used on an alternate day basis for maintenance.

Ichthyosis (fish scale disease)

Cause and pathogenesis

Very rare congenital disorder of keratinisation identified in the dog and cat. It may be equivalent to lamellar ichthyosis in man.

Clinical signs

- No sex predilection. Seen in young dogs and cats.
- Animals are abnormal at birth. Several animals in a litter may be affected.
- Predisposed canine breeds include the West Highland white terrier, golden retriever, cavalier King Charles spaniel, Doberman pinschers, Jack Russell terriers, Norfolk terriers and Yorkshire terriers.
- Animals have generalised grey scales and roughened skin (Figures 14.5).
- Scales will flake off in large sheets (Figure 14.6 and 14.7) or can accumulate as scales on the skin surface.
- Malodorous seborrhoeic skin; secondary infection with Malassezia very common.
- Hyperkeratosis of footpads (Figures 14.8 and 14.9) (especially at the periphery) and nasal planum.

Congenital and hereditary skin diseases 241

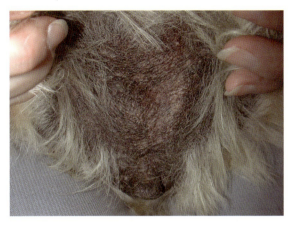

Figure 14.5 Ventral abdomen of West Highland white terrier with ichthyosis showing roughened scale.

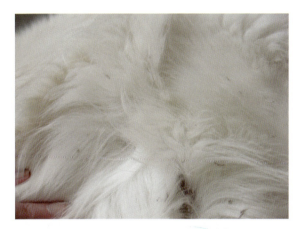

Figure 14.6 Scaly skin in a retriever with ichthyosis.

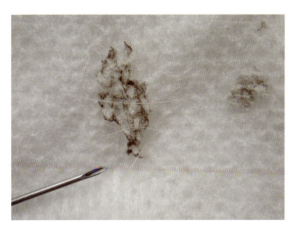

Figure 14.7 Scale from the case in Figure 14.6.

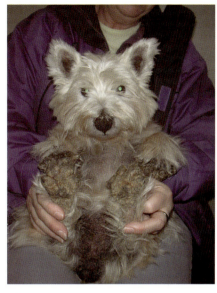

Figure 14.8 Hyperkeratosis of the footpads in a West Highland white terrier with ichthyosis.

Differential diagnosis

- Seborrhoeic skin disease:
    - Primary seborrhoea
    - Other causes of secondary seborrhoea
- Footpad hyperkeratosis:

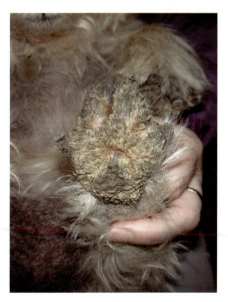

Figure 14.9 Close-up of hyperkeratosis in Figure 14.8.

- Distemper
- Zinc responsive dermatosis
- Pemphigus foliaceus

Diagnosis

- History and clinical signs, especially in predisposed breeds.
- Diagnostic rule outs of other differentials.
- Skin biopsy reveals signs of orthokeratotic hyperkeratosis and hypergranulosis. Keratinocytes contain numerous mitotic figures. Follicular keratosis and plugging are common.

Treatment

- Incurable disease; needs aggressive long-term management.
- Topical treatment:
  - Emollients:
    - May be useful to soften the skin especially footpads.
    - Suitable products contain lactic acid 5% spray or ointment, propylene glycol 50% solution.
  - Antiseborrhoeic shampoo:
    - See therapy of primary seborrhoea.
- Systemic treatment:
  - Essential fatty acid supplementation
  - Retinoids (as primary seborrhoea)
  - Glucocorticoids (as primary seborrhoea)
- In cases where skin changes are severe, animals may be euthanised.

Lichenoid psoriasiform dermatosis of English springer spaniels

Cause and pathogenesis

A rare skin disease occurring in the English springer spaniel. Occasionally it can be seen in other breeds. It is thought to be an exaggerated reaction to a superficial staphylococcal infection.

Clinical signs

- No sex predilection; tends to be recognised in young dogs.
- The disease is characterised by multiple erythematous hyperkeratotic papules that coalesce to form plaques.
- Lesions tend to be roughly symmetrical and found on inner aspect of pinnae, inguinal and abdominal skin and prepuce.
- Chronically the lesions can become generalised.

Differential diagnosis

- Demodicosis
- Dermatophytosis
- Neoplasia – lymphoma

Diagnosis

- History and clinical signs, especially in predisposed breed.
- Skin biopsy reveals signs of regular or papillate epidermal hyperplasia with the formation of blunt-ended rete ridges.

Treatment

- Topical therapy:
  - Antibacterial shampoo using actives such as acetic acid, benzoyl peroxide, chlorhexidine, ethyl lactate.
- Systemic therapy:
  - Antibiotics should be prescribed on the basis of culture and sensitivity.
  - Suitable drugs include the following:
    - Cephalexin 20–25 mg/kg po bid
    - Clavamox 12.5–25 mg/kg po bid/tid
    - Clindamycin 5.5 mg/kg po bid
    - Enrofloxacin 5 mg/kg po bid
    - Marbofloxacin 2 mg/kg po bid
  - Antibiotics should be prescribed for 3–6 weeks and at least 10 days beyond clinical cure.

Schnauzer comedo syndrome

Cause and pathogenesis

Uncommon disease, which has only been recorded in the miniature schnauzers (Figure 14.10). It is thought to be an acne-like developmental abnormality of hair follicles.

Congenital and hereditary skin diseases   243

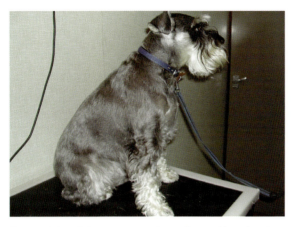

Figure 14.10 Schnauzer comedo syndrome. Note that there are no generalised skin abnormalities.

Clinical signs

- No sex predilection. Seen usually in young dogs.
- Lesions are found almost exclusively on the dorsum.
- In mild cases there is diffuse thinning of the hair coat.
- In severe cases there is alopecia with hyperpigmentation of the skin and comedone formation (Figure 14.11).
- Hair can be easily epilated from affected area and commonly contains follicular casts.
- Secondary bacterial folliculitis is very common.
- Pruritus is mild in uncomplicated cases.

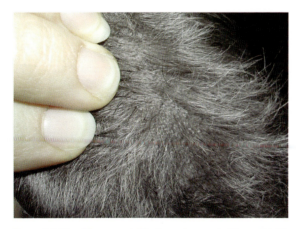

Figure 14.11 Close-up of skin from dorsum in Figure 14.10.

Differential diagnosis

- Dermatophytosis
- Demodicosis
- Endocrine disease especially hypothyroidism, hyperadrenocorticism
- Flea-allergic dermatitis
- Allergy with secondary infection

Diagnosis

- History and clinical signs in predisposed breed.
- Diagnostic rule outs of other differentials.
- Skin biopsy reveals that the superficial portion of the hair follicle is dilated with keratin with an almost 'cyst-like' appearance. Secondary bacterial infection and follicular rupture producing areas of furunculosis are common.

Treatment

- Long-term control requires a combination of topical and often systemic therapy.
- Topical treatment:
  - Shampoo therapy with antiseborrhoeic shampoo. Benzoyl peroxide is particularly useful because it has follicular flushing activity.
- Systemic treatment:
  - Antibiotics for secondary infection based on sensitivity for at least 3 weeks and 10 days beyond clinical cure. Some animals need to stay on long-term antibiotics possibly as pulse therapy to prevent recurrence. In these cases, a full therapeutic dose of antibiotics is given twice weekly to prevent reinfection.
  - Retinoids in the form of isotretinoin 1.0 mg/kg po bid or acitretin 0.5–1.0 mg/kg po sid. Response should be seen within 4 weeks. Dogs should be monitored for liver dysfunction and owners should be made aware of the teratogenic nature of the drug.
  - Vitamin A 8,000–10,000 IU/10 kg po sid may be beneficial.
- Prognosis is good, but animals will need long-term care. Disease is only of cosmetic consideration.

Dermoid sinus

Cause and pathogenesis

Dermoid sinus is a rare congenital abnormality that has not been reported in the cat. It has been recognised in many different breeds but most commonly recognised in the Rhodesian ridgeback. It is a congenital defect due to incomplete separation of skin and neural tube. This produces a blind ending sac or sinus that communicates with the dura mater extending from the dorsal mid-line.

Clinical signs

- No sex predilection. Always seen in young dogs.
- Tufts of hair protrude from single or multiple openings on dorsum.
- Can occur at any site on the dorsum but most commonly over the cervical spine.
- Cord of tissue can occasionally be palpated extending down to spine.
- The sinus may contain sebum, keratin debris or hair and can become secondarily infected.

Differential diagnosis

- Congenital nevus
- Bacterial folliculitis
- Foreign body
- Inclusion cyst

Diagnosis

- History and clinical signs, especially in predisposed breed.
- Fistulogram to delineate extent of tract.
- MRI or CT scan are non-invasive ways to assess the boundaries of the lesion.

Treatment

- Where the sac is blind ending and quiescent it may be removed surgically, but treatment is not usually necessary.
- For draining or cystic tracts complete surgical removal of the sinus is necessary. There is a risk of meningitis associated with surgery.
- Appropriate antibiotic therapy should be given to treat animals prior to surgery.

Aplasia cutis

Cause and pathogenesis

Rare inherited congenital abnormality in the dog and cat. Anomaly leads to a discontinuity of squamous epithelium. Mode of inheritance in the cat and dog is unclear.

Clinical signs

- No sex or breed predisposition. It is present at birth.
- Skin lesions consist of areas of skin ulceration due to loss of epithelium.
- May be seen at any site on the body and deficits may be small or cover an extensive areas.

Differential diagnosis

- Mechanical trauma
- Burns either mechanical, heat or chemical
- Other congenital abnormalities especially epidermolysis bullosa

Diagnosis

- History and clinical signs in a young animal.
- Skin biopsy reveals signs of complete absence of epidermis, hair follicles and glands. Skin to either side of the lesion is normal.

Treatment

- Surgical repair:
    - Primary closure or skin grafting may repair small areas.
    - Where there is extensive skin loss, dehydration and secondary infection is common, leading to death.

Epidermolysis bullosa

Cause and pathogenesis

Rare congenital disease identified in both dogs and cats. Hereditary mechanobullous disease

Table 14.1 Different forms of epidermolysis bullosa.

Disease	Structure affected	Deficient protein
Epidermolysis simplex	Intermediate filaments Hemidesmosomes	K5 or 14 Plectin
Junctional epidermolysis bullosa	Hemidesmosomes Anchoring filaments	Integrin $\alpha 6$ or $\beta 4$ Type XVIII collagen or laminin 5
Dystrophic epidermolysis bullosa	Anchoring fibrils	Type VII collagen

caused through a variety of different faults at the level of the basement membrane zone, which leads to separation of the epidermis from the dermis. The level of splitting cannot be identified on normal histopathological sections but requires electron microscopy or immunohistochemistry.

Three subtypes have been identified in man based on the abnormality and the level of cleavage (see Table 14.1).

Clinical signs

- Signs become apparent at birth or soon afterwards.
- Typical lesions are vesicles and bullae. However, these lesions may be transient and lesions appear as areas of ulceration with crusting.
- Lesions typically seen at mucocutaneous junctions, footpads (Figure 14.12), ventral abdomen (Figure 14.13) and over bony prominences.
- Bacterial paronychia common (Figure 14.14) and claws often slough.
- Defects in tooth enamel and retarded growth can also be seen.

Differential diagnosis

- Dermatomyositis
- Pemphigus vulgaris
- Bullous pemphigoid
- Systemic lupus erythematosus
- Erythema multiforme
- Drug eruption
- Vasculitis

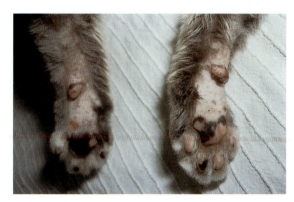

Figure 14.12 Ulceration on paws with epidermolysis bullosa.

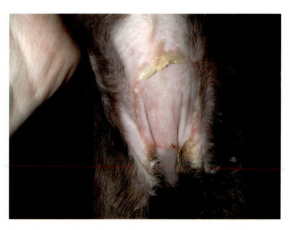

Figure 14.13 Vesicles and ulceration on ventral abdomen of a puppy with epidermolysis bullosa (EB).

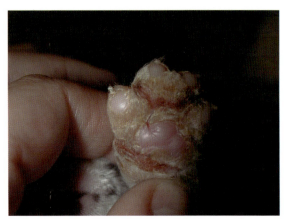

Figure 14.14 Bacterial paronychia in a puppy with EB.

Diagnosis

- History and clinical signs, which are present at birth or soon afterwards.
- Skin biopsy reveals signs of dermal/epidermal separation, which extends to involve hair follicles. There is no apoptosis or hydropic change of the basal layer.
- Electron microscopy and immunohistochemistry are required to determine the level of the cleavage and therefore the subtype of the disease.

Treatment

- No therapy is currently available.
- Environmental management may be helpful to minimise trauma to skin. The use of protective boots and coats may help minimise trauma.
- Antibiotics can be given to help with secondary infection.
- Guarded prognosis: affected animals should not be used for breeding.

Dermatomyositis

Cause and pathogenesis

Uncommon disease only recognised in the dog. Familial history is commonly seen. Aetiology is not fully determined but it is thought that this may be a genetic predisposition that invokes an immune mediated disease. Drug reactions, infections (especially viral) toxins, internal neoplasia may contribute.

Clinical signs

- No sex predilection. It is commonly seen in dogs <6 months of age.
- Predisposed breeds include the collie and Shetland sheepdog.
- Cutaneous lesions:
    - Lesion progression variable but dogs usually deteriorate up to the age of 12 months after which regression may occur.
    - Lesions occur at sites of mechanical trauma (bony prominences), face (bridge of nose, lips, periocular, Figure 14.15), ear and tail tips (Figure 14.16).
    - Footpad ulcers can occur but are rare.
    - Primary lesions are papules and vesicles but are uncommon.
    - Dogs usually present with alopecia, erythema, scaling and crusting.
    - Lesions are aggravated by trauma and ultraviolet light.
    - Non-pruritic lesions that wax and wane.

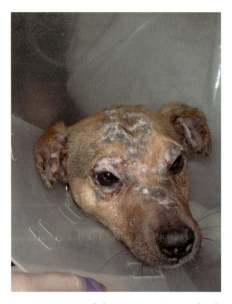

Figure 14.15 Lesions of dermatomyositis on the face of a dog.

Congenital and hereditary skin diseases

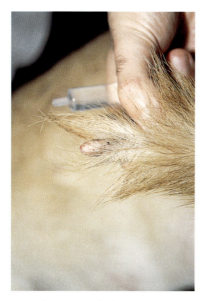

Figure 14.16 Ulceration and alopecia of tail tip in a collie with dermatomyositis.

- Non-cutaneous lesions:
  - Myositis variable, not always present.
  - Most commonly asymptomatic atrophy of muscles of mastication and distal limbs.
  - In Severe cases, problems with drinking, chewing, swallowing (megaoesophagus), high stepping gait.

Differential diagnosis

- Demodicosis
- Staphylococcal folliculitis
- Dermatophytosis
- Discoid lupus erythematosus
- Epidermolysis bullosa
- Vasculitis

Diagnosis

- History and clinical signs, especially in predisposed breed.
- Skin and muscle biopsy may be non-diagnostic:
  - Skin biopsy reveals signs of scattered epidermal basal cell degeneration, perifollicular lympho-histiocytic infiltrates. Follicular basal cell degeneration and follicular atrophy 'faded follicles'.
  - Muscle biopsy reveals signs of multifocal accumulations of inflammatory cells, myofibril degeneration and myofibre atrophy.
- Electromyography produces signs of fibrillation potentials and bizarre high-frequency discharges.

Treatment

- Symptomatic therapy to remove crust and scale from the skin.
- Minimise trauma and exposure to ultraviolet light.
- Therapy of any secondary infection.
- Neutering is advised as oestrous and pregnancy exacerbate the disease, and neither sex should be used for breeding.
- Moderate/mild cases:
  - Vitamin E 400–800 IU po sid; improvement may take 2–3 months.
  - Essential fatty acids/cold marine oil supplements.
  - Prednisolone 1.0 mg/kg po sid initially to produce clinical improvement (7–10 days) and then cut to lowest possible alternate day dosage.
  - Pentoxifylline 25 mg/kg po tid with food; improvement may take 1–3 months.
- Prognosis is very variable. Dogs with mild to moderate disease can resolve spontaneously or be controlled with medication. They can be left with some scarring. Severe cases are often unresponsive to therapy and animals are euthanised.

Hereditary lupoid dermatosis of German short-haired pointers

Cause and pathogenesis

A very rare disease, only seen in the German short-haired pointer. Aetiology is unknown but a definite familial predisposition has been recognised.

Clinical signs

- No sex predisposition. Affects young dogs approximately 6 months of age.

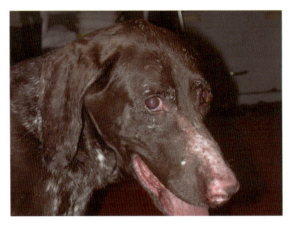

Figure 14.17 Crusting and scaling on the face of a German short-haired pointer with hereditary lupoid dermatosis.

- Initial lesions are seen on the face (Figure 14.17), ears and dorsum.
- Chronically the disease becomes more generalised.
- Crusting and scaling is seen on the dorsum (Figure 14.18).
- Hyperkeratosis and ulceration of the planum nasale commonly seen.
- Cyclical disease whose clinical signs wax and wane.

Differential diagnosis

- Sebaceous adenitis
- Systemic lupus erythematosus
- Pemphigus foliaceus
- Dermatophytosis
- Zinc responsive dermatosis

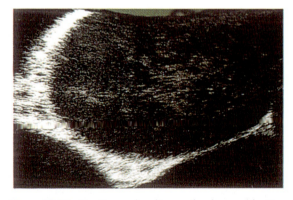

Figure 14.18 Crusting and scaling on the dorsum of a German Shorthaired Pointer with hereditary lupoid dermatosis.

Diagnosis

- History and clinical signs, especially in predisposed breed.
- Skin biopsy reveals signs of moderate acanthosis with orthokeratotic and parakeratotic hyperkeratosis. Hydropic degeneration of basal cells and individual keratinocytes show signs of apoptosis.

Treatment

- Disease is often poorly responsive to therapy.
- Topical treatment:
  - Antiseborrhoeic shampoos especially those containing ethyl lactate, salicylic acid, sulphur and tar.
  - Emollient and humectant sprays.
- Systemic treatment:
  - Essential fatty acid supplementation; minimal benefit.
  - Glucocorticoids even at immunosuppressive dosages of 2 mg/kg po sid daily produce poor results.
  - Other immunosuppressive therapy produces variable results, i.e. cyclosporine, azathioprine, chlorambucil.

Congenital and hereditary disorders of hair and hair growth

See Chapter 12.

Congenital and hereditary disorders of pigmentation

See also Chapter 15.

Chediak–Higashi syndrome

Cause and pathogenesis

Inherited autosomal recessive disease seen in blue Persian cats. Not been recorded in dogs.

Affected cats have giant lysosomes in the cells of numerous tissues including neutrophils and macrophages. Abnormal neutrophils exhibit delayed intracellular killing, leading to increased susceptibility to infection.

Clinical signs

- No sex predilection. Affected animals tend to be young kittens.
- Breed incidence exclusively found in blue smoke, yellow-eyed Persian cats.
- Cutaneous signs:
  - Dilute pigmentation of the coat, which is a blue smoke colour.
  - Cats have an increased risk of bacterial and fungal infection (especially dermatophytic pseudomycetoma).
- Ocular signs:
  - Cats show signs of a partial ocular albinism; their iris is yellow compared to the normal copper coloured iris typical of blue Persians.
  - Animals show signs of photophobia.
  - There is reduced fundic pigmentation, which appears red compared to the normal yellow/green colour.
  - An increased incidence of congenital cataracts is seen.
- Haematological signs:
  - Abnormal platelet function is seen leading to increased bleeding tendency.

Differential diagnosis

Little else present with this range of clinical signs in this breed and colour of cat.

Diagnosis

- History and clinical signs.
- Trichography of hairs reveals that hair shafts contain multiple large irregular clumps of melanin (macromelanosomes).
- Blood smear reveals that neutrophils and macrophages contain large eosinophilic granules (giant lysosomes).
- Platelet counts are normal as this tends to be a thrombocytopathy rather than thrombocytopaenia.

Treatment

- Nothing is available.
- In view of the heritability of the disease, affected animals should be removed from any breeding programme.

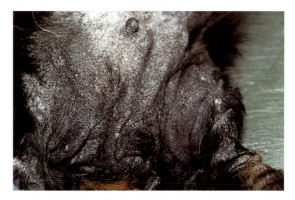

Figure 14.19 Primary idiopathic acanthosis nigricans in a dachshund.

Acanthosis nigricans

Cause and pathogenesis

Multiple causes exist for this disease, which can occur as a primary entity or secondary to other inciting factors:

- Primary idiopathic acanthosis nigricans is seen especially in dachshunds and is thought to be genetically determined (Figure 14.19).
- Secondary acanthosis nigricans can be seen in any breed and can be associated with the following:
  - Conformation defects leading to intertrigenous disease.
  - Allergy, especially self-inflicted trauma, due to chronic pruritus (Figure 14.20).
  - Endocrinopathy leading to pigment change especially, e.g. hypothyroidism.

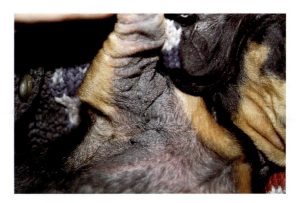

Figure 14.20 Secondary acanthosis nigri.

Clinical signs

- Primary acanthosis nigricans:
  - No sex predilection is seen in young dogs less than 1 year of age.
  - Acute lesions present with hyperpigmentation, bilaterally in the axilla.
  - Chronically lesions become lichenification with accompanying seborrhoea and can spread to involve larger areas on the ventral abdominal skin.
  - Secondary infection with both yeast and bacteria is common.
- Secondary acanthosis nigricans presents with similar signs on the ventrum plus signs associated with any underlying disease, e.g. pedal pruritus and otitis externa in cases of atopy or bilateral flank alopecia in hypothyroidism.

Differential diagnosis

Causes of secondary acanthosis nigricans for primary disease.

Diagnosis

- History and clinical signs as well as predisposed breeds for primary acanthosis nigricans.
- Laboratory rule outs of underlying causes.
- Skin biopsy reveals a non-diagnostic picture of hyperplastic superficial perivascular dermatitis with focal parakeratotic hyperkeratosis. Epidermal melanosis is present with pigmentary incontinence and follicular keratosis.

Treatment

- Secondary acanthosis nigricans:
  - Treatment of underlying disease and secondary infection is important. In many cases the lesions will resolve often without any other therapy. Where they persist, treatment should be undertaken as primary acanthosis nigricans.
- Primary acanthosis nigricans:
  - Topical therapy:
    - Antibacterial/antiyeast shampoos.
    - Glucocorticoid cream for short-term use, provided infection is controlled.
    - Antiseborrhoeic shampoos (see 'Primary Seborrhoea' section in this chapter).
  - Systemic treatment:
    - Melatonin 2 mg/per dog po sid for 3–5 days, then weekly or monthly as required.
    - Prednisolone 1 mg/kg po sid 7–10 days, then lowest possible alternate day dosage.
    - Vitamin E 200–400 IU po bid 30–60 days, then as required; improvement is variable and can take several months.

Canine cyclic haematopoiesis (grey collie syndrome)

See Chapter 4.

Acquired aurotrichia in miniature schnauzers

Cause and pathogenesis

Unknown aetiology, but there is thought to be a genetic influence.

Clinical signs

- No age or sex predilection.
- Primary guard hairs turn from silver or black to gold especially seen on the dorsal, thorax and abdomen (Figure 14.21).
- Hair coat is diffusely thinned.
- Non-pruritic disease.

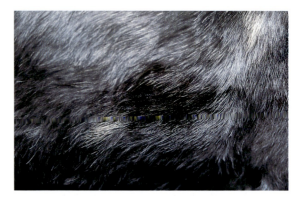

Figure 14.21 Acquired aurotrichia in a miniature schnauzer.

Differential diagnosis

- Endocrine skin disease especially hypothyroidism
- Follicular dystrophy

Diagnosis

- History and clinical signs in a predisposed breed.
- Trichography of hair mounted in liquid paraffin to demonstrate changes in pigment in hairs.
- Skin biopsy reveals no signs of inflammatory change in affected areas. Secondary hairs in these sites are decreased and guard hairs show signs of pigmentary changes.

Treatment

- Disease is a cosmetic only.
- No treatment is successful.

Congenital and hereditary disorders of collagen

Ehlers–Danlos (cutaneous asthenia, dermatosparaxis)

Cause and pathogenesis

Rare syndrome recorded in both the dog and cat. Ehlers–Danlos is a group of inherited congenital defect in collagen formation. The disease results in a reduction of the tensile strength of the skin of 10–40-fold so that the skin will tear easily. Both dominant and recessive modes of inheritance have been recognised. The disease has been reported in many different breeds.

Clinical signs

- No sex predilection. Seen in young animals.
- Predisposed feline breeds include domestic short-haired, long-haired and Himalayan cats.
- No breed predisposition in the dog.
- Cutaneous signs:
  - Skin soft, hyperextensible (Figure 14.22), usually thin.

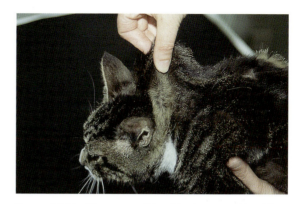

Figure 14.22 Hyperextensible skin in cat with Ehlers–Danlos.

  - Often hangs loosely in folds especially legs and throat.
  - Tears easily to produce large gaping wounds (Figure 14.23) but heals quickly leaving 'cigarette paper' scars; minimal bleeding.
  - Widening of bridge of nose may be seen.
- Non-cutaneous signs:
  - Joint laxity, dislocations and hygromas.
  - Ocular changes, e.g. lens luxations, cataract.

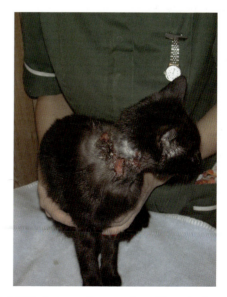

Figure 14.23 Large gaping wounds on the neck of a cat with Ehlers–Danlos.

Differential diagnosis

- No real differentials in the dog.
- Feline-acquired skin fragility (cat) due to the following:
  - Diabetes mellitus
  - Spontaneous hyperadrenocorticism
  - Hepatic lipidosis
  - Overadministration of glucocorticoids

Diagnosis

- History and clinical signs are very characteristic.
- Extensibility index of dorsolumbar skin
$$= \frac{\text{vertical height dorsal lumbar skin fold}}{\text{body length occipital crest to tail base}} \times 100$$
- Affected cat greater than 19.0 %, affected dog greater than 14.5 %.
- Skin biopsy can appear normal. In some cases dermis may be thinned and collagen bundles may be abnormal; special collagen stains may be useful.
- Electron microscopy is diagnostic, showing disordered collagen bundles or else reduction in collagen (Figures 14.24 and 14.25).

Treatment

- Important that animals are prevented from breeding.
- Environmental modification can help to reduce trauma to the skin, e.g. padded beds, removal of objects with sharp or rough edges.

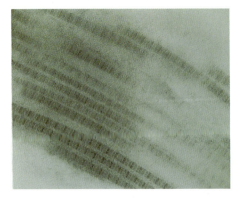

Figure 14.24 Electron microscopy of well-ordered collagen bundles from a normal cat.

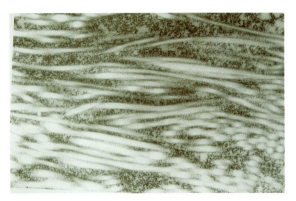

Figure 14.25 Electron microscopy of disorganised abnormal collagen bundles from cat in Figure 14.22.

- Careful restraint of the animal is important to avoid tearing the skin.
- Cats should be declawed to prevent self-traumatisation.
- Strict ectoparasite control should be practiced to eliminate any pruritic insults to the skin.
- Vitamin C therapy may produce some possible benefit: 50 mg/cat/dog po sid.

Focal metatarsal fistulation in German shepherd dogs

Cause and pathogenesis

Rare disease, only recognised in the dog. It is almost exclusively seen in German shepherd dogs and German shepherd dog crosses. The aetiology is unknown but may be a familial disease of collagen.

Clinical signs

- No sex predilection, commonly seen in young dogs 2–4 years of age.
- Well-demarcated fistulae seen on the area proximal to the metatarsal/carpal pads (Figure 14.26).
- Fibrous tract extends to deeper tissue.
- Sero-sanguineus discharge is seen but can become purulent if secondary infection occurs.
- Lesions confined exclusively to the lower legs and no other sites on the body are involved.
- Lesions do not tend to be pruritic but can be painful.

Congenital and hereditary skin diseases

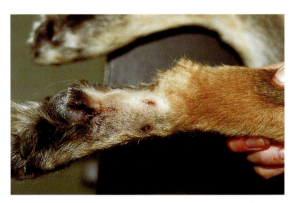

Figure 14.26 Focal metatarsal fistula in a German shepherd dog.

Differential diagnosis

- Penetrating foreign body
- Focal infection with bacteria or fungus

Diagnosis

- History and clinical signs in a predisposed breed.
- Cytology of exudate reveals signs of pyogranulomatous inflammation often with secondary infection.
- Skin biopsy for histopathology and tissue culture are useful. Biopsy reveals signs of deep nodular to diffuse dermatitis with fibrosis and fistulous tracts.

Treatment

- Surgical resection produces only temporary remission.
- Topical therapy:
  - In non-infected lesions some response has been seen with topical tacrolimus.
- Systemic therapy:
  - Antibiotics for secondary infection based on culture and sensitivity.
  - Prednisolone 1.0–2.0 mg/kg po sid then tapering to alternate day or withdrawal if possible.
  - Vitamin E 400–800 IU/dog po bid helps in some cases.

Lymphoedema

Cause and pathogenesis

Can occur as both a primary and secondary disease. It has been recorded in both the dog and cat:

- Primary disease is caused by developmental defect in lymphatic system.
- Secondary disease is caused through lymphatic obstruction due to inflammation, trauma or neoplasia.

Clinical signs

- Primary disease:
  - No breed predilection in cats; in dogs it has been described in the English bulldog, German shepherd dog, Borzoi, Belgian Tervuren, Old English sheepdog, Labrador retriever, Great Dane and poodle.
  - Young dogs <3 months of age.
  - Skin over hind limbs thickened and pits on pressure (Figure 14.27).
  - Can also affect front limbs, ventrum, tail and pinnae.

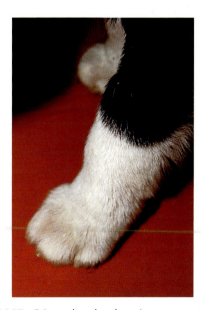

Figure 14.27 Primary lymphoedema in a young collie.

- Secondary infection can occur in many cases.
- Secondary disease:
  - Clinical signs similar to primary disease but lesions will tend to localise to the area of insult to the lymphatic.

Differential diagnosis

Oedema due to obstruction, inflammation or hypoproteinaemic causes.

Diagnosis

- History and clinical signs.
- Laboratory rule outs of other differentials.
- Skin biopsy reveals signs of subcutaneous and dermal oedema; lymphatics are usually dilated and hyperplastic. Chronic cases may show signs of fibrosis and epidermal hyperplasia.

Treatment

- Mild cases often require no treatment.
- Moderate/severe cases:
  - Bandages to reduce swelling
  - Surgical resection of oedematous tissue
  - Surgery to reconstruct lymphatics
  - Amputation of affected area if possible

Acrodermatitis

Cause and pathogenesis

Acrodermatitis is an inherited autosomal recessive disease of bull terriers. The precise defect remains unknown but is thought to be related to abnormal zinc metabolism.

Clinical signs

- Present from birth.
- Cutaneous signs:
  - Hyperkeratosis of footpads, leading to interdigital pyoderma and paronychia then onychodystrophy (Figure 14.28).
  - Ulcerated exudative lesions on ears and muzzle (Figure 14.29).

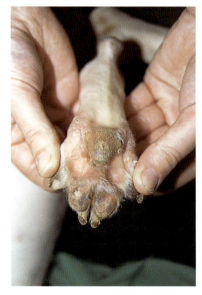

Figure 14.28 Hyperkeratosis of footpads in an English bull terrier with lethal acrodermatitis.

  - Secondary bacterial and yeast infections common.
- Non-cutaneous signs:
  - Weak puppies, difficulty chewing and swallowing.
  - Retarded growth.
  - Initially dogs are aggressive but become lethargic, somnolent.
  - Diarrhoea, respiratory infections.
- Average survival time 7 months.

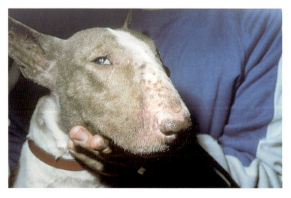

Figure 14.29 Ulcerative lesions on the face in an English bull terrier with lethal acrodermatitis. (Source: Picture courtesy of S. Shaw.)

Differential diagnosis

- Atopy
- Distemper
- Pemphigus foliaceus
- Primary keratinisation disorder

Diagnosis

- History and clinical signs, especially in a predisposed breed.
- Skin biopsy reveals signs of diffuse parakeratotic hyperkeratosis with focal crusting and intraepidermal pustules. The superficial epidermis may show signs of laminar pallor suggestive of necrolytic migratory erythema; however, keratinocytes in acrodermatitis are viable.

Treatment

- Symptomatic treatment for secondary infection is helpful, especially where yeast infection is present. Ketoconazole has been reported to be of good benefit.
- Zinc supplementation is unrewarding.
- No relatives of affected dogs should be used for breeding.

Acral mutilation syndrome

Cause and pathogenesis

Hereditary sensory neuropathy caused through inadequate development and slows progressive post-natal degeneration of sensory neurones. A very rare disease, which has only been reported in dogs. It is thought to be inherited in an autosomal recessive manner.

Clinical signs

- Predisposed breeds include German shorthaired pointer, English springer spaniel and English pointer. No sex predilection.
- Affected pups from 3 months of age.
- As toes become cold and insensitive dogs start to bite and lick paws.
- Severe self-mutilation occurs of toes, especially hind legs (Figure 14.30).

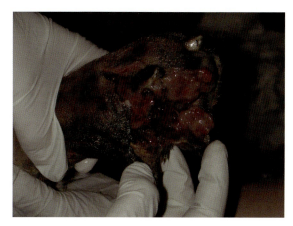

Figure 14.30 Acral mutilation syndrome in an English pointer.

- Neurological examination shows normal proprioception, tendon reflex and motor and cutaneous function.

Differential diagnosis

- Vasculitis
- Frost bite

Diagnosis

- History and clinical signs in predisposed breeds.
- Histopathology of nerve tissue at necropsy.

Treatment

- Attempts to stop the dogs self-mutilating with either physical means (collars, muzzles) or chemical restraints (sedatives) are of little benefit.
- Euthanasia is usually the only option in severe cases.
- Relatives of affected pups should not be used for breeding.

Canine Chiari-like malformation and syringomyelia

Cause and pathogenesis

Chiari-like malformation (CM) is a condition characterised by a disparity between the caudal fossa volume and its contents, the cerebellum and brainstem. This results in neural structures being displaced into the foramen magnum obstructing cerebrospinal fluid (CSF) movement. This leads to syringomyelia (SM) where fluid-filled cavities develop within the spinal cord. CM is most commonly recognised in the cavalier King Charles spaniel but has been reported in other breeds and cats.

Clinical signs

- Cutaneous signs:
  - Most dogs present with unilateral pruritus.
  - Itching commonly occurs when the dog is walking and often without skin contact, so-called 'phantom' scratching.
  - Scratching can be triggered by excitement, touching an area or wearing a collar.
- Non-cutaneous signs:
  - SM may cause thoracic limb weakness, muscle atrophy and pelvic limb ataxia and weakness.
  - Seizures, facial nerve paralysis and deafness may also be seen.
  - CM causes facial pain, especially ear and facial rubbing/scratching.

Differential diagnosis

Cutaneous signs:

- Allergy – atopy, food intolerance, flea allergy
- Ectoparasitic disease

Non-cutaneous signs:

- Intervertebral disc disease
- Granulomatous meningoencephalomyelitis
- Discospondylitis

Diagnosis

- History and clinical signs, especially in a predisposed breed.
- MRI, which reveals that the cerebellum and medulla extend into or through the foramen magnum, which is occluded with little or no CSF around the neural structures.

Treatment

- Surgical therapy using cranial/cervical decompression.
- Medical therapy has been undertaken with a wide range of different medications. Often the best results are seen combining two drugs:
  - Furosemide 1.0–2.0 mg/kg po bid
  - Non-steroidal anti-inflammatory drugs, e.g. carprofen 4 mg/kg po sid
  - Gabapentin 10–20 mg/kg po bid
  - Prednisolone 0.5 mg/kg po sid

Cutaneous mucinosis

Cause and pathogenesis

Can be seen as an idiopathic disease possibly related to overproduction of mucin, which is part of the normal dermal ground substance. It can be seen in other diseases such as hypothyroidism, acromegaly, dermatomyositis and systemic lupus.

Clinical signs

- No sex predilection. Most commonly seen in young dogs.
- Shar-peis have more mucin in their skin than normal dogs and seem to be overpredisposed to developing mucinosis.
- Exaggerated swollen skin folds, especially head (Figure 14.31) and extremities, appear as wrinkles down the dog's legs (Figure 14.32) and on the ventrum.

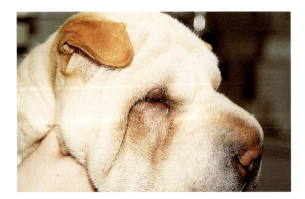

Figure 14.31 Cutaneous mucinosis in a shar-pei.

Diagnosis

- History and clinical signs, especially in a predisposed breed.
- Mucin prick test can be performed by carefully pricking the skin with a fine sterile needle and withdrawing it. A positive test produces a thick sticky liquid exudes from vesicles.
- Skin biopsy reveals non-specific and often minimal changes in the skin except excessive production of mucin.

Treatment

- Where mucin production is secondary to an underlying disease, the identification of concurrent disease, e.g. hypothyroidism needs to be identified and treated.
- Natural resolution of lesions can occur in some shar-peis as they grow so that they rarely need treatment.
- Recalcitrant cases or those with oropharyngeal signs may benefit from the following:
  - Prednisolone 2.0 mg/kg 7–10 days then tapered off over a month.
  - Pentoxifylline 25 mg/kg po tid for 4–6 weeks then tapered to the lowest possible alternate day dose aiming to withdraw if possible.

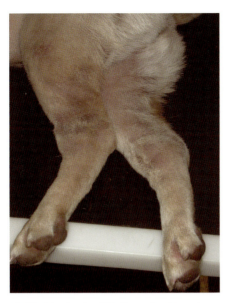

Figure 14.32 Mucinosis of the legs of a shar-pei.

- Mucinous vesiculation (Figure 14.33) can be seen on affected areas often with secondary infection.
- Oropharyngeal involvement leads to snoring and snorting.

Differential diagnosis

- Amyloidosis
- Epitheliotropic lymphoma
- Cutaneous histiocytosis

Selected references and further reading

Cummings, J.F. et al. (1981) Acral mutilation and nociceptive loss in English Pointer dogs. *Acta Neuropathol*, **53**, 119

Kwochka, K.W. (1993) Keratinisation abnormalities: understanding the mechanisms of scale formation. In: Ihrke, P.J. et al. (ed) *Advances in Veterinary Dermatology*. Vol. 2. pp. 91–93. Pergamon, New York

Matousek, J.L. (2004) Disorders of collagen and elastin. In: Campbell, K.L. (ed) *Small Animal Dermatology Secrets*. pp. 105–111. Hanley and Belfus, Philadelphia

Matousek, J.L. (2004) Miscellaneous congenital and hereditary disorders. In: Campbell, K.L. (ed) *Small Animal Dermatology Secrets*. pp 119–125. Hanley and Belfus, Philadelphia

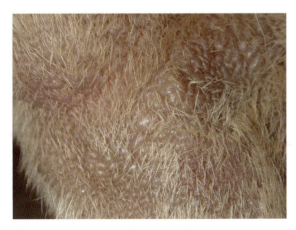

Figure 14.33 Close-up of mucinous blisters.

Medleau, L. and Hnilica, K. (2006) Congenital disease. In: *Small Animal Dermatology: A Color Atlas and Therapeutic Guide.* 2nd edn. pp. 1275–283. WB Saunders, Philadelphia

Olivry, T. et al. (1997) Heterogenicity of canine autoimmune subepidermal blistering diseases: identification of target antigens defines novel clinicopathological entities. *Proc Annu Memb Meet Am Acad Vet Dermatol Coll. Vet Dermatol*, **13**, 80–81

Olivry, T. and Mason, I.S. (1998) Genodermatoses: inheritance and management. In: Kwochka, K.W. et al. (ed) *Advances in Veterinary Dermatology III.* pp. 365–367. Butterworth-Heinemann, Boston

Paciello, O. et al. (2003) Ehlers Danlos-like syndrome in two dogs: clinical, histologic and ultrastructural findings. *Vet Clin Pathol*, **32**, 13–18

Rees, C.A. (2004) Inherited vesiculobullous disorders. In: Campbell, K.L. (ed) *Small Animal Dermatology Secrets.* pp. 112–118. Hanley and Belfus, Philadelphia

Rushbridge, C. et al. (2000) Syringohydromyelia in Cavalier King Charles spaniels. *J Am Anim Hosp Assoc*, **36**, 34

Scott, D.W. et al. (2001) *Congenital and Hereditary Defects Muller and Kirk's Small Animal Dermatology.* 6th edn. pp. 913–1004. WB Saunders, Philadelphia

Pigment abnormalities

Increases in pigment

- Hyperpigmentation – increased pigment in skin or hair
- Melanoderma – excessive pigment in skin
- Melanotrichia – excessive pigment in hairs

Genetic causes of hyperpigmentation

Lentigo (pl. lentigines)

Cause and pathogenesis
Asymptomatic flat macular areas of melanosis. Common disease of dogs; uncommon disease of cats. Unknown aetiology.

Clinical signs
- Dogs:
  - No breed or sex predisposition but generally seen in middle aged to old dogs. Lesions appear as macular to patchy areas of hyperpigmented skin usually on the ventrum.
  - Lesions can increase in numbers and size, often spreading.
  - Lentiginosis profuse is a hereditary form of lentigo seen in pugs.
- Cats:
  - Breeds affected include domestic short-haired and long-haired orange cats.
  - Most commonly seen in cats <1 year old.
  - Lesions found commonly on the lips, also nose (Figure 15.1), gingiva and eyelids.
  - Small uniformly black macules (1–10 mm in diameter) that enlarge and proliferate with time.
  - Asymptomatic, non-pruritic, do not ulcerate.
- Do not undergo neoplastic transformation.

Differential diagnosis
Pigmented neoplasms, e.g. melanoma, basal cell tumour.

Diagnosis
- History and clinical signs especially in particularly coloured cats.
- Skin biopsy reveals signs of epidermal hyperplasia with hyperpigmentation and increased numbers of melanocytes.

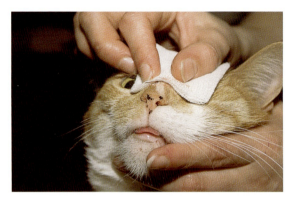

Figure 15.1 Macular melanosis of planum nasale in orange cat.

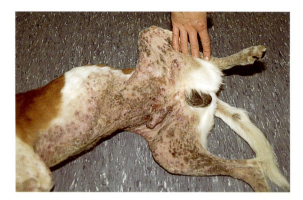

Figure 15.3 Patchy hyperpigmentation on the abdomen of a dog with chronic bacterial infection.

Treatment

No treatment is necessary as this is a cosmetic defect.

Acquired causes of hyperpigmentation

Post-inflammatory hyperpigmentation

Cats uncommonly produce post-inflammatory hyperpigmentation.

Can been seen secondary to

- infection bacterial/fungal (Figure 15.2),
- chronic pruritus secondary to allergy or ectoparasites,
- endocrine imbalance.

Dogs commonly produce signs of hyperpigmentation. Different reaction patterns are recognised:

- Lattice-like appearance seen with infection (bacterial/fungal, Figure 15.3) and chronic allergy (Figure 15.4).
- Comedone formation can be seen as confluent comedones producing blue/grey patches of hyperpigmentation in demodicosis (Figure 15.5) and hyperadrenocorticism.
- Diffuse hyperpigmentation/macular hyperpigmentation can be seen in endocrine disease, e.g. hypothyroidism (Figure 15.6),

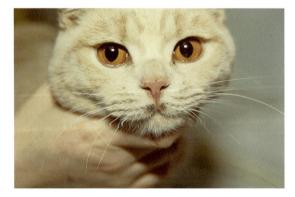

Figure 15.2 Post-inflammatory hyperpigmentation on nose.

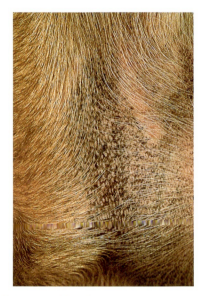

Figure 15.4 Lattice-like hyperpigmentation in a dog with chronic atopy.

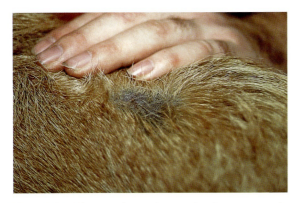

Figure 15.5 Blue–grey hyperpigmentation in squamous demodicosis.

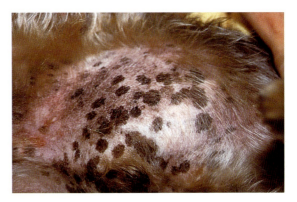

Figure 15.7 Macular hyperpigmentation in a dog with hyperadrenocorticism.

Sertoli cell tumour and hyperadrenocorticism (Figure 15.7).

Acanthosis nigricans

Primary and secondary acanthosis nigricans; see Chapter 14.

Tumour hypermelanosis

Many different tumours can appear as pigmented lesions including the following:

- Melanoma
- Basal cell tumour
- Mastocytosis (Urticaria pigmentosa)
- Epidermal nevi

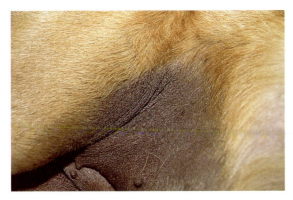

Figure 15.6 Diffuse hyperpigmentation in a dog with hypothyroidism.

Melanotrichia

Uncommon finding when the hair becomes hyperpigmented. It has been recognised in dogs. It is associated with the following:

- Healing of deep inflammatory lesions, e.g. vasculitis, panniculitis.
- Resolution of endocrine or metabolic disease, e.g. hyperadrenocorticism.

Feline acromelanism

- This is the naturally occurring coloration of the extremities, and is seen in particular breeds such as the Siamese, Burmese, Himalayan and Balinese.
- A temperature-dependent enzyme involved in melanin synthesis, which controls the colour.
- High environmental temperatures produce light hair, and low temperatures dark hair.
- Physiological factors such as inflammation and alopecia can also influence colour (Figures 15.8 and 15.9).
- Many of these cats will regrow dark hair over an area that has been clipped for surgery.
- Hair will return to its normal colour after the next hair cycle.

Decreases in pigmentation

- Hypopigmentation – decreased pigment in skin or hair coat

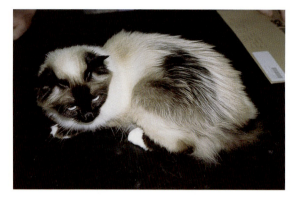

Figure 15.8 Dark hair regrowth on the flanks after successful therapy of flank alopecia due to atopy.

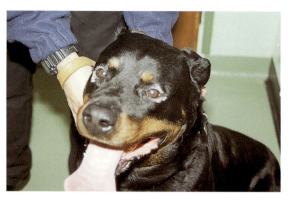

Figure 15.10 Vitiligo in a Rottweiler.

- Leukoderma – lack of pigment in skin
- Leukotrichia – lack of pigment in hair

Genetic causes of hypopigmentation

Chediak–Higashi syndrome

See Chapter 14.

Vitiligo

Cause and pathogenesis
Rare autoimmune reaction thought to selectively destroy epidermal melanocytes leading to loss of pigment in the affected areas. Uncommon disease in dogs and rare in the cat.

Clinical signs
- Dogs:
  - No sex predilection; commonly seen in young dogs.
  - Predisposed breeds include Belgian Tervurens, German shepherd dogs, collies, Rottweilers, Doberman pinschers, Giant schnauzers.
  - One or more areas of macular depigmentation of the skin (leukoderma) or hair (leukotrichia, Figure 15.10).
  - Found especially on nose, lips (Figure 15.11), buccal mucosa and facial skin.
  - Depigmentation may be temporary or permanent.
- Cats:
  - No sex predilection; commonly seen in young animals.

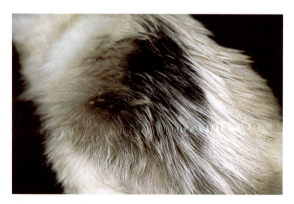

Figure 15.9 Close-up of hair in Figure 15.8.

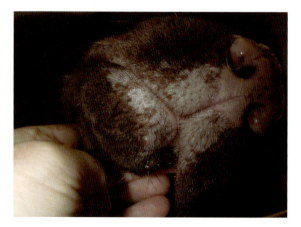

Figure 15.11 Vitiligo of nose and lips of a Labrador.

- Siamese cats appear to be predisposed.
- Similar signs and distribution of lesions in cats and dogs.

Differential diagnosis
- Uveo-dermatologic syndrome
- Discoid lupus erythematosus
- Epitheliotropic lymphoma

Diagnosis
- History and clinical signs.
- Skin biopsy reveals a lack of melanocytes in lesional skin without inflammatory or degenerative changes.

Treatment
- Therapy is unsuccessful.
- The prognosis remains good for dogs and cats as this is a benign disease. Occasionally some animals will completely repigment.

Waardenburg–Klein syndrome (WKS)

Cause and pathogenesis
WKS is caused by the failure of migration and/or differentiation of melanoblasts. It is an autosomal-dominant mode of inheritance with incomplete penetrance.

Clinical signs
- No sex predisposition; occurs in young animals.
- Overrepresented breeds include bull terriers, Sealyham terriers, collies and Dalmatians.
- WKS has also been recorded in cats.
- Cutaneous lesions:
  - Complete lack of pigment in the hair and skin (white animals).
- Other lesions:
  - Deafness
  - Blue or heterochromia of irides

Differential diagnosis
Albinism

Diagnosis
- History and clinical signs.
- Skin biopsy reveals lack of melanocytes.

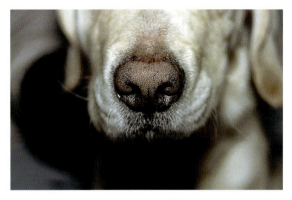

Figure 15.12 Hypopigmentation of the nose in a Labrador.

Treatment
- No therapy is available.
- Animal should not be used for breeding.

Nasal depigmentation 'Dudley nose'

Cause and pathogenesis
This may be a localised form of vitiligo where the depigmentation of skin is confined to the nose.

Clinical signs
- No sex predilection; young dogs affected.
- Predisposed breeds include yellow Afghan hound, Samoyed, Siberian husky, Labrador retrievers, white German shepherd dog, golden retrievers, poodles, Dobermans, Irish setters and pointers.
- Pigment on the nose fades from black to chocolate brown/white from puppy hood (Figure 15.12).
- Some animals will recover spontaneously.

Differential diagnosis
As vitiligo.

Diagnosis
- History and clinical signs.
- Skin biopsy is usually not necessary unless crusting or ulceration present. Dudley nose is typically a non-inflammatory disease; if lesions are present biopsies are indicated to rule out other differentials.

Treatment

Nothing is successful.

Canine cyclic haematopoiesis

See Chapter 4.

Albinism

Cause and pathogenesis

Animals have normal numbers of melanocytes but lack ability to produce melanin and hence pigment. Albinism is a hereditary defect, which is an autosomal recessive. Very rare disease seen in the dog.

Clinical signs

- No sex predilection; seen in young animals from birth.
- The hair, skin and mucous membranes are unpigmented.
- Ocular changes tend to be mild. Unlike humans where the iris in albinos is pink; in the dog it is usually blue.

Diagnosis

- History and clinical signs.
- Skin biopsy reveals no signs of inflammation in the skin. Melanocytes are present in the skin but they appear as clear cells as they do not contain any melanin.

Treatment

- None available.
- Affected animals should be removed from any breeding programme.

Uveo-dermatologic syndrome

Vogt–Koyanagi–Harada-like syndrome (VKH)

Cause and pathogenesis

The precise aetiology is unknown. VKH is thought to be an immune mediated disease with hereditary components. Autoantibodies produced to melanocytes in the skin and eye lead to extensive cutaneous and ocular damage. It is a rare disease in dogs and has not been recorded in cats.

Clinical signs

- No sex predilection; young adult and middle-aged dogs are overrepresented.
- The Akita is a highly predisposed breed; however, the Samoyed, Siberian husky, chow chow, Irish setter, dachshund, fox terrier, Shetland sheepdog, St Bernard and Old English sheepdog are also commonly affected.
- Non-cutaneous:
  - Acute onset anterior uveitis.
  - Reduced or absent pupillary light reflex.
  - Blepharospasm, photophobia, hyphaema.
  - Conjunctivitis, ocular discharge.
  - Retinal detachment, glaucoma and blindness.
  - Neurological signs – rare in dog.
- Cutaneous lesions:
  - Depigmentation of nose, lips, eyelids (Figure 15.13).
  - Occasionally footpads, palate, scrotum and anus.
  - Erosions; ulcerations can occur but rare.
  - In some dogs generalised depigmentation of hair coat can occur.

Differential diagnosis

- Ocular lesions:

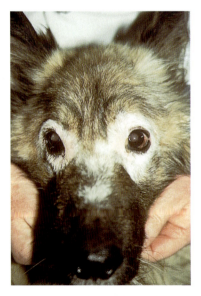

Figure 15.13 Depigmentation of the eyelids and periocular areas in an Akita with uveo-dermatologic syndrome.

- Other causes of uveitis including infection, trauma, neoplasia, immune mediated disease and toxins.
- Cutaneous lesions:
  - Vitiligo
  - Discoid lupus erythematosus
  - Pemphigus erythematosus/foliaceus
  - Epitheliotropic lymphoma

Diagnosis
- History and clinical signs, especially in predisposed breeds.
- Diagnostic rule out of other differentials.
- Ophthalmic signs in addition to cutaneous lesions.
- Skin biopsy reveals signs of a lichenoid interface dermatitis consisting of histiocytes, small mononuclear cells and multi-nucleate giant cells.

Treatment
- Uveitis:
  - Early aggressive treatment is essential to save dog's eyesight.
  - Topical or subconjunctival glucocorticoids (prednisolone, dexamethasone, triamcinolone) and cycloplegics (1% atropine ophthalmic solution) should be used until uveitis resolves.
  - Eyes must be checked regularly for recurrence.
- Cutaneous lesions:
  - Control of skin lesions easier than uveitis.
  - Variety of treatment protocol can be used:
    - Glucocorticoids according to Table 11.1 can be used as sole form of therapy.
    - Combination treatment with prednisolone or methyl prednisolone (see Table 11.1) plus azathioprine (see Table 11.1) is often successful. Intensive therapy is usually required for 4–8 weeks to achieve remission, then tapered down to lowest possible alternate day maintenance dose.
    - Other non-steroid immunosuppressive therapies that can be used alone or as steroid sparing drugs include oxytetracycline and niacinamide, cyclosporine and cyclophosphamide.

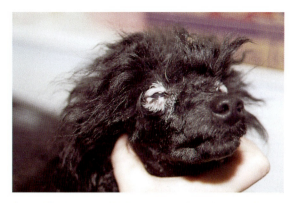

Figure 15.14 Periocular hypopigmentation in a poodle after cryosurgery for distichiasis.

Acquired causes of hypopigmentation

Hypopigmentation can occur secondary to any agent that destroys melanocytes or inhibits their ability to produce pigment. It can occur as a sequela to any underlying skin disease. It is a common finding in the dog and rare in the cat.

Causes in the dog and cat include the following:

- Trauma.
- Burns – chemical, heat, cold (especially cryosurgery (Figure 15.14, irradiation).
- Infection – fungal, bacterial (Figure 15.15, protozoal).
- Drugs – especially glucocorticoids.
- Nutritional deficiencies especially copper.
- Neoplasia – epitheliotropic lymphoma (Figures 15.16 and 15.17), squamous cell carcinoma.

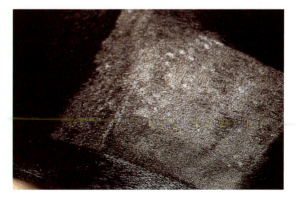

Figure 15.15 Patchy hypopigmentation of post-bacterial infection.

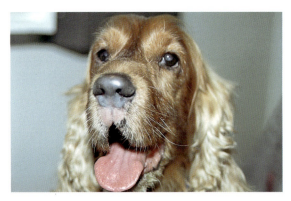

Figure 15.16 Patchy hypopigmentation of the planum nasale in a dog with epitheliotrophic lymphoma.

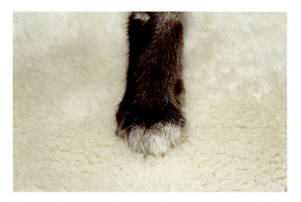

Figure 15.18 Post-inflammatory hyperpigmentation of pedal hair after successful therapy for pemphigus foliaceus.

- Immune mediated disease, e.g. lupus erythematosus, uveo-dermatologic syndrome, pemphigus foliaceus (Figure 15.18).

Animals with nasal hypopigmentation will be predisposed to solar dermatitis.

Idiopathic periocular leukotrichia

Cause and pathogenesis
Pigmentation is lost from the periocular area in cats. Its precise cause is unknown.

Precipitating factors include the following:

- Oestrous
- Pregnancy
- Dietary deficiency
- Systemic illness (upper respiratory tract disease)

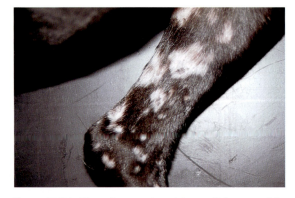

Figure 15.17 Hypopigmentation of the medial aspect of the hock in a dog with epitheliotrophic lymphoma.

Clinical signs
- No sex or age predisposition.
- Siamese cats appear to be predisposed.
- Most commonly seen in females.
- Patchy or complete loss of hair pigment is seen around both eyes to produce a halo-like appearance.

Differential diagnosis
- Post-inflammatory hypopigmentation
- Vitiligo
- Aguirre syndrome
- Systemic/discoid lupus erythematosus

Diagnosis
- History and clinical signs.
- Skin biopsy non-diagnostic; reveals non-specific signs but may be useful as a diagnostic rule out.

Treatment
- Therapy of any underlying systemic trigger.
- No treatment of skin disease is necessary; the hair will repigment within two hair cycles.

Aguirre syndrome

Cause and pathogenesis
A rare disease of unknown aetiology characterised by unilateral periocular depigmentation It is often associated with Horner's syndrome.

Clinical signs
- No age or sex predisposition.
- Siamese cats appear to be predisposed.
- Cutaneous lesions:
  - Unilateral periocular depigmentation
- Non-cutaneous lesions:
  - Horner's syndrome
  - Corneal necrosis
  - Upper respiratory tract infections

Differential diagnosis
As idiopathic periocular leukotrichia.

Diagnosis
History and clinical signs in a predisposed breed.

Treatment
- Symptomatic therapy of concurrent disease.
- Specific therapy of the periocular pigment loss has not been described.

Selected references and further reading

Guaguere, E. and Alhaidari, Z. (1991) Disorders of melanin pigmentation in the skin of dogs and cats. *Proc World Small Anim Vet Assoc*, 8, 47

MacDonald, J.M. (1993) Uveodermatologic syndrome in the dog. In: Griffin, C.E. et al. (eds) *Current Veterinary Dermatology Mosby-Year book.* pp. 217–218. Mosby, St Louis

Medleau, L. and Hnilica, K. (2006) Pigmentary abnormalities. In: *Small Animal Dermatology: A Color Atlas and Therapeutic Guide.* 2nd edn. pp. 287–293. WB Saunders, Philadelphia

Scott, D.W. et al. (2001) *Pigmentary Abnormalities Muller and Kirk's Small Animal Dermatology.* 6th edn. pp. 1005–1024. WB Saunders, Philadelphia

Stokking, L.B. and Campbell, K.L. (2004) Disorders of pigmentation. In: Campbell, K.L. (ed) *Small Animal Dermatology Secrets.* pp. 352–363. Hanley and Belfus, Philadelphia

Psychogenic skin disease

Psychogenic skin disease is overdiagnosed in the cat and the dog. True psychogenic disease is rare. Usually cats and dogs have a primary inciting trigger, which is often a skin problem; however, a stressful environmental or medical factor superimposed on the primary disease can lead to the development of any one of a variety of different problems discussed in the following pages. Anxiety is usually the underlying psychogenic trigger and can be induced by a variety of factors including the following:

- Introduction of a new pet, relative, baby to the house.
- House move.
- Boarding in cattery.
- Enforced confinement due to illness, especially orthopaedic problems.
- Death of a companion human or another pet.
- 'Bullying' by a dominant cat/dog in external environment.
- Overgrooming, where a chronic skin disease or local area of pain/abnormal sensation is left undiagnosed/untreated.

To deal with any of these problems, three factors need to be addressed:

(1) A vigorous search should be made for a primary trigger, which should be identified and treated.
(2) Infection should be treated.
(3) Behavioural component of the disease should be treated using a combination of behaviour-modifying drugs and environmental modification.

Acral lick dermatitis 'lick granuloma'

Cause and pathogenesis

This is a common disease in the dog but rare in the cat. Lesions are formed through repetitive licking. Typical histopathological features have been described (see diagnosis below). Lesions that mimic lick granuloma, i.e. resemble it macroscopically but histopathologically, are consistent with another primary disease process that has subsequently been traumatised are better described as pseudo lick granulomas. Although histopathologically these lesions are different, e.g. neoplastic lesions or primary infections such as mycetoma, they can still lead to stereotypic behaviour. More than 90% of

Table 16.1 Dermatological triggers for lick granuloma.

Dermatological triggers – may be localised or generalised and true or pseudo lick granuloma lesions

Localised skin disease	True or pseudo lick granuloma
1 Traumatic injury (penetrating foreign body, bite wound)	True
2 Neoplasia (mast cell tumour, basal cell tumour)	Pseudo
3 Parasites (demodex, localised tick reaction)	Pseudo
4 Infection (bacterial – atypical mycobacteria, fungal infection, e.g. dermatophytic kerion)	Pseudo
5 Others (pressure point granuloma, calcinosis cutis)	Pseudo

Generalised skin disease – usually a primary inciting factor, e.g. trauma leads to focusing of the generalised disease

1 Parasites (sarcoptes, demodex, cheyletiella, lice)	True
2 Allergy (atopy, food intolerance/allergy, flea allergy)	True
3 Endocrine disease (hypothyroidism, hyperadrenocorticism)	True

lick granulomas are infected. Investigation in all cases should thus be aimed at identification of the underlying cause, appropriate therapy for the infection based on cultures and behaviour modification to break the obsessive–compulsive cycle. Triggers may be dermatological (Table 16.1), orthopaedic (Table 16.2) or neurological (Table 16.3).

Table 16.2 Orthopaedic triggers for lick granuloma.

Orthopaedic triggers – animal will lick over an area of pain; these tend to be true lick granulomas

1. Infection – osteomyelitis
2. Joint pain – septic or immune mediated arthritis, OCD lesions
3. Reaction to orthopaedic implant or suture material
4. Neoplasia – soft tissue or bone incl. metastatic disease
5. Trauma – fracture, dislocation

Table 16.3 Neurological triggers for lick granuloma.

Neurological triggers – area of lick granuloma may match the area of cutaneous innervation

1. Road traffic accident
2. Spinal or nerve root neoplasia
3. L/S degenerative stenosis
4. Neuritis

Clinical signs

- Most animals are <3 years of age; males are affected twice as frequently as females.
- Predisposed breeds are generally large attention-seeking dog breeds, e.g. Dobermans (Figure 16.1), Rottweilers, Labrador retrievers, German shepherd dogs and Irish setters, and when it occurs in cats (Figure 16.2) oriental breeds appear to be predisposed.
- Lesions in the dog are usually 2–6 cm single, unilateral, chronically thickened plaque or nodules often with ulcerated surface (Figure 16.3).
- A surrounding halo of hyperpigmentation is common.
- Usually seen over cranial carpal or metacarpal area.
- Usually a localised lymphadenopathy.

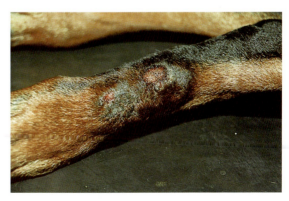

Figure 16.1 Lick granuloma in a Doberman with underlying hypothyroidism.

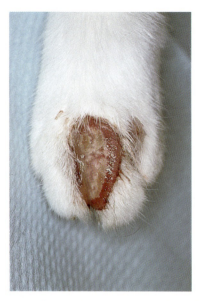

Figure 16.2 Lick granuloma on foot of flea allergic cat (Source: Picture courtesy of D. Crossley.)

Differential diagnosis

Important to differentiate a 'true' lick granuloma from a 'pseudo' lick granuloma.

Diagnosis

- History and clinical signs, including a behavioural history.

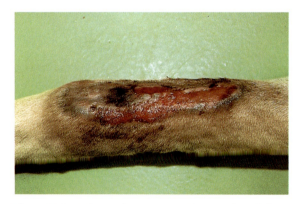

Figure 16.3 Lick granuloma in a Great Dane with underlying orthopaedic problem.

- Diagnostic tests to investigate underlying orthopaedic, neurological and dermatological disease where the history and clinical signs are suggestive.
- Basic core tests should be performed in every case and include skin scrapings, hair pluckings, fine needle aspirates and impression smears, biopsy and tissue culture. Biopsy specimens should be obtained by punch biopsy from non-ulcerated areas.
- Skin biopsy reveals signs of compact hyperkeratosis and multifocal parakeratosis with severe irregular acanthosis of epidermal and superficial follicular epithelium. Superficial dermal fibrosis leads to a 'vertical streaking' pattern between intact follicles. Distinctive plasmacytic periadnexal inflammation is seen. Hair follicles appear larger thickened and elongated.

Treatment

General treatment:

- Therapy of any underlying orthopaedic, neurological or dermatological disease.
- Antibiotic therapy based on culture and sensitivity. Usually antibiotics for 3–4 months are needed as a minimum.
- Environmental modification to reduce stress, decrease boredom.
- Behaviour-modifying therapy may be useful (Table 16.4). A full description of all these drugs is beyond the scope of this text. The prescribing clinician should be aware of the potential side effects of these drugs, together with appropriate use of drugs via the veterinary cascade. There is a lag phase with most drugs before benefit is seen.

Other treatment modalities can be directed at specific lesional treatment. This should never replace a proper work-up but includes the following:

- Physical prevention of licking with collars, socks, bandages, side braces, etc.
- Topical treatment:

Table 16.4 Drugs suitable for behavioural therapy in the dog and cat.

Drug	Oral dose rate
Tricyclic antidepressants – potential side effects include sedation, antimuscarinic and antihistaminic effect; contraindicated in hepatic or renal disease	
Amitriptyline	Dog final dose 1–4 mg/kg po bid, start 1–2 mg/kg bid and increase to full dose over 4 weeks Cat final dose 0.5–1.0 mg/kg po bid, start 0.5 mg/kg bid and increase to full dose over 4 weeks
Doxepin	Dog final dose 1–5 mg/kg bid, start 1 mg/kg bid and increase to full dose over 4 weeks
Clomipramine	Dog final dose 1–3.5 mg/kg po bid, start 1 mg/kg bid and increase to full dose over 4 weeks Cat final dose 0.5–1.0 mg/kg po bid, start 0.5 mg/kg bid and increase to final dose over 4 weeks
Fluoxetine	Dog and cat final dose 1 mg/kg po sid/bid; allow 4–6 weeks for clinical trial
Sertraline	Dog final dose 1 mg/kg po sid; allow 4–6 weeks for clinical trial
Anxiolytics – potential side effects can include disinhibition, interference with memory, ataxia, depression and paradoxical excitement; phenobarbitone should not be used in animals with hepatic disease; hydroxyzine has antihistaminic effects	
Diazepam	Dog and cat 0.55–2.2 mg/kg po sid/bid as needed
Alprazolam	Dog 0.05–0.25 mg/kg po sid/bid
Lorazepam	Dog 0.025–0.25 mg/kg po sid/bid
Oxazepam	Dog 0.2–1.0 mg/kg po sid/bid
Clonazepam	Dog 0.05–0.25 mg/kg po sid/bid
Phenobarbitone	Dog and cat 2.2–6.8 mg/kg po bid
Hydroxyzine	Dog 2.2 mg/kg po tid
Endorphin blocker	
Naltrexone	Dog 2.2 mg/kg po sid
Endorphin substitute	
Hydrocodone	Dog 0.25 mg/kg po tid

- Topical glucocorticoids – short-term use only; never use when infection is present.
- Bad-tasting topical applications, e.g. bitter apple.
- Topical analgesics.
- Surgical removal – not recommended as it tends to produce short-term remission and lesions are often reproduced at same site.
- Radiation therapy has a limited usage.
- Cryosurgery can be successful as it denervates the area.
- Laser ablation is useful as it sterilises the area as well as denervates it.

Tail biting

Cause and pathogenesis

Dogs that chase and bite their tails; thought to be a behavioural problem but a rigorous search should be made for underlying disease.

Clinical signs

- No sex predilection; generally seen in young dogs.

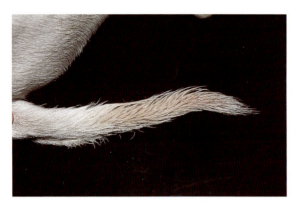

Figure 16.4 Traumatisation of the tail tip due to psychogenic tail biting in an English bull terrier.

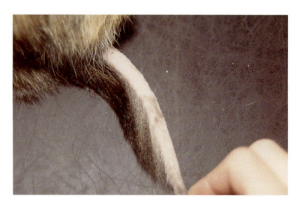

Figure 16.5 Tail licking in a cat with chronic diarrhoea.

- Hyperexcitable breeds such as Staffordshire bull terriers and English bull terriers may be predisposed.
- Self-inflicted trauma to the tail tip caused as the animal circles to grab the tail (Figure 16.4).

Differential diagnosis

- Tail pruritus caused by allergy, parasites especially fleas.
- Abnormal tail sensation due to lumbosacral disease or tail dock neuroma.

Diagnosis

- History and clinical signs.
- Diagnostic rule outs of other differentials.

Treatment

- Anxiolytics or tricyclic antidepressants using the same dosage regime as for acral lick dermatitis.

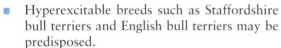

Cause and pathogenesis

Cats that sit and suck their tails (Figure 16.5). It is usually associated with boredom or enforced confinement, but rigorous steps should be taken to ensure that there is no underlying clinical condition.

Clinical signs

- No sex or age predilection.
- Predisposed breeds include oriental breeds especially the Siamese.
- Distal 2–3 cm of the tail is wet due to sucking but no other clinical lesions are present.

Differential diagnosis

- Conditions causing pruritus or pain to the tail
- Allergy
- Parasites
- Traumatic injury to tail base

Diagnosis

- History and clinical signs.
- Diagnostic rule outs of other conditions.

Treatment

- Anxiolytics or tricyclic antidepressants – dosage as for acral lick dermatitis.

Psychogenic skin disease

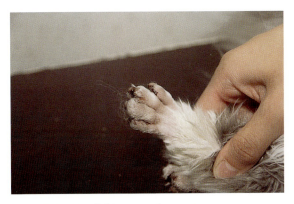

Figure 16.6 Foot licking secondary to atopy.

Foot licking

Cause and pathogenesis

Foot licking is a very common problem in both the dog and cat. However, it is rarely a psychogenic problem. In the cat, it is usually associated with paronychial problems. Underlying causes include the following:

- Infection especially bacteria, Malassezia.
- Allergy especially atopy (Figures 16.6 and 16.7) or food.
- Autoimmune disease, e.g. pemphigus foliaceus.

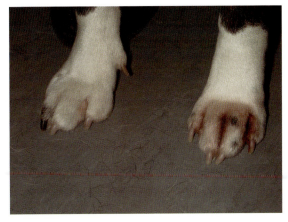

Figure 16.7 Foot licking in an atopic dog. The unilateral nature of the lesion is suggestive of a possible behavioural component.

- Neoplasia especially metastatic bronchial carcinoma.

Similar triggers are recognised in the dog including the following:

- Infection – bacterial, *Malassezia*
- Pododemodicosis
- Allergy especially atopy or food

Clinical signs

- Wetness of the feet due to licking often with associated hair loss.
- In white-haired animals brown pedal saliva staining is obvious.
- No primary lesions, no exudate from nail beds is seen in psychogenic disease.

Differential diagnosis

Medical causes of paronychia and pododermatitis.

Treatment

- Treatment of underlying causes.
- Anxiolytic drug or tricyclic antidepressants as acral lick dermatitis.

Flank suckers

Cause and pathogenesis

Animals that suck their flanks. May be associated with 'comfort sucking' in dogs that have been separated from their dam at an early age.

Clinical signs

- No age or sex predilection.
- Doberman pinscher may be predisposed.
- Dogs rarely cause obvious clinical signs other than wetting of the hair coat on the flanks.

Differential diagnosis

Cause of pruritus of flanks especially allergy.

Diagnosis

- History and clinical signs.
- Diagnostic rule out to ensure that the animal is not sucking due to an underlying painful or pruritic condition.

Treatment

Anxiolytic or tricyclic antidepressant drugs as acral lick dermatitis.

Self-nursing

Cause and pathogenesis

Recognised in dogs (usually bitches) that suckle their own nipples. Not been reported in cats. Thought to be a behaviour problem; may be associated with premature removal from dam.

Clinical signs

Dogs rarely cause obvious clinical signs other than wetting of the ventral abdominal skin around their nipples (Figure 16.8).

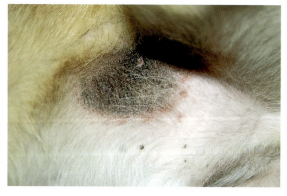

Figure 16.8 Lichenification and erythema due to self-nursing in a Labrador. The dog had induced a secondary malassezia dermatitis.

Differential diagnosis

- Causes of ventral pruritus especially allergy
- Mastitis

Diagnosis

- History and clinical signs.
- Diagnostic rule out to ensure that the animal is not sucking due to an underlying painful or pruritic condition.

Treatment

Anxiolytic or tricyclic antidepressant drugs as acral lick dermatitis.

Anal licking

Cause and pathogenesis

Animals that either lick or drag/scoot themselves along on their perianal skin. May be a behavioural problem but is more commonly associated with underlying disease. In the same way as dermatological disease can lead on to lick granuloma, there is no doubt perianal irritation can develop into anal self-traumatisation with a strong behavioural component. Seen in dogs (licking and scooting) and cats (licking only).

Clinical signs

- No age or sex predilection.
- Poodles seem to be predisposed.
- Lesions vary from mild perianal saliva staining to chronic lichenification with self-inflicted trauma of the perianal area.

Differential diagnosis

- Causes of perianal irritation:
  - Mucocutaneous pyoderma
  - *Malassezia* infection

- Allergy – flea allergic dermatitis, atopy, food intolerance
- Contact allergy/irritancy
- Anal sac disease, colonic disease

Diagnosis

- History and clinical signs.
- Diagnostic rule out of concurrent disease.

Treatment

- Identification and treatment of any underlying trigger.
- Anxiolytic drug and tricyclic antidepressants as acral lick dermatitis.

Psychogenic dermatitis (neurodermatitis)

Cause and pathogenesis

Anxiety is the most common trigger for true psychogenic dermatitis. Stress may lead to increases in adrenocorticotrophic hormone and melanocyte-stimulating hormone causing increased endorphin production. Endorphins are thought to protect the animal from stressful situations, although their production may reinforce the overgrooming activity. Obsessive grooming may be an extension of overgrooming induced by primary skin disease.

Clinical signs

- No age or sex predilection is recognised.
- Breed predisposition is seen most commonly in oriental breeds especially Siamese.
- In mild cases, alopecia is the only finding often with no associated inflammation.
- In severe cases, alopecia is accompanied by marked self-inflicted trauma in the form of ulceration, often with the formation of eosinophilic plaques and secondary infection.

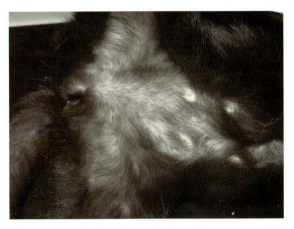

Figure 16.9 Ventral psychogenic alopecia in a cat responded completely to improved flea control.

- Distribution patterns of alopecia:
  - Ventral alopecia (Figure 16.9)
  - Bilateral flank alopecia
  - Medial forelegs
- Chronic lesions become lichenified and hyperpigmented.

Differential diagnosis

- Causes of traumatic alopecia:
  - Ectoparasites (fleas, cheyletiella, otodectes, lice, demodex)
  - Allergy (atopy, food),
  - Dermatophytosis
  - Seborrhoeic dermatitis (malassezia)
- Causes of non-pruritic alopecia:
  - Hypothyroidism (very rare)
  - Hyperadrenocorticism (very rare)
  - Telogen defluxion
  - Anagen defluxion
  - Acquired symmetrical alopecia

Diagnosis

- These cases require an extensive work up to rule out both traumatic and non-pruritic causes of alopecia.
- Investigations should include the following:
  - Skin scrapings.
  - Fungal cultures.

- ☐ Allergy work-up including exclusion diets, intradermal testing.
- ☐ Blood count – if there is an eosinophilia present then the condition is not psychogenic.
- ☐ Skin biopsy of non-lesional areas reveals normal skin.
- ☐ Ectoparasite therapy.
- ☐ Endocrine function tests.

Treatment

- Therapy of any underlying diseases.
- Psychological drug therapy as acral lick dermatitis.

Selected references and further reading

Dodman, N.D. et al. (1988) Use of narcotic antagonists to modify and stereotypic self-licking, self chewing and scratching behaviour in dogs. *J Am Vet Med Assoc*, **193**, 815–819

Doering, G.G. (1974) Acral lick dermatitis: medical management. *Canine Pract*, **55**, 21–25

Luescher, A.U. (2003) Diagnosis and management of compulsive disorders in dogs and cats. *Vet Clin North Am Small Anim Pract*, **33**, 253–267

Medleau, L. and Hnilica, K. (2006) Feline psychogenic alopecia. In: *Small Animal Dermatology: A Color Atlas and Therapeutic Guide*. 2nd edn. pp. 271–273. WB Saunders, Philadelphia

Patterson, A.P. (2004) Psychocutaneous disorders. In: Campbell, K.L. (ed) *Small Animal Dermatology Secrets*. pp. 324–331. Hanley and Belfus, Philadelphia

Scott, D.W. et al. (2001) *Psychogenic Skin Diseases Muller and Kirk's Small Animal Dermatology*. 6th edn. pp. 1055–1071. WB Saunders, Philadelphia

Virga, V. (2003) Behavioural dermatology. *Vet Clin North Am Small Anim Pract*, **33**, 231–251

White, S.D. (1990) Naltrexone for treatment of acral lick dermatitis in dogs. *J Am Vet Med Assoc*, **196**, 1073–1076.

Keratinisation defects

Seborrhoea

This is defined as abnormal formation of the cornified layer of the skin leading to scaling, and abnormal sebum production.
Seborrhoea oleosa describes greasy seborrhoea.
Seborrhoea sicca describes dry seborrhoea.
Neither term is a diagnosis but a description of a clinical finding.
Different diseases and breeds produce different types of seborrhoea.

Primary seborrhoea
Rare disease; covered in Chapter 14. This is a diagnosis of exclusion.

Secondary seborrhoea
Almost any skin disease can produce seborrhoea. Commonly seen with the following:

- Endocrine disease especially hypothyroidism (dog, Figure 17.1), hyperthyroidism (cat, Figure 17.2), hyperadrenocorticism.
- Nutritional factors such as inappropriate diet (malabsorption, maldigestion syndromes, zinc responsive dermatosis).
- Allergy such as flea (Figure 17.3), atopy, food (Figure 17.4), contact allergy.
- Environmental factors, e.g. central heating, harsh shampoo therapy.
- Infection with bacteria (Figure 17.5), *Malassezia* spp., dermatophytes, leishmaniasis.
- Ectoparasitism including demodicosis, sarcoptes (Figure 17.6), cheyletiella, pediculosis.
- Immune mediated disease such as pemphigus foliaceus (Figure 17.7), systemic lupus erythematosus.
- Neoplasia especially epitheliotropic lymphoma (Figure 17.8).
- Systemic disease in the cat FeLV, FIV, FIP.
- Inability to groom especially in cats with dental disease, hypervitaminosis A.

Clinical signs

- Abnormal scaliness of the coat; tends to be more pronounced in dogs than cats as cats grooming activity removes much of the scale.
- Signs variable and can include dry, lustreless hair coat with excessive scaling, follicular casts, scaly seborrhoeic patches and plaques with greasy malodorous skin.

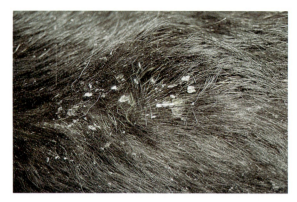

Figure 17.1 Seborrhoea secondary to hypothyroidism.

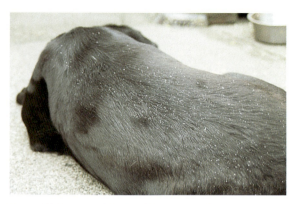

Figure 17.4 Generalised scaling in a Labrador with food intolerance.

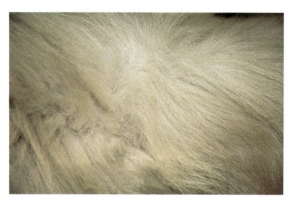

Figure 17.2 Generalised seborrhoea oleosa in a hyperthyroid cat.

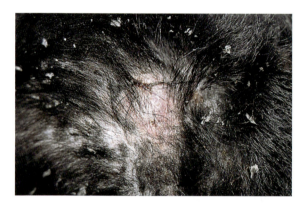

Figure 17.5 Scaling due to superficial bacterial infection.

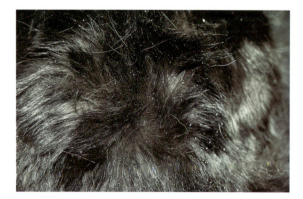

Figure 17.3 Dorsal seborrhoea secondary to flea allergy.

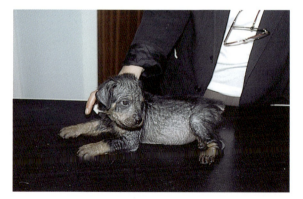

Figure 17.6 Generalised seborrhoea due to sarcoptic mange.

Keratinisation defects 279

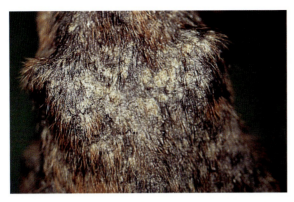

Figure 17.7 Scaling on the dorsum of a dog with pemphigus foliaceus.

- Ceruminous otitis externa common.
- Precise signs and distribution depend on underlying diseases and species and breed.

Diagnosis

- History and clinical signs.
- Identification of underlying disease. Investigation of seborrhoea is time consuming and expensive. It is important to run a basic screen (see diagnostic tests) to include skin scrapes, tape strips, hair plucks, impression smears, cytology of any primary lesions and fungal culture. A food trial, ectoparasite therapy and bloods including endocrine function tests may also be indicated.

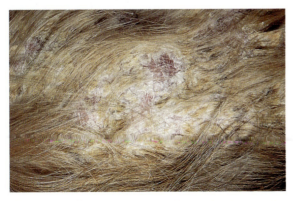

Figure 17.8 Thick crusting and scaling on the skin of a dog with epitheliotrophic lymphoma.

- Skin biopsy especially with allergic, endocrine and systemic disease is often non-specific. In the case of other differentials, histopathology may be diagnostic, e.g. zinc responsive disease.

Treatment

- Correction of underlying disease will allow seborrhoea to control itself in 1–2 months.
- Antibiotics or antiyeast treatment for secondary infections.
- Topical treatment (see primary seborrhoea, Chapter 14.)
- Dogs and cats need to be continually re-assessed but skin condition will change as primary disease is controlled.

Ichthyosis

See Chapter 14.

Canine acne

See Chapter 4.

Feline acne

Cause and pathogenesis

Common idiopathic disorder of follicular keratinisation and glandular hyperplasia seen in cats.
Contributory factors may include the following:

- Poor grooming habits.
- Abnormal sebum production.
- Primary keratinisation defects.
- Stress associated with illness especially viral effects.
- Immunosuppression.

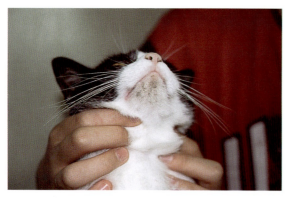

Figure 17.9 Comedones on chin with feline acne.

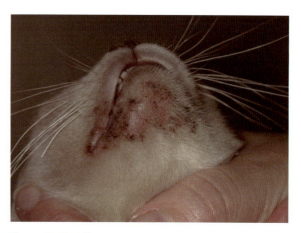

Figure 17.10 Chronic acne in a cat.

- Hormonal factors are not thought to be important.

Clinical signs

- No breed, sex or age predisposition.
- Lesions can occur as a single episode; appear cyclical or are constant.
- Early lesions:
    - Comedones on chin and lips (often asymptomatic) (Figure 17.9).
    - Papules and pustules develop later.
    - Pruritus mild in uncomplicated cases.
- Chronic severe cases:
    - Secondary infection leads to folliculitis, furunculosis and cellulitis (Figure 17.10).
    - Pathogens include *Pasteurella multocida*, B-haemolytic streptococcus and coagulase positive staphylococcus.
    - Chronic lesions are more pruritic.
    - Oedema with overlying skin thickened, cystic and scarred.

Differential diagnosis

- Sebaceous adenitis
- Eosinophilic granuloma complex
- Dermatophytosis
- Demodicosis
- Allergy (food, atopy)
- Malassezia

Diagnosis

- History and clinical signs.
- Diagnostic rule out by skin scrapings, fungal culture, cytology.
- Skin biopsy reveals comedone formation with glandular hyperplasia and perifolliculitis. Folliculitis, furunculosis and cellulitis can be seen when secondary infection is present.
- Culture and sensitivity may be useful to identify secondary infection.

Treatment

- Asymptomatic cases are essentially a cosmetic problem and can be left untreated.
- Topical therapy may be used every 1–3 days as required:
    - Antiseborrhoeic shampoos:
        - Mild degreasing products include those containing sulphur and salicylic acid.
        - Where additional antibacterial/yeast action is required acetic acid, boric acid, chlorhexidine and ethyl lactate based products may be beneficial.
        - Benzoyl peroxide has excellent degreasing and follicular flushing activity but can be irritating to some cats.

- Antibacterial creams/lotions containing clindamycin, fucidin, erythromycin or tetracycline may also be useful where secondary infection is present.
- Topical vitamin A as 0.01–0.025% tretinoin cream or lotion may be useful but irritancy can occur.

■ Systemic therapy:
- Antibiotics based on culture and sensitivity for a minimum of 3 weeks.
- Essential fatty acid supplementation may be useful in some cases.
- Steroids rarely indicated but may be given as a short course in sterile cases (1–2 mg/kg daily by mouth).
- Retinoid therapy can be given in severe cases – isotretinoin 1.0–2.0 mg/kg po sid for up to 1 month, then every other day. These drugs are potent teratogens and should be dispensed with care, especially to female owners of childbearing age. Monitoring of the feline patient should include routine haematology, biochemistry especially liver function, triglycerides and cholesterol.

Tail gland hyperplasia

Cause and pathogenesis

Cats:
The tail gland in the cat is located along a dorsal line on the tail; it is rich in sebaceous and apocrine glands. Hyperplasia of the gland leads to the accumulation of waxy secretion on the surface of the skin. It is a condition commonly seen in entire males as 'stud tail' but hormonal link is unclear as can be seen in neutered cats and females.

Dogs:
Tail gland is an area 2.5–5.0 cm distal to the anus on dorsal surface of the tail. Hair follicles at this site are simple. The area contains both sebaceous and hepatoid glands. Hyperplasia occurs secondary to other diseases, e.g. primary or secondary seborrhoea, elevated androgen levels.

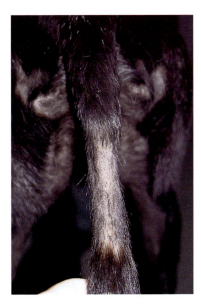

Figure 17.11 Greasy seborrhoea on dorsum of tail 'stud tail'.

Clinical signs

Cats:

- No breed or age predilection; entire males may be overrepresented.
- More commonly seen in catteries/cats that are confined.
- Greasy band of excessive secretions with scale and crust seen along dorsum of tail (Figure 17.11).
- Overlying hair coat may be thinned, skin often hyperpigmented.
- Often asymptomatic and no other areas affected.
- Secondary infection is a rare complication.

Dogs:

- Oval bulging alopecic areas seen just below the tail head on dorsum of tail.
- Overlying skin scaly, greasy and hyperpigmented.
- Secondary infection can occur leading to pustular eruptions (Figure 17.12).
- Where the tail gland hyperplasia is seen associated with generalised seborrhoeic skin disease other lesions are present on distant sites.

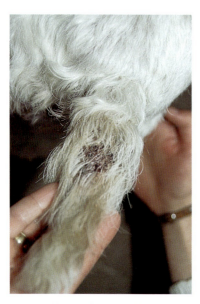

Figure 17.12 Tail gland hyperplasia secondary to hypothyroidism.

Differential diagnosis

- Little else presents at this site with this clinical appearance, unlikely differentials therefore include the following:
  - Demodicosis
  - Dermatophytosis
  - Superficial pyoderma
  - Neoplasia

Diagnosis

- History and clinical signs.
- Bacteriological culture, tape strippings where secondary infection is present.
- Skin biopsy reveals signs of sebaceous gland hyperplasia.

Treatment

- Systemic antibiotics where secondary infection is present.
- Where generalised seborrhoeic skin disease is present, this needs to be addressed.

- Topical shampoo with salicylic acid, sulphur or benzoyl peroxide based products.
- Cats:
  - Self-grooming should be encouraged by reduction of periods of confinement and increased owner interaction. Owner may have to groom cats that will not self-groom.
  - Castration of entire males may only produce partial improvement or only stop further progression of the disease
- Dogs:
  - Castration may be beneficial in entire males to produce partial of complete remission.
  - Where large unsightly lesions are present surgery resection of the gland may be possible. This requires skilled surgery as the area is difficult to close post-operatively. However, regression lesions can be seen with 18 months to 3 years.

Vitamin A responsive dermatosis

Cause and pathogenesis

Vitamin A responsive dermatosis is a rare disease of dogs of unknown aetiology. Its response to vitamin A does not indicate a deficiency state.

Clinical signs

- Occurs in any age of dog but young dogs of 2–3 years appear to be overrepresented.
- Predisposed breed is the American cocker spaniel.
- Follicular plugs and hyperkeratotic plaques with crusting seen on ventral and lateral chest and abdomen especially around the nipples (Figure 17.13).
- Footpad hyperkeratosis may also be seen (Figure 17.14).
- Pruritus is mild to moderate.
- Ceruminous otitis common.
- Hair coat easily epilated, malodorous rancid body smell.

Keratinisation defects 283

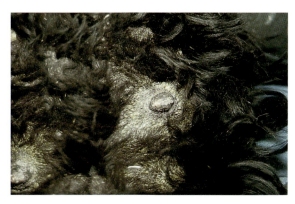

Figure 17.13 Vitamin A responsive dermatosis showing hyperkeratotic plaques around the nipples.

Differential diagnosis

- Primary seborrhoea
- Secondary seborrhoea (multiple causes of this)
- Sebaceous adenitis
- Zinc responsive dermatosis

Diagnosis

- History and clinical signs, especially in predisposed breeds.

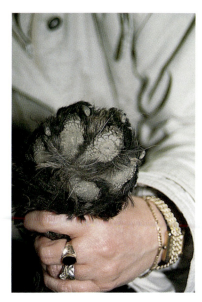

Figure 17.14 Footpad hyperkeratosis in a case of vitamin A responsive dermatosis.

- Trichography of hairs mounted in liquid paraffin reveals prominent follicular casts.
- Skin biopsy reveals signs of disproportionate follicular orthokeratotic hyperkeratosis with only minimal epidermal hyperkeratosis.
- Response to vitamin A.

Treatment

- Topical therapy:
  □ Symptomatic relief is possible using antiseborrhoeic shampoos, especially those containing sulphur, salicylic acid, benzoyl peroxide and tar.
- Systemic therapy:
  □ Vitamin A (retinol) 8,000–10,000 IU po/10 kg sid with a fatty meal. Improvement should be seen within 4–6 weeks and clinical remission within 8–10 weeks. Vitamin A toxicity is possible.
  □ Response to therapy is usually good but lifetime treatment is required.

Nasodigital hyperkeratosis

Cause and pathogenesis

This disease is characterised by the formation of excessive footpad and nasal keratin. Common condition in old dogs. This can occur in two forms:

- Idiopathic disease in old dogs.
- As a component of other disorders. In these diseases, it is uncommon for other clinical signs *not* to be present in addition to the nasodigital lesions. Conditions include the following:
  □ Ichthyosis
  □ Distemper
  □ Leishmaniasis
  □ Pemphigus foliaceus
  □ Systemic lupus erythematosus
  □ Zinc responsive dermatosis
  □ Generic food dermatosis
  □ Cutaneous lymphoma
  □ Superficial necrolytic migratory erythema
  □ Familial footpad hyperkeratosis

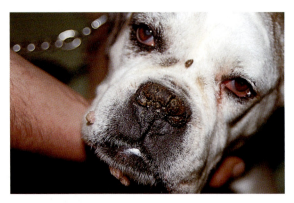

Figure 17.15 Idiopathic nasal hyperkeratosis.

Clinical signs

Idiopathic nasodigital hyperkeratosis:

- Keratin builds up on the dorsum of the nose and the edge of the footpads.
- Nasal planum is hard, dry, rough and hyperkeratotic (Figure 17.15).
- Footpads show similar signs and are also hard, cracked and hyperkeratotic (Figure 17.16). The signs are most pronounced at the edges of weight-bearing pads where horny growths cause pain by their pressure against the other pads, making it difficult for the dog to walk.
- If ulcers, erosions or fissures are present, it is suggestive of an immune mediated problem such as vasculitis or pemphigus foliaceus.
- Parasympathetic dysfunction can be seen concurrently leading to loss of nasal gland secretions and exacerbating the problem.
- In idiopathic disease dogs are otherwise fit.

Differential diagnosis

All of the other causes of nasodigital hyperkeratosis listed above.

Diagnosis

- History and clinical signs.
- Diagnostic rule outs of other conditions.
- Skin biopsy in cases of idiopathic disease reveals signs of epidermal hyperplasia with marked orthokeratotic or parakeratotic hyperkeratosis.

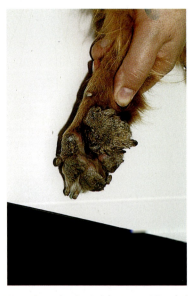

Figure 17.16 Idiopathic hyperkeratosis of footpads in an old dog.

Treatment

- Mild asymptomatic cases:
    - Need little therapy only observation.
- Moderate to severe cases:
    - Trim excessive keratin (scissors or razor blade).
    - Hydration of pads is best achieved by soaking them in water. The application of compresses to the nose for 5–10 minutes helps hydrate the planum nasale.
    - Application of keratolytic/softening agent, e.g. 50% propylene glycol, petroleum jelly, lanolin, tretinoin gel, ichthammol ointment after hydration.
    - Intensive daily treatment for 7–10 days, then maintenance once or twice weekly.

Benign disease with a good prognosis; dogs may need symptomatic therapy to keep them comfortable.

Hereditary nasal parakeratosis of labrador retrievers

Cause and pathogenesis

Uncommon keratinisation problem seen in Labrador retrievers and their crosses that causes hyperkeratosis of the planum nasale. An autosomal recessive mode of inheritance has been proposed.

Clinical signs

- No sex predilection; the disease is seen in young dogs 6–12 months of age.
- Thick, hard, hyperkeratotic crust accumulates on the dorsal aspect of the planum nasale (Figure 17.17).
- Crusts, erosions, ulcerations, fissures and depigmentation may develop (Figure 17.18).
- Lesions are not pruritic or painful.
- The disease can wax and wane.
- Rare to see any other signs of the animal's body.
- Some reports have suggested that there can be involvement of the haired dorsal planum nasale as well as footpads.

Differential diagnosis

- Ichthyosis
- Distemper
- Leishmaniasis
- Pemphigus foliaceus
- Systemic lupus erythematosus
- Zinc responsive dermatosis
- Generic food dermatosis
- Cutaneous lymphoma

Diagnosis

- History and clinical signs in a predisposed breed.
- Diagnostic rule outs of other causes of nasal hyperkeratosis.

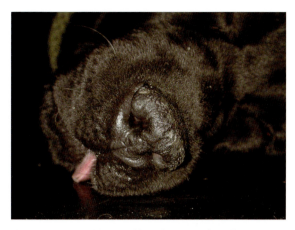

Figure 17.17 Mild case of hereditary nasal parakeratosis.

- Skin biopsy reveals signs of parakeratosis with multifocal accumulations of proteinaceous fluid between keratinocytes within the stratum corneum and stratum spinosum 'protein lakes'. Lymphocystic and neutrophilic exocytosis with some pigment incontinence.

Treatment

- No specific therapy is recorded; therapy as for nasodigital hyperkeratosis is useful.
- Other topical treatment, which may produce benefits if applied twice daily, includes the following:
  - Petroleum jelly.
  - Vitamin E cream.

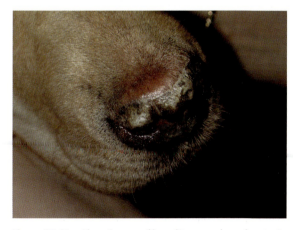

Figure 17.18 Chronic case of hereditary nasal parakeratosis.

- ☐ Propylene glycol 50:50 in water.
- ☐ Frequency of application can be decreased once a response has been seen.
- Prognosis is poor for a cure. However, dogs can be kept comfortable for what is a benign disease with topical symptomatic therapy.

Familial footpad hyperkeratosis

Cause and pathogenesis

A rare familial keratinisation disorder that results in severe hyperkeratosis of the footpads in young dogs of certain breeds. Disease has a tardive onset so that the dogs are born with normal pads but the disease develops over the first 6 months of age. An autosomal recessive mode of inheritance is thought to exist in Irish terriers.

Clinical signs

- No sex predilection; the disease first becomes evident in dogs of 5–6 months of age.
- Predisposed breeds include Irish terriers, Dogue de Bordeaux and Kerry blue terriers.
- Footpads become thickened, hyperkeratotic, hard and cracked (Figure 17.19).
- Horny growths and expanding fissures develop as the disease becomes more chronic.
- Secondary infection is very common.
- Dogs will become very lame due to the horny growths putting pressure on adjacent pads and the infection.
- Irish terriers have accompanying nail abnormalities but no other skin changes are noted in cases.

Differential diagnosis

- Ichthyosis
- Distemper
- Pemphigus foliaceus
- Systemic lupus erythematosus
- Zinc responsive dermatosis
- Superficial necrolytic migratory erythema

Diagnosis

- History and clinical signs.
- Diagnostic rule outs of other differentials.
- Skin biopsy of footpads reveals signs of orthokeratotic hyperkeratosis with mild to severe epidermal hyperplasia.

Treatment

- No specific treatment regime has been described but therapy as described for idiopathic nasodigital hyperkeratosis may be useful.
- Topical daily foot soaks with 50% propylene glycol and filing of the excessive keratin from the footpads can help to keep dogs comfortable.
- Retinoid therapy with isotretinoin at a dose of 1 mg/kg po sid may be beneficial in some cases. Monitoring is necessary due to hepatotoxicity and owners should be made aware of teratogenicity of the drug.
- The prognosis for a cure is poor but with a dedicated owner the dogs can be kept comfortable. Owners should be made aware that animals will need lifetime therapy.

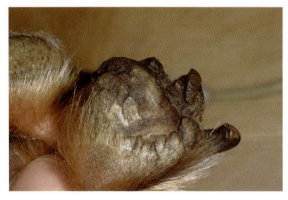

Figure 17.19 Familial footpad hyperkeratosis in a Dogue de Bordeaux. (Picture courtesy Dr. S. Shaw.)

Schnauzer comedone syndrome

See Chapter 14.

Sebaceous adenitis

Cause and pathogenesis

The precise aetiology of sebaceous adenitis is unclear. Different mechanisms may be responsible for disease in different breeds. Uncommon disease in the dog and rare disease in the cat. Possible underlying triggers include the following:

- Developmental/inherited defects leading to sebaceous gland destruction.
- Immune mediated attack against components of sebaceous gland.
- Keratinisation disorder.
- Abnormality of lipid metabolism.

Clinical signs

- Breed predilection Vizla, Akita, Samoyed, standard poodle (Figure 17.20), springer spaniel. An autosomal recessive mode of inheritance is recognised in the poodle and the Akita. No breed predilection is recognised in the cat.

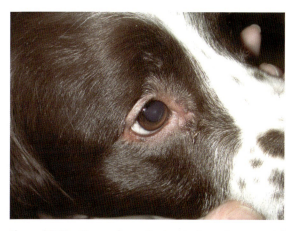

Figure 17.21 Fine scale on the head of a springer spaniel with sebaceous adenitis.

- No sex predilection; affects young, middle-aged animals.
- Lesions may be focal, multifocal or generalised. Initial lesions found on head (Figure 17.21), pinnae and neck.
- Cutaneous lesions depend on coat type. Scaling usually affects the dorsum (Figure 17.22), top of head, face, ear pinnae and tail.
- Cats:
  - Multifocal annular areas of crust and scale; hairs epilate easily and contain prominent follicular casts on hairs.
- Short-haired dog:
  - May be asymptomatic annular areas of alopecia with fine scale, which is

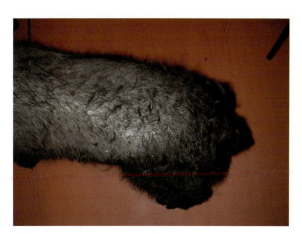

Figure 17.20 Sebaceous adenitis in a poodle.

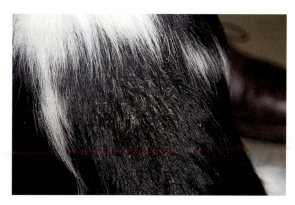

Figure 17.22 Sebaceous adenitis in a springer spaniel showing diffuse fine scaling.

non-adherent. Secondary infection with bacteria and yeast can occur.
- Long coated:
  - Generalised scale is evident. Matted hairs easily epilated and prominent follicular casts with diffuse alopecia are seen. The primary hairs are usually retained but the soft undercoat is lost. Secondary infection is common. Some Akitas are profoundly affected and be febrile with weight loss.
- Pruritus variable in both cases.

Differential diagnosis

- Bacterial folliculitis
- Demodicosis
- Dermatophytosis
- Follicular dystrophy
- Endocrinopathy especially hypothyroidism

Diagnosis

- History and clinical signs, especially in predisposed breeds.
- Laboratory rule outs of other conditions.
- Trichography of plucked hairs mounted in liquid paraffin reveals prominent follicular casts.
- Skin biopsy reveals signs of discrete granulomas in the areas of the sebaceous glands. In chronic lesions sebaceous glands are completely lost and replaced with fibrosis.

Treatment

- Response to treatment can be disappointing and often difficult to assess as sebaceous adenitis can be cyclical in nature.
- Secondary bacterial infection needs to be treated with systemic antibiotics based on sensitivity. In many cases pulse therapy with antibiotics, i.e. full therapeutic doses of antibiotic therapy given twice weekly, is needed to prevent re-infection.
- Yeast infection can be managed using topical therapy. Shampoo containing miconazole or boric acid or rinses containing enilconazole or lime sulphur may be used.
- Topical treatment:
  - Mild cases:
    - Antiseborrhoeic shampoos containing salicylic acid, sulphur and ethyl lactate plus emollient rinses (see treatment for primary seborrhoea, Chapter 14).
  - Severe cases:
    - Potent antiseborrhoeic shampoos containing tar and benzoyl peroxide.
    - Propylene glycol 50–75% in water as a rinse as required.
- Systemic treatment:
  - Essential fatty acids as oral administration of omega 6 and omega 3 containing fatty acids have been shown to be useful in some cases.
  - Prednisolone 1–2 mg/kg daily for 10–14 days, then alternate day tapering to lowest possible dose.
  - Cyclosporine 5 mg/kg po sid for up to 4 weeks or until maximal benefit, whichever occurs first. Then taper to lowest possible alternate or twice weekly dose rate.
  - Asparaginase 10,000 IU im weekly for 2–3 treatments, then as required.
  - Retinoids:
    - Isotretinoin 1 mg/kg po sid/bid until improvement is seen (up to 6 weeks), then 1 mg/kg po every other day for 6 weeks tapering down to lowest possible maintenance dose rate. Monitoring is necessary due to hepatotoxicity and owners should be made aware of teratogenicity of the drug.
    - Acitretin 1 mg/kg po sid/bid until improvement is seen (up to 6 weeks), then 1 mg/kg po every other day for 6 weeks tapering down to lowest possible maintenance dose rate.
- Removal of dogs from breeding programmes is important.
- Prognosis is variable, but tends to be best for short-coated breeds and those diagnosed early in the course of their disease.

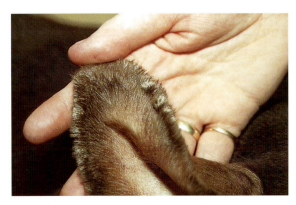

Figure 17.23 Thick adherent crust on the periphery of the ear pinna in a dog with hypothyroidism.

Ear margin dermatosis

Cause and pathogenesis

Idiopathic seborrhoeic disease of the margins of the pinna seen in dogs with pendulous ears.
 Clinical signs can be recognised as components of other diseases including

- vasculitis,
- hypothyroidism (Figure 17.23),
- head flapping secondary to otitis externa or pinnal pruritus (scabies, atopy etc.).

Clinical signs

- No sex or age predilection; dachshunds appear to be predisposed.
- Early cases present with soft greasy seborrhoea with erythema (Figure 17.24) affecting the margins of the pinnae.
- In chronic cases, thick, hard crust accumulates on the margins leading to a cracked, ulcerated and fissured appearance.
- The condition may be painful leading to head shaking and further trauma.

Differential diagnosis

- Scabies
- Vasculitis

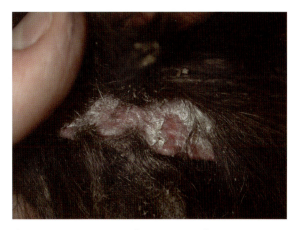

Figure 17.24 Ear margin dermatosis in a flat coat retriever.

- Neoplasia especially squamous cell carcinoma
- Hypothyroidism

Diagnosis

- History and clinical signs, especially in predisposed breeds.
- Diagnostic rule outs of other differentials.
- Skin biopsy reveals signs of orthokeratotic or parakeratotic hyperkeratosis with follicular keratosis.

Treatment

- Topical therapy:
  - Antiseborrhoeic shampoos containing sulphur, salicylic acid, benzoyl peroxide may be used to remove crust and seborrhoeic discharge. Shampoos are applied daily until crusts and scale removed then decreased to maintenance levels.
  - Topical moisturisers may be used after shampoo therapy.
- Systemic therapy:
  - Pentoxifylline 10–15 mg/kg po tid may be helpful in some animals. Drug is slow to work, taking 4–12 weeks.
  - Essential fatty acid supplementation may be useful in some cases.

- Therapy with tetracycline, niacinamide, doxycycline or vitamin E has been shown to produce improvement in some dogs (for doses see Table 11.1).
- Prednisolone may be used for severely inflamed pinnae at a dose of 1 mg/kg po sid for 7–10 days then tapered down and withdrawn where possible.
- Surgical therapy:
  - In cases where ear fissuring is severe and unresponsive to medical therapy, surgical resection in the form of an ear crop may be indicated.

Idiopathic facial dermatitis in Persians cats

Cause and pathogenesis

Uncommon variable pruritic facial disease seen in the Persian cat. Aetiology is unknown but it is thought this may represent a keratinisation disorder in that cats may have a sebaceous gland abnormality. A genetic basis of the disease may be possible.

Clinical signs

- Young Persian and Himalayan cats of either sex appear predisposed.
- Highest incidence in older kittens and young adult cats.
- Lesions confined to the head and neck.
- Erythema, alopecia and marked self-inflicted trauma.
- Thick black exudation with crusting of hairs around the eyes, mouth and chin (Figure 17.25).
- Ceruminous otitis seen as thick black waxy debris in the canals; seen in approximately 50% of cases.
- Secondary bacterial and yeast infection common (Figure 17.26), which leads to increased pruritus.
- A mucoid ocular discharge is common and herpetic eye disease may be present concurrently.

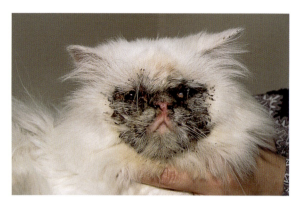

Figure 17.25 Idiopathic facial dermatitis in a Persian.

Differential diagnosis

- Allergy (atopy, food, fleas)
- Demodicosis
- Dermatophytosis
- Idiopathic sterile pyogranulomatous disease

Diagnosis

- History and clinical signs in a predisposed breed.
- Cultures for bacteria and yeasts are secondary problems but need to be treated.
- Other findings include negative FeLV, FIV assays, dermatophyte cultures.

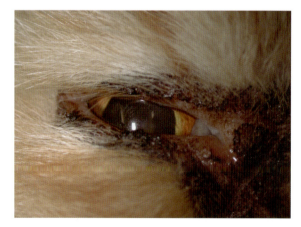

Figure 17.26 Periocular infection in a Persian with idiopathic facial dermatitis.

- Occasional positive skin test reactivity but cats rarely show a response to allergen-specific immunotherapy.
- Skin biopsy reveals signs of acanthosis, superficial crusting, hydropic degeneration of basal cells with occasional dyskeratotic keratinocytes. Sebaceous hyperplasia presents with a mixed superficial dermal infiltrate.

Treatment

- Guarded prognosis; mild to moderate cases can be managed but therapy is usually labour intensive and requires a dedicated owner.
- Topical therapy:
  - Crusts and debris removal with antiseborrhoeic shampoos containing sulphur, salicylic acid and ethyl lactate.
  - Antibacterial/antiyeast washes and wipes containing acetic acid, boric acid, chlorhexidine, ethyl lactate, miconazole, EDTA tris to help control secondary infection.
  - Ear treatment using ceruminolytic agents to remove wax from the ears plus topical therapy based on cytology/culture of discharge.
  - Eye cleansers to remove the discharge and then antibacterial agents if infection is present.
  - Anti-inflammatory therapy should only be used once all infection has been adequately treated. Topical glucocorticoids, cyclosporine and tacrolimus may be used sparingly for short periods to effect.
- Systemic therapy:
  - Antibiotics and antiyeast therapy where appropriate to deal with secondary infection. Pulse therapy may be needed for maintenance, i.e. full therapeutic dosage of drugs given twice weekly as preventative therapy once infection has resolved.
  - Anti-inflammatory therapy should only be used once infection has been treated:
    - Prednisolone 1–3 mg/kg po sid for 14–21 days then tapered to lowest possible alternate day maintenance dose rate.
    - Cyclosporine 5–7 mg/kg po sid to achieve clinical improvement then tapered to lowest possible maintenance dose rate. Cats should be assessed for suitability of cyclosporine therapy with routine bloods including a viral screen.
- Prognosis is guarded and many cats are euthanised due to lack of owner commitment, resources or failure to respond to therapy.

Selected references and further reading

Bond, R. et al. (2000) An idiopathic facial dermatitis of Persian cats. *Vet Dermatol*, **11**, 35–41

Kuhl, K. (2004) Disorders of keratinisation. In: Campbell, K.L. (ed) *Small Animal Dermatology Secrets*. pp. 91–98. Hanley and Belfus, Philadelphia

Medleau, L. and Hnilica, K. (2006) Keratinisation and seborrhoeic disorders. In: *Small Animal Dermatology: A Color Atlas and Therapeutic Guide*. 2nd edn. pp. 295–325. WB Saunders, Philadelphia

Page, N. et al. (2003) Hereditary nasal parakeratosis in Labrador retrievers. *Vet Dermatol*, **14**, 103–110

Paradis, M. (1992) Footpad hyperkeratosis in a family of Dogue de Bordeaux. *Vet Dermatol*, **3**, 75–78

Paradis, M. (2001) Primary hereditary seborrhoea oleosa. In: August, J.R. (ed) *Consultations in Feline Internal Medicine 4*. pp. 202–207. WB Saunders, Philadelphia

Reichler, I.M. et al. (2001) Sebaceous adenitis in the Akita: clinical observations, histopathology and hereditary. *Vet Dermatol*, **12**, 243–253

Rybnicek, J. et al. (1998) Sebaceous adenitis: an immunohistological examination. In: Kwochka, K. et al. (eds) *Advances in Veterinary Dermatology*. Vol. 3. pp. 539–540. Butterworth-Heinemann, Oxford

Scott, D.W. et al. (2001) *Keratinisation defects Muller and Kirk's Small Animal Dermatology*. 6th edn. pp. 1025–1053. WB Saunders, Philadelphia

Miscellaneous skin diseases in the dog

Subcorneal pustular dermatosis

Cause and pathogenesis

Very rare sterile pustular disease identified in the dog. No clear cause has been identified; it may be an immune mediated disease. Some sources have suggested that it is a variant of pemphigus foliaceus.

Clinical signs

- Has been identified in many different breeds but miniature schnauzers appear to be predisposed.
- No age or sex predilection.
- Lesions may be multifocal or generalised, appearing as non-follicular pustules especially on the head and trunk (Figure 18.1).
- Pustules transient so that secondary lesions often more prominent as alopecia, scale, crust, epidermal collarettes (Figure 18.2).
- Peripheral lymphadenopathy is an inconsistent finding.
- Footpads, mucous membranes, mouth rarely affected.
- Dogs usually systemically well.

Differential diagnosis

- Pemphigus foliaceus
- Sterile eosinophilic pustulosis
- Bacterial impetigo/folliculitis
- Systemic lupus erythematosus
- Superficial pyoderma

Diagnosis

- History and clinical signs.
- Diagnosis by exclusion of other diseases.
- Cytology of pustules reveals non-degenerate neutrophils, occasionally acanthocytes. In uncomplicated cases bacteria are not present.
- Cultures, if taken carefully, are usually sterile.
- Skin biopsy reveals signs of subcorneal pustules containing non-degenerate neutrophils. Acanthocytes are an inconsistent finding.

Treatment

- Therapy as for pemphigus foliaceus may be successful in some cases (see Chapter 11).
- Dapsone 1 mg/kg po tid until a response is seen, which can take 1–4 weeks. The dose is then tapered to daily treatment twice weekly.

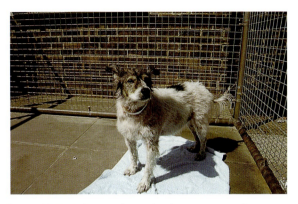

Figure 18.1 Subcorneal pustular dermatosis in a dog.

Haematology and liver enzymes levels should be monitored during treatment.
- Sulphasalazine 10–20 mg/kg po tid until controlled, then as required. It is important to monitor tear function in these dogs.

Sterile eosinophilic pustulosis

Cause and pathogenesis

Rare skin disease only recorded in the dog. It is thought to be an immune mediated disease.

Clinical signs

- No age, breed or sex predilection.
- Primary lesions are of follicular and non-follicular papules and pustules.

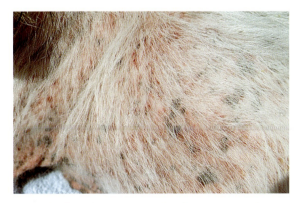

Figure 18.2 Subcorneal pustular dermatosis – close-up showing scaling and crusting.

- Chronically lesions progress to annular erosions with epidermal collarettes and target lesions.
- Distribution variable but often starts on the trunk.
- Lesions are usually pruritic.
- Dogs usually systemically well, but concurrent lymphadenopathy, depression, anorexia or pyrexia may be seen.

Differential diagnosis

- Bacterial folliculitis/impetigo
- Pemphigus foliaceus
- Dermatophytosis
- Demodicosis
- Subcorneal pustular dermatosis
- Ectoparasitic disease
- Drug eruption

Diagnosis

- History and clinical signs.
- Haematology usually reveals signs of a peripheral eosinophilia.
- Cytology of pustule content reveals eosinophils, non-degenerate neutrophils, occasional acanthocytes but no bacteria.
- Cultures, if taken carefully, are sterile.
- Skin biopsy reveals signs of eosinophilic intraepidermal pustules with folliculitis and furunculosis.

Treatment

- Systemic glucocorticoids in the form of prednisolone 2.0–4.0 mg/kg po sid until lesions resolve, which can takes up to a month. Once remission has been achieved then prednisolone should be switched to an alternate day regime at the lowest possible dose rate.
- Dapsone may be used as described under subcorneal pustular dermatosis.
- The prognosis for these cases remains very poor. Some animals can be kept comfortable with low dose alternate day prednisolone.

Idiopathic sterile granuloma and pyogranulomas

Cause and pathogenesis

Uncommon skin disease only recognised in dogs. It is thought to be an immune-mediated disease.

Clinical signs

- Any age, sex or breed.
- Predisposed breeds include the Boxer, golden retriever, collie, Great Dane and any other large short-coated breed.
- Lesions appear as multiple asymptomatic dermal papules and nodules.
- Lesions can be identified at any site but the head (bridge of nose, Figure 18.3, muzzle, pinnae), paws, and scrotum appear to be areas commonly affected.
- Chronic lesions can become alopecic, ulcerated and secondarily infected (Figure 18.4).

Differential diagnosis

- Infectious granulomas, (bacteria, mycobacteria, fungal)
- Parasites (leishmania, tick bites)
- Foreign body granulomas
- Neoplasia

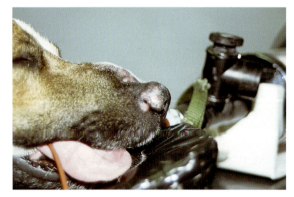

Figure 18.3 Idiopathic sterile pyogranulomas on the nose of a German shepherd dog.

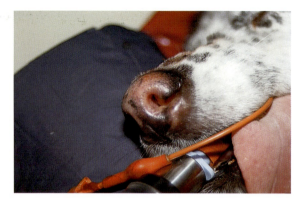

Figure 18.4 Ulcerated depigmented lesions on a collie with advanced idiopathic sterile pyogranulomas.

Diagnosis

- History and clinical signs.
- Laboratory rule out of other conditions.
- Cytological examination of fine needle aspirate reveals a pyogranulomatous inflammatory infiltrate with no evidence of micro-organisms.
- Microbial culture of tissue via biopsy or discharge via swab is usually negative.
- Skin biopsy reveals signs of nodular to diffuse sterile granuloma/pyogranuloma. Special stains fail to reveal signs of micro-organisms.

Treatment

- Solitary lesions:
  - Surgical excision.
- Multiple lesions:
  - Systemic treatments:
    - Prednisolone 2.0–4.0 mg/kg po sid. Remission can take 2–6 weeks. However, dose rate should be tapered 10–14 days into therapy to an alternate day regime to prevent glucocorticoid side effects due to long-term use. Once remission has been achieved the steroid dose rate should be tapered to the lowest possible alternate day regime.
    - Other therapeutic options include azathioprine, L-asparaginase, doxycycline/niacinamide, oxytetracycline/niacinamide; for dose rates, see Table 11.1.

- Prognosis is good for the majority of dogs as remission can be achieved in most cases. However, many dogs need lifetime therapy.

Localised scleroderma (morphea)

Cause and pathogenesis

Rare disease, identified in domestic species of dogs. It has an unknown aetiology but may be due to

- vascular damage,
- abnormal collagen metabolism,
- autoimmune disease.

Clinical signs

- No age, sex or breed predilection.
- Lesions tend to be asymptomatic and present as shiny alopecic sclerotic plaques.
- Lesions are most commonly found on the trunk and limbs.
- Animals are generally systemically well.

Diagnosis

- History and clinical signs.
- Skin biopsy reveals signs of a fibrosing dermatitis.

Treatment

Benign disease often undergoes spontaneous remission and so does not generally require any specific therapy.

Eosinophilic granuloma

Cause and pathogenesis

Unknown aetiology, but may represent a hypersensitivity reaction to environmental allergens especially arthropod bites or stings, which leads to collagen degeneration.

Clinical signs

- Usually dogs less than 3 years of age.
- Males seem to be predisposed. Higher incidence of lesions seen in Siberian husky and cavalier King Charles spaniel.
- Lesions are plaques and proliferative nodules often ulcerated, found in oral cavity and on the skin:
  - Oral cavity lesions found on tonsils, palate and tongue. Oral plaques can be painful leading to halitosis as the presenting complaint.
  - Cutaneous lesions found on ventral abdomen, prepuce and flanks. Lesions on the skin are usually asymptomatic. Dogs are systemically well.

Differential diagnosis

- Infectious granulomas (fungal/bacterial)
- Sterile granulomas
- Neoplasia

Diagnosis

- History and clinical signs, especially in predisposed breeds.
- Skin biopsy reveals signs of eosinophilic/ histiocytic granulomas with collagen degeneration.
- Haematology often unremarkable but on occasions an eosinophilia may be present.
- Carefully taken cultures submitted for both aerobic and anaerobic plus mycobacterial culture are sterile.

Treatment

- Solitary lesions may undergo spontaneous regression and do not require therapy.
- Glucocorticoids needed for multiple or oral lesions. Prednisolone 0.5–2.0 mg/kg po sid for 10–14 days or until clinical remission, then

tapered to lowest possible maintenance dose rate aiming to withdraw.
- On the rare occasions where glucocorticoids are unsuccessful other anti-inflammatory medication suitable for therapy of atopy (see Chapter 10) can be employed.
- In most cases complete remission is achieved with therapy and no further treatment is required. Prognosis is good.

Juvenile cellulitis (puppy strangles, big head disease)

Cause and pathogenesis

A disease of unknown aetiology, which may be immune mediated. A familial tendency is often seen so that the disease can affect more than one puppy in a litter.

Clinical signs

- Commonly seen in young puppies 3 weeks to 6 months of age.
- Predisposed breeds include the golden retriever, dachshund, beagle, pointer and Gordon setter.
- Cutaneous signs:
    - Acute onset swollen face, submandibular lymphadenopathy.
    - Vesicles, papules, pustules with purulent exudate progressing to fistulae (Figure 18.5).
    - Lesions are found on lips, muzzle and eyelids (Figure 18.6).
    - Ear pinnae can be swollen and exudative and commonly a sterile discharge is produced from the ear canal.
    - In rare cases the anus and prepuce can be involved.
    - Lesions are painful but not pruritic.
- Non-cutaneous signs:
    - Lethargic, anorexic, pyrexic.
    - Joint pain due to a sterile suppurative arthritis is seen in 25% of cases.

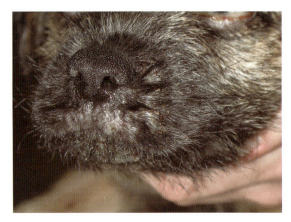

Figure 18.5 Papules and pustules on the face of a puppy with juvenile cellulitis.

Differential diagnosis

- Angioedema
- Demodicosis
- Drug eruption
- Deep bacterial pyoderma
- Distemper

Diagnosis

- History and clinical signs.
- Laboratory rule outs of other conditions.
- Impression smears from the exudative lesions from skin or the ear reveal macrophages, with non-degenerate neutrophils. Microorganisms are not usually seen.

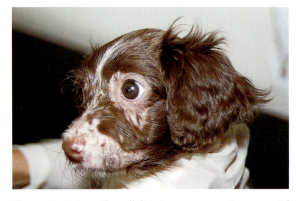

Figure 18.6 Juvenile cellulitis in a young springer spaniel puppy.

- Skin biopsy reveals diffuse granulomatous to pyogranulomatous inflammation. Infectious agents are rarely seen.
- Culture, if taken carefully, are sterile. In chronic cases secondary infection may be identified but appropriate therapy based on cultures or cytology rarely leads to a significant improvement.

Treatment

- Early treatment is important to avoid scarring.
- Topical therapy:
  - Warm water soaks, and gentle emollient baths to remove crust and scale.
- Systemic therapy:
  - Prednisolone 2 mg/kg po sid until remission 7–28 days, then cut to an alternate day regime for a further 14–21 days, then taper further aiming to withdraw. If medication is decreased too quickly then relapse will occur.
  - Broad spectrum antibiotics therapy may be given during the treatment period in the form of cephalexin 25 mg/kg po bid or clavamox 22 mg/kg po bid/tid.
- Although the disease is fatal if not treated, the prognosis is good and recovery without scarring is possible if early treatment with appropriate antibiotics and glucocorticoid is undertaken.

Symmetrical lupoid onychodystrophy

Cause and pathogenesis

Condition of unknown aetiology, possibly an immune mediated disease that leads to sloughing of the claws. It is an uncommon disease in the dog.

Clinical signs

- Principally affects young to middle-aged dogs.

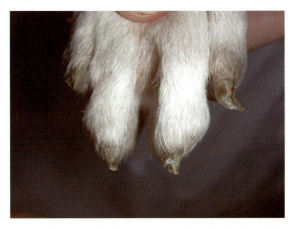

Figure 18.7 Onychorrhexis and onychomalacia of nails in symmetrical lupoid onychodystrophy.

- Predisposed breeds include German shepherd dogs and Rottweilers although it can be recognised in any breed.
- All four feet are affected but often front feet most severe.
- Initial signs are confined to one or two claws, which are lost; however, the problem will eventually affect all of the claws to some degree.
- No other cutaneous lesions.
- Onychomalacia and onychorrhexis (Figure 18.7) often followed by onychomadesis (Figure 18.8). Nails that are shed are replaced with misshapen nails that are of a similar soft or brittle quality.

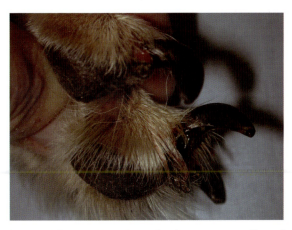

Figure 18.8 Onychomadesis of nails in symmetrical lupoid onychodystrophy.

- Dogs feet are often swollen and painful.
- Paronychia is uncommon.

Differential diagnosis

- Other causes of onychodystrophy:
  - Onychomycosis
  - Systemic lupus erythematosus
  - Pemphigus vulgaris
  - Bullous pemphigoid
  - Vasculitis

Diagnosis

- History and clinical signs.
- Laboratory rule outs of other diseases.
- Skin biopsy of skin around nail produces a non-specific pattern. Diagnostic histopathology is only possible if the nail is submitted with the nail bed; however, in many cases the third phalanx has to be removed and submitted to achieve this, unless the nail can be split longitudinally. Biopsy reveals hydropic basal cell degeneration with apoptosis of individual keratinocytes in the basal cell layer. Pigmentary incontinence and a lichenoid infiltrate are also common.

Treatment

- Surgical therapy:
  - Although medical therapy can be implemented without the removal of all the damaged nails, it is rarely successful. Removal of all of the nails under general anaesthetic is important to remove damaged, deformed nails to allow new nails to grow through (Figure 18.9).
  - Nail removal is undertaken by manual removal using haemostats taking care not to leave remnants of nails behind. The nail beds bleed profusely after removal (Figure 18.10) and sterile dressing should be applied for the first 24–48 hours in combination with antibiotic therapy and painkillers. After this the dog can be left undressed but should wear an Elizabethan collar to prevent traumatisation.
  - In recurrent cases or severe cases P3 amputation may be a useful surgical option to medical therapy.
- Medical therapy:
  - Antibiotics for secondary infection based on culture and sensitivity.
  - Post nail removal a range of therapeutic regimes have been described with varying success (see Table 18.1). Drugs listed below in the table may be used in isolation or as combinations. The author favours a combination of biotin, GLA and pentoxifylline.

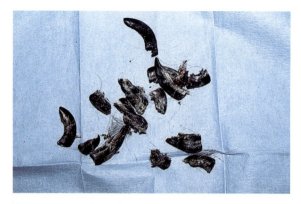

Figure 18.9 Deformed nails removed under general anaesthetic in a dog with lupoid onychodystrophy.

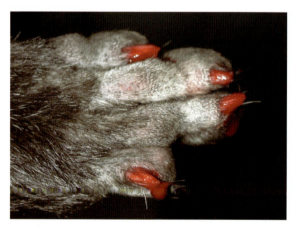

Figure 18.10 Appearance of nail beds after removal of damaged nails.

Table 18.1 Drug therapies for onychodystrophy.

Drug	Dosage	Details
Essential fatty acid	Dosage differs with individuals EPA 400 mg/10 kg GLA 100 mg/10 kg	Improvement will take up to 3 months
Biotin	2.5 mg/dog po sid	Improvement as above
Tetracycline /niacinamide	Dogs <10 kg, 250 mg po tid of each drug Dogs >10 kg, 500 mg po tid of each drug	Give tid until noticeable nail growth is seen 3–6 months Then give bid for 2 months, then sid for maintenance
Pentoxifylline	10–25 mg/kg po bid/tid	Improvement will take up to 3 months
Prednisolone	1–2 mg/kg po bid	Give bid for 2–4 weeks then sid for 2–4 weeks, then taper to lowest possible alternate day dosage
Azathioprine	2 mg/kg po sid	Improvement will take 2–3 months, then taper to alternate day medication for maintenance; drug needs to be monitored (see Chapter 11.)

Anal sac disease

Cause and pathogenesis

Anal sacs are two small structures located between the internal and external anal sphincter muscles. They are found at the four and eight o'clock positions. Each of the sacs in lined with both sebaceous and apocrine glands. In a normal dog the sac empties via a short, narrow duct to the surface of the perianal skin on the edge of the anus. The secreted substance is a semi-oily, foul-smelling brownish fluid. Recurrent anal sac disease can be associated with abnormalities of anal gland secretion, anatomical defects or underlying disease (Table 18.2). It is a common disease, but it is principally seen in dogs.

Clinical signs

- No age or sex predilection. Large breeds are underrepresented. Small breeds especially poodles, Chihuahuas, and Lhasa apsos have an increased risk.
- Dogs scoot along the floor or bite or lick their perianal skin.
- Some animals can cause severe damage to the skin leading to lichenification, hyperpigmentation and ulceration (Figure 18.11).
- Secondary infection with both yeast and bacteria are common.

Table 18.2 Causes of anal sac impaction.

Cause of impaction	Details
Abnormal anal gland secretion	Dogs that produce thick or dry discharge that cannot be naturally expelled
Abnormal anal gland ducts	Dogs with congenitally narrow ducts, dogs with acquired damage to the ducts due to perianal infections, trauma, allergies
Perianal disease	Food allergy or atopy that causes perianal irritation

Table 18.3 Anal sac contents.

Sac contents – disease status	Appearance of contents	Microscopic examination
Normal sac	Clear or pale yellow straw/brown coloured fluid	Corneocytes and basophilic material; bacteria predominantly Gram positive cocci, with a few Gram positive rods and rare Gram negative rods; rare neutrophils and yeast (Figure 18.12)
Impacted anal sac	Thick yellow or brown and pasty consistency	As above
Anal sacculitis	Creamy yellow or yellow green exudate variable consistency	Corneocytes and basophilic bacteria as above; large numbers of bacteria of varying types; neutrophils in large numbers often with intracytoplasmic bacteria (Figure 18.13)
Anal gland abscess (Figure 18.14)	Reddish brown exudate – necrotic/purulent exudate	As above for anal sacculitis, often large numbers of erythrocytes and necrotic debris

- Some dogs also show signs of faecal tenesmus, tail chasing and areas of acute moist dermatitis.

Differential diagnosis

- Anal sac neoplasia
- Perianal fistula
- Tapeworms

- Contact irritant/hypersensitivity
- Food allergy

Diagnosis

- History and clinical signs.
- Digital palpation of distended anal sac.
- Expression of anal sac contents can reveal a variety of clinical findings (see Table 18.3).

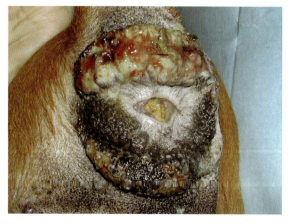

Figure 18.11 Severe perianal damage due to self-inflicted trauma.

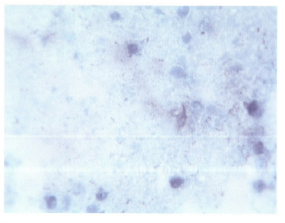

Figure 18.12 Cytology of normal anal gland secretion.

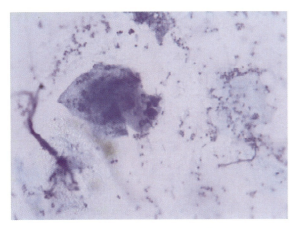

Figure 18.13 Cytology of abnormal anal gland secretion.

Treatment

- Identification and therapy of any underlying disease.
- Anal sac impaction manual evacuation may be sufficient; owners can be instructed as to how to empty glands on future occasions.
- Anal sacculitis requires manual evacuation and lavage of the sacs with either chlorhexidine (0.025%), povidone iodine (0.4%) or EDTA tris. The sacs can then be packed based on culture and sensitivity with an antibiotic and glucocorticoid combination in the form of a cream or ear drops. Systemic antibiotics may be necessary for 10–14 days.
- Anal sac abscess is treated in a similar way to the sacculitis with flushing, topical instillation and systemic antibiotics on the basis of culture and sensitivity.
- For recurrent or severe disease, excision of the affected gland may be necessary.
- Prognosis is moderate, provided that the initial problem can be resolved and owners can be educated as to how to express their pets' glands on a long-term basis.

Anal furunculosis

Cause and pathogenesis

Cutaneous disease affecting the perianal, anal and perirectal skin. The precise aetiology of anal furunculosis is unknown but it is thought to be in part due to anatomical factors and also due to immune mediated disease. In some cases food allergy has been implicated as a contributory factor. Uncommon disease of dogs.

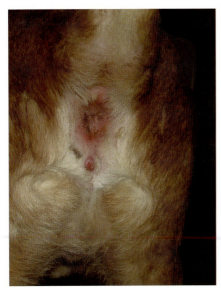

Figure 18.14 Anal gland abscess.

Clinical signs

- No sex predilection. Middle-aged German shepherd dogs and their crosses seem to be at increased risk.
- Lesions vary from small pinpoint draining sinuses with ulceration and fistula formation to deep areas of ulceration and furunculosis.
- Rectal examination reveals a thickened fibrotic colonic mucosa.
- Anal sacs are rarely involved.
- Area is swollen and painful and animals resent examination of the site.
- Other signs include perianal licking, anorectal discharge, faecal tenesmus, low tail carriage, weight loss and decreased exercise tolerance.
- Some animals may have concurrent inflammatory bowel disease.

Differential diagnosis

- Anal gland neoplasia
- Anal gland abscess
- Deep perianal bacterial or fungal infection

Diagnosis

- History and clinical signs.
- Skin biopsy reveals signs of hidradenitis, necrosis of the epithelium of the follicular infundibulum and a mixed inflammatory infiltrate.

Treatment

- Treatment of any concurrent disease, e.g. food allergy or colitis.
- Medical therapy:
  - Topical treatment:
    - Clipping and cleansing of the area with chlorhexidine.
    - Topical anti-inflammatory therapy should only be used where bacterial infection has been adequately treated.
    - Glucocorticoid creams applied every 12–24 hours for 2–3 weeks then tapered aiming to withdraw.
    - Tacrolimus applied every 12 hours to achieve remission then tapered to every 48–72 hours.
  - Systemic treatment:
    - Antibiotic therapy should be used based on culture and sensitivity to resolve infection for 14–21 days before starting immunomodulating therapy.
    - Cyclosporine 5 mg/kg po sid for 3–5 months and for at least 4 weeks beyond clinical cure. Some dogs require lifetime therapy. In these dogs the cyclosporine should be cut to the lowest possible dose to maintain remission. Ketoconazole at a dose of 5–10 mg/kg po sid may be added to reduce the cost and dose of cyclosporine. Liver function should be monitored in dogs on long-term therapy. Prednisolone 2 mg/kg po sid for 2 weeks, then 1 mg/kg po sid for 4 weeks, then 1 mg/kg po every 48 hours for maintenance.
    - Azathioprine 1.5 mg/kg po sid with metronidazole 11–13 mg/kg po sid may be used in refractory cases for 4–8 weeks prior to surgery to debride lesions followed by similar therapy for a further 3–6 weeks.
- Surgical treatment:
  - Surgery to debride ulcers and remove fistulae may be effective. Best results are often seen when medical therapy is combined with surgical intervention. Surgical procedures include cryosurgery, laser surgery and chemical cautery. Multiple surgeries are usually required and post-surgical complications include recurrence of fistulae, anal stenosis and faecal incontinence.
- The prognosis is best for dogs that are treated early in the course of their disease. A combination of cyclosporine and ketoconazole with laser debridement seems to offer the best success rate.

Selected references and further reading

Angus, J.C. (2004) Diseases of the claw and claw bed. In: Campbell, K.L. (ed) *Small Animal Dermatology Secrets*. pp. 332–340. Hanley and Belfus, Philadelphia

Auxilia, S.T. et al. (2001) Canine symmetrical lupoid onychodystrophy: a retrospective study with particular reference to management. *J Small Anim Pract*, **42**, 82–87

Crow, D. (2004) Idiopathic sterile granuloma and pyogranuloma syndrome. In: Campbell, K.L. (ed) *Small Animal Dermatology Secrets*. pp. 227–230. Hanley and Belfus, Philadelphia

Day, M.J. (1993) Immunopathology of anal furunculosis in the dog. *J Small Anim Pract*, **34**, 381–389

Marks, S.L. (2004) Perianal fistula disease. In: Campbell, K.L. (ed) *Small Animal*

Medleau, L. and Hnilica, K. (2006) Diseases of eyes, claws, anal sacs and ear canals. In: *Small Animal Dermatology: A Color Atlas and Therapeutic Guide*. 2nd edn. pp. 359–392. WB Saunders, Philadelphia

Medleau, L. and Hnilica, K. (2006) Miscellaneous cutaneous disorders of the dog. In: *Small Animal Dermatology: A Color Atlas and Therapeutic Guide*. 2nd edn. pp. 327–342. WB Saunders, Philadelphia

Dermatology Secrets. pp. 341–343. Hanley and Belfus, Philadelphia

Mueller, R.S. and Olivry, T. (1999) Onychobiopsy without onychectomy: description of a new biopsy technique for canine claws. *Vet Dermatol*, **10**, 55–59

Patricelli, A.J. et al. (2002) Cyclosporine and ketoconazole for the treatment of perianal fistulas in dogs. *J Am Vet Med Assoc*, **220**, 1009–1016

Scott, D.W. et al. (2001) *Miscellaneous Skin Diseases; Muller and Kirk's Small Animal Dermatology*. 6th edn. pp. 1125–1185. WB Saunders, Philadelphia

Miscellaneous skin diseases in the cat

Feline plasma cell pododermatitis

Cause and pathogenesis

Feline plasma cell pododermatitis is an inflammatory disease of the footpads in cats characterised by a plasma cell infiltrate; the precise aetiology is unknown. Clinical findings, which include tissue plasmacytosis and hypergammaglobulinaemia, together with the cat's response to immune modulating drugs suggest an immune mediated cause. Some cases show a seasonal pattern. It is a rare disease in the cat.

Clinical signs

- No breed, sex or age predilection is recognised.
- Cutaneous signs.
- Early/mild signs:
  - Soft painless swellings of multiple footpads on multiple paws (Figure 19.1).
  - Central metatarsal or metacarpal pads usually affected.
  - Surface of pads often appears purple with white cross-hatching.
  - Pads feel soft and spongy.
- Severe signs:
  - Cats are lame and footpads become very painful.
  - Pads may become ulcerated, often burst open (Figure 19.2).
  - Secondary infection is common.
- Other signs:
  - Plasmacytic dermatitis affecting the bridge of the nose.
  - Plasma cell stomatitis.
  - Immune mediated glomerulonephritis.
  - Renal amyloidosis.

Differential diagnosis

- Infectious causes of pyogranulomatous disease include the following:
  - Bacterial infections such as
    - Bacterial pseudomycetoma
    - Mycobacteria
    - Actinomycosis
    - Actinobacillosis
    - Nocardiosis
  - Dermatophytic pseudomycetoma
  - Fungal mycetoma
  - Viral disease:

Miscellaneous skin diseases in the cat 305

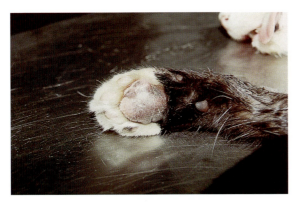

Figure 19.1 Plasma cell pododermatitis showing purple cross-hatching of pad.

- Calici virus
- Herpes virus
- Pox virus
■ Sterile causes of nodular skin disease:
    □ Neoplasia.
    □ Foreign body.
    □ These all usually only affect a single footpad.

Diagnosis

■ History and clinical signs.
■ Fine needle aspirates reveal numerous plasma cells with small numbers of lymphocytes and neutrophils.

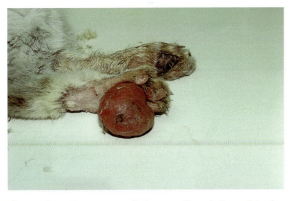

Figure 19.2 Severe case of plasma cell pododermatitis after the pad has split.

- Biopsy reveals signs of a perivascular to diffuse dermatitis with heavy plasma cell infiltrate and Mott cells (plasma cells that contain immunoglobulin and stain pink).
- Cultures usually negative.
- Blood samples hypergammaglobulinaemia.
- ANA, FeLV, FIV occasionally positive but inconsistent finding.

Treatment

- Benign neglect in non-painful cases as regression can occur spontaneously.
- Medical treatment can be used with the following:
    □ Prednisolone 2.0 mg./kg po bid:
        • Taper down to lowest possible alternate day levels once clinical remission has occurred. Usually takes about 2–3 weeks to see benefits; maximal improvement is seen in 10–14 days.
    □ Doxycycline 5–10 mg/kg po bid:
        • Can take 4–8 weeks for improvement and should be continued until pads have completely healed. It may be tapered, withdrawn or continued indefinitely depending on the cat's response and dependency on it.
    □ Cyclosporine 5–10 mg/kg sid po:
        • Use in the same way as prednisolone, tapering once benefits are seen.
- Surgical treatment:
    □ In severe cases that are unresponsive to therapy badly affected footpads may have to be amputated.
- Prognosis is good in uncomplicated cases; where stomatitis or renal disease is present the outlook is more guarded.

Idiopathic sterile granuloma and pyogranulomas

Cause and pathogenesis

Sterile granulomatous lesions usually found on the head of cats. Aetiology is unknown but it

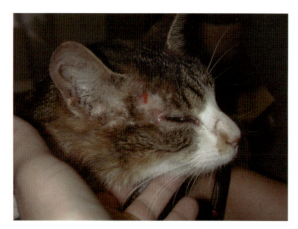

Figure 19.3 Preauricular plaques in a cat.

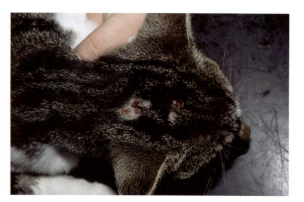

Figure 19.4 Sterile papulonodular lesions on head.

is thought to be an immune mediated disease. Underlying allergy especially flea hypersensitivity has been identified in some cases.

Clinical signs

- Two syndromes are recognised.
- Preauricular plaques:
  - No breed predilection; older males may be predisposed.
  - Papules coalesce to form orange yellow well-circumscribed plaques (Figure 19.3).
  - Pruritus variable; may be moderate to severe.
  - Palpation of lesions leads to red/purple discoloration.
- Papulonodular lesions:
  - No breed predilections; young females may be predisposed.
  - Pruritic papules and nodules on the head and pinnae (Figure 19.4).
  - Lesions erythematous to violaceous; variable pruritus.

Differential diagnosis

- Infectious granulomas, (bacterial, fungal)
- Foreign body granulomas
- Neoplasia
- Eosinophilic granuloma
- Granulomatous sebaceous adenitis

Diagnosis

- History and clinical signs.
- Tissue culture to include fungal; aerobic and anaerobic bacteriological culture is negative.
- Skin biopsy:
  - Preauricular plaques biopsies reveal a diffuse granulomatous dermatitis with a narrow Grenz zone containing multinucleate giant cells.
  - Papulonodular lesions biopsies reveal a perifollicular pyogranulomatous dermatitis.

Treatment

- Solitary lesions – surgical excision
- Multiple lesions
  - Prednisolone 2.0–4.0 mg/kg po sid until regression occurs; usually 10–14 days. Prednisolone should then be tapered to the lowest possible alternate day dose with a view to withdrawal.
  - Cyclosporine 5 mg/kg po sid until regression, then as glucocorticoids.
- Many cats' lesions resolve spontaneously over 6–9 months without therapy. Remission can be long lived.

Hypereosinophilic syndrome

Cause and pathogenesis

A rare disease manifesting with persistent idiopathic eosinophilia with diffuse infiltration of the skin and internal organs. Aetiology is unknown but it may be an immune mediated disease.

Clinical signs

- No age, breed or sex predilection.
- Cutaneous lesions are uncommon:
  - Maculopapular eruptions with erythema, severe pruritus, and excoriation at any site.
- Systemic signs are common:
  - Typically there is infiltration of bone marrow, lymph nodes, liver, spleen and gastrointestinal tract.
  - Diarrhoea, vomiting and weight loss frequent finding.

Differential diagnosis

- Cutaneous lesions:
  - Eosinophilic granuloma complex
  - Idiopathic sterile granulomatous disease
  - Ectoparasitic infestation
  - Allergy (food, atopy)

Diagnosis

- History and clinical signs.
- Haematology shows signs of a peripheral eosinophilia; biochemical abnormalities will be present depending on the degree of involvement of internal organs.
- Cytology of skin lesions reveals a large number of eosinophils with basophils.
- Skin biopsy reveals signs of a superficial and deep eosinophilic perivascular dermatitis.

Treatment

- Poor prognosis; the disease is poorly responsive to therapy and systemic disease is rapidly fatal.
- Where cutaneous lesions predominate, the prognosis is better and cats will survive 2–4 years. In these cases high doses of steroids may be beneficial.

Ulcerative dermatitis with linear subepidermal fibrosis

Cause and pathogenesis

An idiopathic ulcerative skin disease of the cat of unknown aetiology. It is not thought to be caused by trauma, injection reactions, infection or foreign bodies. It may be some form of vascular insult that leads to the production of a non-healing ulcer.

Clinical signs

- No sex, age or breed predilection.
- Lesions are solitary and occur over the dorsal neck and shoulder area (Figure 19.5).
- Non-painful; pruritus variable.
- Non-healing ulcer initially 0.5–1.0 cm in diameter, enlarges over several weeks.

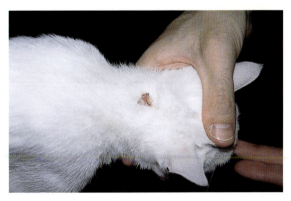

Figure 19.5 Idiopathic ulcerative dermatitis affecting the back of the neck.

- Thick adherent crusting over the surface with peripheral thickened skin.
- Cats are systemically well.

Differential diagnosis

- Injection reaction
- Trauma especially bite wound
- Panniculitis (infectious or sterile)
- Neoplasia especially squamous cell carcinoma
- Burn (cold, heat, chemical)

Diagnosis

- History and clinical signs.
- Carefully performed cultures are negative.
- Skin biopsy reveals signs of epidermal ulceration and superficial dermal necrosis with only minimal dermal inflammation. A linear subepidermal band of superficial fibrosis is seen extending from the periphery of the ulcer in chronic lesions.

Treatment

- Identification and therapy of any underlying disease is important.
- Restraint devices such as soft collars, bandages etc. may be helpful to prevent the cat mutilating the area.
- Glucocorticoid therapy may be useful in some cases:
    - Prednisolone 2–4 mg/kg po sid until clinical remission, then tapering to alternate day and withdrawal. If no response is seen within 4 weeks surgical excision should be undertaken.
- Antihistamine therapy (see Chapter 10) or behaviour modifying drugs (see Chapter 16) may be useful in some cases.
- Wide surgical excision carries a moderate prognosis; recurrence can occur.
- Laser ablation may be useful in some cases.
- Prognosis is guarded to poor as many cases fail to respond to medical therapy and are too extensive for surgical intervention.

Perforating dermatitis

Cause and pathogenesis

Unusual rare hyperkeratotic condition of the cat of unknown aetiology. In man these conditions are often associated with internal malignancy, diabetes mellitus or chronic renal failure. No such association has been identified in the cat. Lesions thought to be caused by some abnormality in collagen metabolism.

Clinical signs

- Any site can be affected but often on the dorsum.
- Lesions consist of multiple, firm, conical, hyperkeratotic yellow/brown masses, 2–7 mm in diameter.
- Appear often in clusters, forming lines.
- Non-pruritic, non-painful.
- Lesions cannot be scraped or pulled off.

Differential diagnosis

- Cutaneous horn
- Dermatophytosis

Diagnosis

- History and clinical signs.
- Routine haematology and biochemistry to check for internal disease.
- Skin biopsy reveals signs of a conical exophytic mass containing keratin and degenerate collagen. Transepidermal elimination of collagen fibres is seen into the base of the mass.

Treatment

- Where concurrent disease such as allergy is present, management of this can lead to improvement in the perforating dermatitis.

- Ascorbic acid (vitamin C) 100 mg po bid may be useful leading to resolution within 30 days. Cats may need long-term therapy.

Acquired skin fragility

Cause and pathogenesis

A rare disease of the cat characterised by thin fragile skin. It is a multifactorial disease and can be associated with a range of underlying diseases:

- Hyperadrenocorticism
- Iatrogenic Cushing's syndrome
- Diabetes mellitus
- Hepatic/renal disease
- Overuse of progestational compounds
- Idiopathic

Clinical signs

- No sex or breed predilection, although middle-aged to old cats appear to be predisposed.
- Skin is thin and fragile and easily torn by only minor trauma.
- Irregular tears of the skin occur and large sheets of skin can be lost.
- Partial alopecia often present; unlike cutaneous asthenia a major differential diagnosis the skin is not hyperextensible.

Differential diagnosis

- Cutaneous asthenia
- Hyperadrenocorticism
- Iatrogenic Cushing's syndrome
- Pancreatic paraneoplastic alopecia

Diagnosis

- History and clinical signs.
- Clinical signs.
- Routine blood profile to check for internal disease and where appropriate dynamic function tests to rule out endocrine disease.
- Skin biopsy is difficult to achieve because of the fragility of the skin. The dermis is severely atrophic leading to folding and twisting of the sample. Dermal collagen fibres are thin and disorganised. Panniculus is not normally present in biopsy samples.

Treatment

- Even if an underlying cause is identified, skin changes appear to be irreversible.
- Cats are impossible to handle without causing severe skin damage.
- Surgical repair unsuccessful.
- Very poor prognosis.

Feline orofacial pain syndrome (FOPs)

Cause and pathogenesis

An uncommon facial pain/mutilation syndrome recently recognised in the cat that shows similarities to trigeminal neuralgia in people.

Clinical signs

- No age or sex predilection.
- Predisposed breeds include the Burmese and occasionally domestic short-haired cats, Burmilla and Siamese.
- Cats present with exaggerated licking and chewing movements and pawing at their mouth and will often traumatise their face (Figure 19.6).
- Signs are usually unilateral and may be episodic or continuous.
- Episodic signs may be brought on by eating.
- Cats often anorexic.
- Some cases seem to be associated with oral disease and will improve when the

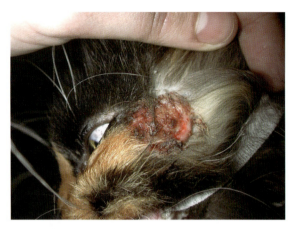

Figure 19.6 Suspected case of FOPS.

underlying disease process resolves. Four groups are recognised:
- Mouth ulceration especially secondary to calici virus infection or vaccination.
- Cutting permanent teeth.
- Dental disease.
- Routine dental procedures including extraction.

Differential diagnosis

- Allergy (atopy, food allergy)
- Sarcoptic mange
- Dental disease
- Epilepsy
- Poisoning
- Encephalitis

Diagnosis

- History and clinical signs.
- Diagnostic rule outs especially of dental disease with good quality dental radiographs.
- Neurological assessment including MRI scan and CSF analysis, which are normal in FOPS.

Treatment

Therapy of any underlying disease especially dental disease, gingivitis.

Drugs that may be useful in FOPS are listed in Table 19.1.

Eosinophilic allergic syndrome

Eosinophilic allergic syndrome is not a specific disease entity but a spectrum of cutaneous reaction patterns exhibited by the cat to a wide variety of different disease processes.

There can therefore be no one drug that can be used to control the clinical signs.

Eosinophilic allergic syndrome encompasses both the eosinophilic granuloma complex and also miliary dermatitis so that it can be subdivided into four categories:

(a) Indolent ulcer (eosinophilic ulcer, rodent ulcer)
(b) Eosinophilic plaque

Table 19.1 Drugs that may be useful in FOPS.

Drug	Dose rate	Details
Phenobarbitone	2–3 mg/kg po bid	Life-long therapy may be needed; assess serum levels: after 2 weeks levels should be 20–25 mg/l; regular hepatic assessment is needed
Carbamazepine	25 mg po bid (100 mg/5 ml stock solution)	Haematological monitoring is required
Gabapentin	2.5–5.0 mg/kg po bid/tid	
Selegiline	1.0 mg/kg po sid	

Note: None of these drugs are licensed for use in the cat.

(c) Allergic miliary dermatitis
(d) Eosinophilic granuloma (linear granuloma, collagenolytic granuloma)

Miliary dermatitis has been included in the grouping as it is now widely accepted as being part of the same disease process. Histologically, lesions of miliary dermatitis can be indistinguishable from those of the eosinophilic plaques.

Any of the different lesions of the complex can occur in the same cat concurrently.

Each disease will be described for cause and pathogenesis, clinical signs, differential diagnosis and diagnosis. Investigation of all four diseases to determine the underlying cause is very similar and will be dealt with in a separate section at the end of the chapter, as will therapy.

Indolent ulcer

Cause and pathogenesis

Cutaneous, mucocutaneous, or oral lesions. Many have underlying immune mediated aetiologies including allergies; other lesions may be a manifestation of excessive grooming leading to a purely mechanical trauma to the area.

Clinical signs

- No age, breed or sex predilection (females may be at higher risk).
- Usually found on the upper lip unilaterally (bilaterally less commonly, Figure 19.7).

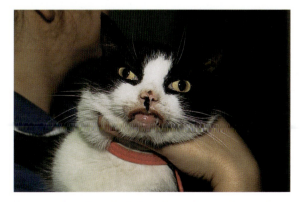

Figure 19.7 Bilateral indolent ulcers affecting the top lips.

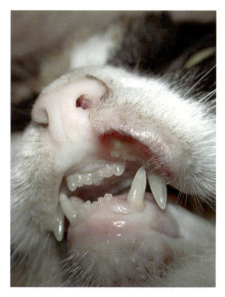

Figure 19.8 Indolent ulcer on upper lip of cat.

- Other lesions found in oral cavity.
- Lesions are well circumscribed, red to brown in colour.
- Alopecic with a raised border, 2 mm to 5 cm in size (Figure 19.8).
- Usually asymptomatic and are rarely pruritic or painful.
- Peripheral lymphadenopathy common.

Differential diagnosis

- Infectious ulcers (bacterial, viral, fungal)
- Trauma
- Neoplasia (squamous cell carcinoma, mast cell tumour)

Diagnosis

- This should initially be aimed at confirming the lesion as an indolent ulcer.
- Once this has been established investigation should be as for all four diseases to identify an inciting cause (see later in the chapter).
- Impression smears stained with Diff-Quik to assess degree of infection.
- Cultures, if carefully performed, are sterile.
- Haematology is usually unremarkable; eosinophilia is a rare finding.

- Biopsies useful only as a diagnostic rule out. Biopsy should be taken as a deep wedge or punch biopsy of margin of ulcer to include normal skin if possible. Results reveal a nonspecific picture of a superficial perivascular to interstitial dermatitis often with fibrosing dermatitis. Eosinophils an inconsistent finding.

Eosinophilic plaque

Cause and pathogenesis

Common cutaneous reaction pattern seen in cats. Most cats have underlying allergic conditions. Overlap occurs between miliary dermatitis lesions and eosinophilic plaques. The former condition can not be easily differentiated from the latter histologically. Miliary dermatitis represents a multifocal distribution of lesions. Eosinophilic plaques represent the same disease process in a localised form.

Clinical signs

- No breed predilection, females may be predisposed.
- Can occur in any age but young adults to middle-aged cats are predisposed.
- Most occur on the ventral abdomen and medial thighs, although occasionally they can be identified at mucocutaneous junctions.
- Lesions may be single or multiple (Figure 19.9) and are usually highly pruritic.

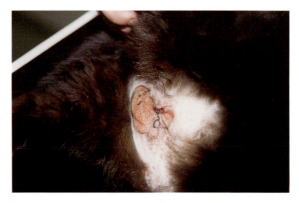

Figure 19.10 Well-demarcated eosinophilic plaque on the ventral abdomen.

- Raised round to oval well-demarcated erythematous lesions (Figure 19.10).
- Lesions often exudative and ulcerated and may be secondary infected (Figure 19.11).
- Vary in size from 0.5–5.0 cm in diameter.
- Regional lymphadenopathy common.

Differential diagnosis

- Infectious granulomas (bacterial, viral, fungal).
- Neoplasia (mast cell tumour, metastatic mammary carcinoma, lymphoma).

Diagnosis

- To confirm the lesion as an eosinophilic plaque.

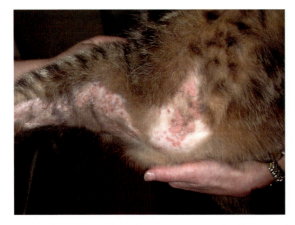

Figure 19.9 Eosinophilic plaque on the ventral abdomen of a cat.

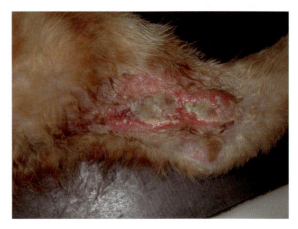

Figure 19.11 Infected plaque on the leg of a cat.

- Impression smears may be stained with Diff-Quik to assess cell infiltrate and degree of secondary infection. Usually eosinophil rich but will contain neutrophils and bacteria if secondarily infected.
- Cultures, if carefully performed, are sterile.
- Haematology reveals eosinophilia as a constant finding.
- Biopsies are diagnostic. A biopsy should be taken from an erythematous plaque with minimal erosion or self-inflicted trauma. Results reveal a hyperplastic superficial and deep perivascular dermatitis with eosinophilia. Eosinophilic microabscesses may be seen.

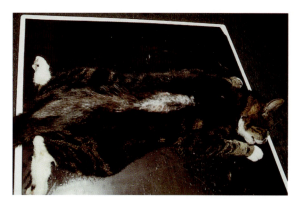

Figure 19.13 Miliary dermatitis showing the typical distribution on the dorsum.

Allergic miliary dermatitis

Cause and pathogenesis

Miliary dermatitis is a multifactorial cutaneous reaction pattern. It is produced by cutaneous hypersensitivity reactions; these may be to environmental allergens, ectoparasites or drugs, so-called allergic miliary dermatitis. Histopathologically there is overlap between this disease and eosinophilic plaques, which are thought to be a more localised form of the same disease. Common lesion in the cat.

Clinical signs

- No breed, age or sex predilection has been identified.
- Multiple discrete erythematous papules with adherent brown/black crust (Figure 19.12).

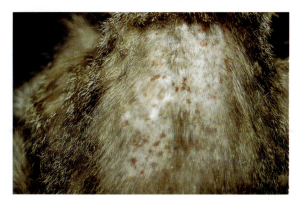

Figure 19.12 Multiple discrete lesions of miliary dermatitis.

- The crusted papules represent primary lesions, not the product of self-inflicted trauma; often there is limited associated alopecia and lesions are identified by feel.
- Lesions typically found on dorsal lumbosacral area (Figure 19.13), caudo-medial thighs and neck.
- Pruritus moderate to severe.
- Chronic resolving lesions may appear as small melanotic macules.

Differential diagnosis

- Pemphigus foliaceus
- Dermatophytosis
- Staphylococcal folliculitis
- Dietary imbalances (biotin, fatty acid deficiency)
- Feline poxvirus

Diagnosis

- To confirm the lesion as miliary dermatitis.
- Impression smears may be stained with Diff-Quik to assess cellular infiltrate, which is usually eosinophil rich, and degree of infection.
- Cultures taken carefully for bacteria and fungi are sterile.
- Haematology reveals an eosinophilia as a consistent finding, often with basophilia.
- Biopsies are non-diagnostic but help as a diagnostic rule out. A biopsy should be taken from non-traumatised recently erupted papules, especially between the shoulder blades. Results

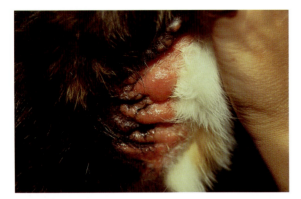

Figure 19.14 Eosinophilic granuloma on the caudal thigh.

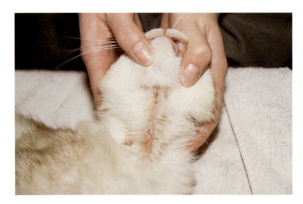

Figure 19.16 Eosinophilic granuloma showing typical configuration on the neck.

reveal a superficial and deep perivascular to interstitial dermatitis with eosinophilic infiltrate accompanied by mast cells.

Eosinophilic granuloma

Cause and pathogenesis

A common cutaneous, mucocutaneous and oral mucosal lesion, which is thought to be a manifestation of allergic disease.

Clinical signs

- No age or breed predilection, although females may be at higher risk.
- Lesions most commonly seen on caudal thighs (Figure 19.14), face and oral cavity, but may be seen on any site (Figure 19.15).
- Appear as well-circumscribed, raised yellow to pink plaques with a linear configuration (Figure 19.16).
- Ulcerated surface can be covered in pinpoint white foci of collagen degeneration.
- Peripheral lymphadenopathy variable.
- Pruritus usually mild.
- Chin oedema, an asymptomatic swelling of the lower lip, is commonly caused by eosinophilic granuloma (Figure 19.17).

Differential diagnosis

- Infectious granulomas (bacterial, viral, fungal).
- Neoplasia (mast cell tumour, metastatic mammary carcinoma, lymphoma).

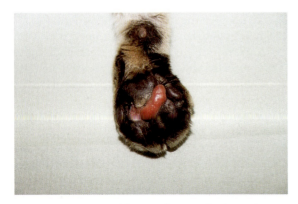

Figure 19.15 Eosinophilic granuloma on the footpad.

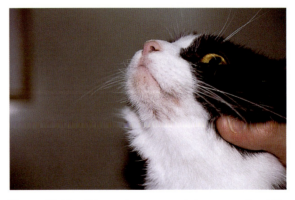

Figure 19.17 Chin oedema caused by an eosinophilic granuloma.

Diagnosis

- To confirm the lesion as an eosinophilic granuloma.
- Impression smears may be stained with Diff-Quik to assess the cellular infiltrate, which is eosinophil rich with occasional neutrophils and bacteria if secondary infection is present.
- Cultures, if carefully performed, are sterile.
- Haematology reveals an eosinophilia as a consistent finding.
- Biopsies are diagnostic. A wedge biopsy should be taken from an ulcerated area with white foci with minimal erosion or self-inflicted trauma to include a normal margin of skin. Results reveal a nodular to diffuse granulomatous dermatitis with multifocal areas of collagen degeneration. Eosinophils and multinucleated giant cells are common.

Investigation of eosinophilic allergic syndrome

When the cat has been identified as having one or more of the following:

- Indolent ulcer
- Eosinophilic plaque
- Allergic miliary dermatitis
- Eosinophilic granuloma

The following protocol should be undertaken in all cases of eosinophilic allergic syndrome, but definitely in all cases that are

- poorly responsive to anti-inflammatory therapy,
- recurrent, and
- severe/multiple (i.e. more than one component of the syndrome is present).

Ectoparasite assessment

- Wet paper test for fleas.
- Acetate tape from coat for superficial parasites, e.g. *Cheyletiella*, *Otodectes*, *Trombicula*, lice, fur mites and flea faeces.
- Skin scrapings for parasites as above plus *Sarcoptes*, *Notoedres* and *Demodex*.

- Empirical therapy for ectoparasites should be undertaken even if no evidence is found on samples. The fastidious grooming habits of the cat can efficiently remove most parasites from the coat. For specific therapeutic agents, see regimes under parasites in Chapter 7. Minimally a rapid acting flea adulticide should be used, an acaricide and a trial period with lime sulphur.

Food trial

This can be started at the same time as the ectoparasite control or after 1 month empirical therapy for parasites.

Food should either be

- home cooked to contain an unusual protein source not normally consumed by the cat, or
- proprietary selected protein hypoallergenic diet (for a more detailed discussion of such diets, see section on food allergy in Chapter 10), and
- food trial should be for a minimum of 4–8 weeks.

Drug withdrawal

Where any drug has been prescribed prior to commencement of the lesions these should, where possible, be discontinued.

Allergy testing

Where specific allergy testing is available this should be undertaken as the next diagnostic step. Intradermal allergy testing or in vitro serum allergy testing may be undertaken. This allows identification of environmental allergens such as house dust mites, pollens, dust, animal danders, and fungal moulds (for a more detailed discussion of such tests, see section on atopy in Chapter 10).

Therapy of eosinophilic allergic syndrome

This ideally should not be undertaken until the cat has had strict parasite control.

However, it can be used in combination with parasite control when the cat is uncomfortable on initial presentation.

Therapy should not replace even the most basic of work-ups. Inflammatory therapy can be started if the lesions are sterile, i.e. negative cultures and no bacteria on impression smears.

Medical therapy:

- Anti-inflammatory therapy should not be given for more than 3–4 weeks at induction dose rates. Therapy should be reassessed if no clinical improvement is seen by this stage. Once lesions have resolved, therapy should be tapered and withdrawn.
- Glucocorticoids should initially be given daily to achieve remission and then cut to an alternate day regime and tapered:
    - Prednisolone 2.0 mg/kg po bid until lesions have resolved
    - Dexamethasone 0.4 mg/kg po sid
    - Triamcinolone 0.8 mg/kg po sid
    - Methylprednisolone acetate 20 mg/cat sq for two injections 2 weeks apart, then maximally every 3 months after that
- Where intradermal allergy testing identifies environmental allergens, specific avoidance therapy or desensitising vaccines can be used.
- Immunomodulating therapy may be used in severe cases that are unresponsive to steroids. For details on monitoring, see section on pemphigus:
    - Chlorambucil 0.1–0.2 mg/kg every 24–48 hours
    - Cyclosporine 5 mg/kg po sid
    - Doxycycline 5–10 mg/kg po bid
- Progestational compounds such as megestrol acetate or medroxyprogesterone acetate are effective in many cases but the side effects of such drugs outweigh any therapeutic benefits and should not therefore be used.
- Essential fatty acid supplementation omega 3 and omega 6 fatty acid containing products have been shown to be useful in some cases of miliary dermatitis and eosinophilic granulomas.

Surgical therapy

- Other modes of therapy that have occasionally been successful in therapy include radiotherapy, cryotherapy, laser therapy, and surgical excision.
- Prognosis is variable depending on the underlying trigger for the disease and whether it can be identified and managed. Where an inciting cannot be identified, cats may need long-term anti-inflammatory therapy.

Selected references and further reading

Bevier, D. (2004) Miliary dermatitis. In: Campbell, K.L. (ed) *Small Animal Dermatology Secrets*. pp. 214–219. Hanley and Belfus, Philadelphia

Guaguere, E. and Prelaud, P. (2000) Efficacy of cyclosporine in the treatment of 12 cases of eosinophilic granuloma complex. *Vet Dermatol*, **11**, 31

Heath, S. et al. (2001) Orofacial pain syndrome in cats. *Vet Rec*, **149**(21), 660

Mason, K. and Burton, G. (2000) Eosinophilic granuloma complex. In: Guaguere, E. and Prelaud, P. (eds) *A Practical Guide to Feline Dermatology*. pp. 12.1–12.9. Blackwell Science, Oxford

Medleau, L. and Hnilica, K. (2006) Miscellaneous cutaneous disorders of the Cat. In: *Small Animal Dermatology: A Color Atlas and Therapeutic Guide*. 2nd edn. pp. 344–358. WB Saunders, Philadelphia

Rees, C. (2004) Feline eosinophilic granuloma complex. In: Campbell, K.L. (ed) *Small Animal Dermatology Secrets*. pp. 220–223. Hanley and Belfus, Philadelphia

Rosenkrantz, W.S. (1993) Feline eosinophilic granuloma complex. In: Griffin, C.E. et al. (eds) *Current Veterinary Dermatology: The Science and Art of Therapy*. pp. 319–324. Mosby, St Louis,

Scott, D.W. (1990) An unusual ulcerative dermatitis associated with linear subepidermal fibrosis in eight cats. *Feline Pract*, **18**, 8–11

Scott, D.W. et al. (2001) *Miscellaneous Skin Diseases Muller and Kirk's Small Animal Dermatology*. 6th edn. pp. 1125–1183. WB Saunders, Philadelphia

Environmental skin diseases

Solar dermatitis

Cause and pathogenesis

Phototoxic reaction seen in poorly pigmented skin of dogs and cats. Initially sun exposure leads to sunburn but with repeated exposure to ultraviolet light pre-neoplastic lesions such as actinic keratoses and squamous cell carcinoma in situ can develop in addition to squamous cell carcinoma.

Clinical signs

- Cats:
  - No sex predilection. Generally seen in older animals and those with poorly pigmented skin and hair, especially those that like to sunbathe.
  - Lesions are found most commonly on ear tips, eyelids, nose and lips (Figure 20.1).
- Dogs:
  - No sex predilection. Skin disease seen on older animals especially outdoor dogs and those that sunbathe.
  - Predisposed breeds include white Boxers, bull terriers, beagles, Dalmatians, Staffordshire bull terriers and German short-haired pointer.
  - Lesions can be found on the nose or on the trunk.
- Nasal disease:
  - Lesions can be found on the planum nasale especially in dogs with non-pigmented sparsely haired skin.
- Truncal disease:
  - Affects the ventral and lateral aspects of the abdomen and inner thighs.
  - Lesions also seen on flanks, tail tip or distal extremities.
- Initial lesions in all cases consist of erythema and scale.
- Chronic lesions show signs of alopecia, exudation, crusting and ulceration.
- Lesions heal with scarring.
- Neoplastic transformation can occur to develop to squamous cell carcinoma.

Differential diagnosis

- Feline lesions:
  - Discoid lupus erythematosus
  - Dermatophytosis
  - Vasculitis

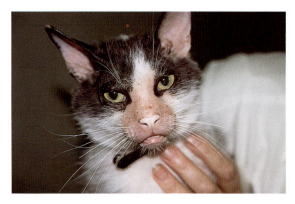

Figure 20.1 Solar dermatitis affecting the nose and ears.

- Canine nasal lesions:
  - Discoid lupus erythematosus
  - Dermatomyositis
  - Pemphigus foliaceus/erythematosus
  - Drug eruption
  - Sterile eosinophilic furunculosis
  - Dermatophytosis
  - Neoplasia
- Canine truncal lesions:
  - Demodicosis
  - Dermatophytosis
  - Superficial pyoderma
  - Drug eruption
  - Neoplasia

Diagnosis

- Clinical signs and history of sun exposure.
- Skin biopsy reveals in early lesions epidermal hyperplasia with non-specific superficial perivascular dermatitis. Vacuolated epidermal cells and dyskeratotic keratinocytes may be seen together with basophilic degeneration of elastin (solar elastosis). In chronic lesions the epidermis changes from hyperplastic to dysplastic but there is no penetration of the basement membrane zone.

Treatment

- Avoid further sun exposure especially between 8.00 a.m. and 5.00 p.m.
- Where secondary infection is present it needs to be treated with appropriate antibiotics for a minimum of 2–3 weeks.
- Photoprotection:
  - Sunblock is useful using zinc oxide or titanium dioxide applied to affected areas twice daily. Preparations should be at least factor 30 and should be waterproof.
- Dogs with severe inflammation often require steroids:
  - Systemic prednisolone 1.0 mg/kg daily.
  - Topical betamethasone, dexamethasone, triamcinolone, prednisolone, hydrocortisone creams, which are best suited for short-term use only; may be used on localised areas.
- Systemic treatment can be employed with the following:
  - Beta carotene 30 mg po bid for 30 days then once daily for life.
  - Vitamin A 8,000–10,000 IU po sid or acitretin 0.5–1.0 mg/kg po sid may be useful.
- Prognosis is very variable depending on lesions and their chronicity. Where repeat exposure and damage occurs, sunlight-induced neoplasms will develop either squamous cell carcinoma or haemangioma/ haemangiosarcoma.

Actinic keratosis

See Chapter 21.

Burns

Burn management is often intensive and specialised.

Only a brief outline of clinical signs and treatment will be provided here. The reader is referred to more detailed text for further information.

Cause and pathogenesis

Types and extent of lesions depend on initial insult. Burns are uncommon in dogs and rare in cats.

Environmental skin diseases 319

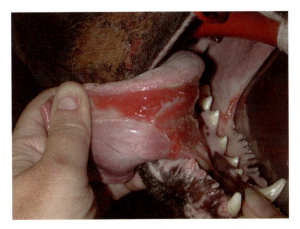

Figure 20.2 Chemical burn on dog's tongue and face.

Inciting factors:

- Strong chemicals (Figure 20.2)
- Electricity
- Solar radiation
- Microwave radiation
- Heat (Figures 20.3 and 20.4)

Categories of burns:

- Partial thickness burns involving epidermis/superficial dermis:

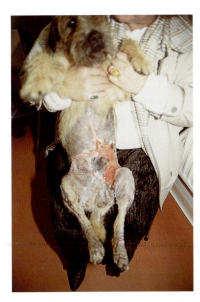

Figure 20.3 Full thickness burns on the ventral abdomen of a dog.

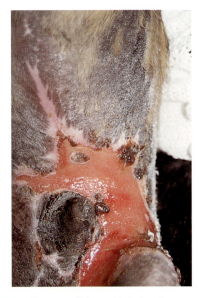

Figure 20.4 Close-up of Figure 20.3 showing tapering areas of coagulation necrosis.

  - Heals without scarring
- Full thickness burns – all cutaneous structures damaged:
  - Extensive scarring without surgical treatment

Clinical signs

- Cutaneous lesions:
  - Often lesions not obvious for 24–48 hours.
  - Skin hard and dry, hair may hide full extent of lesions.
  - Secondary infection with Gram negative organisms especially *Pseudomonas aeruginosa* occurs after 3–5 days leading to suppuration.
  - Typical lesions of a chemical or thermal burn are tapering areas of coagulation necrosis of epidermis.
- Non-cutaneous lesions:
  - These seen when greater than 25% of body involved.
  - Septicaemia, shock, renal failure, anaemia.

Differential diagnosis

- Drug eruption
- Vasculitis
- Erythema multiforme/toxic epidermal necrolysis

Diagnosis

History and clinical signs.

Treatment

- Treatment of the animal:
  - In severe cases (especially >25% body affected) general assessment of the animal is essential with routine haematology and biochemistry including electrolyte levels, renal function and hydrated status. Fluid therapy and supportive nutritional supplements should be given on the basis of blood profiles.
- Treatment of the lesions:
  - Clean with antiseptic agent preferably one with activity against Gram negative bacteria, e.g. EDTA tris.
  - Debride where appropriate to remove necrotic skin.
  - Topical and systemic antibacterials with good activity against Gram negative bacteria, e.g. silver sulphadiazine topically and fluorinated quinolones systemically.
  - Glucocorticoids are contraindicated in most cases.

Frostbite

Cause and pathogenesis

Frostbite is caused through prolonged exposure to low environmental temperature or contact with frozen objects. The degree of damage to the skin is dependent on the insult to the skin and the skin that is affected. Rare disease in domesticated dogs and cats.

Clinical signs

- Lesions tend to be seen on the extremities especially ear and tail tips as well as the digits.
- Skin is pale and cold whilst frozen; once thawed, a progression of clinical signs are recognised ranging from erythema and pain to necrosis and sloughing in severe cases.

Differential diagnosis

Vasculitis especially cold agglutinin disease.

Diagnosis

History and clinical signs.

Treatment

- Rapid thawing of frozen tissue should be performed with warm water to restore the blood supply to the area.
- Any areas of necrosis and sloughing will heal spontaneously.
- In severe cases surgical resection of necrotic tissue may be necessary.
- Further exposure to cold should be avoided to prevent subsequent damage.

Irritant contact dermatitis

Cause and pathogenesis

Irritant contact dermatitis should be distinguished from contact hypersensitivity. Irritant contact dermatitis causes signs in all exposed animals without a previous period of sensitisation. It is seen when cats have fallen into a chemical, e.g. paints, disinfectants. Because cats are fastidious groomers they often ingest large amounts of toxic or corrosive material in attempts to clean their coats. Ingestion of the irritant may not only cause gastrointestinal ulceration including the mouth but may also show signs of systemic poisoning. The reaction pattern that is seen depends on the

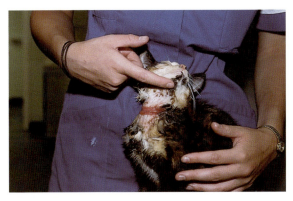

Figure 20.5 Severe contact irritation after application of flea collar.

type of irritant as to whether it is solid, which is less likely to penetrate the hair coat than a liquid.

Types of irritant include the following:

- Corrosive in the form of a strong acid or alkaline:
  - Cause immediate damage, severe reaction often a chemical burn.
- Soaps, detergents, topical insecticides (especially flea collars, Figure 20.5):
  - Prolonged/repeated exposure is required.

Clinical signs

- Irritation occurs on hairless or sparsely haired skin, especially the scrotal skin (Figure 20.6) in entire males and the perianal area.
- Shampoos, creams and other liquids have the ability to penetrate the hair and can cause irritation where they touch the skin (Figure 20.7).
- Lesions consist of papules and erythema, severe pruritus leading to self-inflicted trauma.

Differential diagnosis

- Where the irritant is a liquid, it is usually still present in the coat and there are therefore few other likely causes.
- Where the irritant is non-liquid and affects hairless areas consider

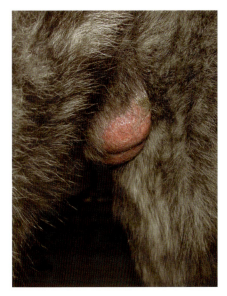

Figure 20.6 Severe contact irritant reaction on scrotal skin.

- intradermal penetration by parasites, e.g. hookworm, Strongyloides,
- allergy (contact, atopy, food).

Diagnosis

- History, especially where multiple animals are affected, and clinical signs.
- Skin biopsy is non-diagnostic except as a rule out. There is overlap histopathologically between contact irritation and hypersensitivity, which produces a superficial perivascular dermatitis.

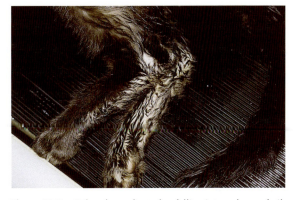

Figure 20.7 Oil on legs of cat after falling into a drum of oil.

- Provocative testing should be avoided especially if there is potential for severe reactions.

Treatment

- Identification of irritant substances plus removal from the animals environment.
- Symptomatic relief with topical or systemic glucocorticoids:
  - Systemic prednisolone 1 mg/kg once daily 7–10 days.
  - Topical steroid creams; short-term use.
- Pentoxifylline at a dose of 10–25 mg/kg bid/tid is useful in cases where there is a hypersensitivity component.

Callus

Cause and pathogenesis

Lesions develop over bony pressure points as a protective response to pressure-induced ischaemia and inflammation. Common in dogs, very rare in cats.

Predisposing factors:

- Giant/large breeds
- Hard bedding/wood, concrete

Clinical signs

- No sex predisposition. Seen in middle-aged to old dogs especially those who are less ambulatory. Dobermans may be predisposed.
- Callus forms over bony prominences especially elbows, hocks and sternum in deep-chested dogs.
- Lesions form as oval hyperkeratotic plaques with associated alopecia (Figure 20.8). In uncomplicated cases there is no ulceration or exudation.
- They are non pruritic and not painful.

Differential diagnosis

- Localised areas of

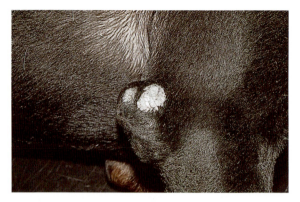

Figure 20.8 Well-circumscribed hyperkeratotic plaque on the elbow of a Doberman typical of callus.

  - dermatophytosis
  - demodicosis
  - sarcoptes
  - neoplasia

Diagnosis

- History and clinical signs.
- Biopsy is inappropriate except where neoplasia is a potential differential diagnosis. It reveals signs of epidermal hyperplasia with orthokeratotic to parakeratotic hyperkeratosis, follicular keratosis and dilated follicular cysts.

Treatment

- Padding either within the environment as a soft bed or on dog as, e.g., elbow pads.
- Surgical removal inadvisable as often healing is poor and lesions will reform.

Callus dermatitis

Cause and pathogenesis

- Callus formed over a pressure point is continually traumatised leading to secondary infection.
- Predisposing factors as callus.

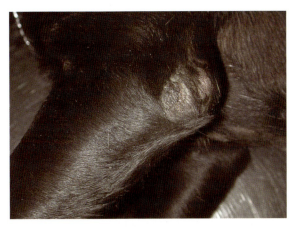

Figure 20.9 Callus dermatitis over elbow.

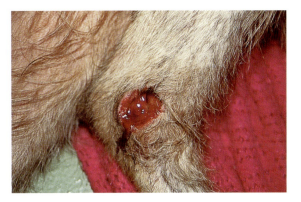

Figure 20.11 Callus dermatitis in a recumbent Great Dane.

Clinical signs

- No sex predisposition. Seen in middle-aged to old dogs especially those who are less ambulatory.
- Callus forms over bony prominences especially elbows (Figure 20.9), hocks and sternum (Figure 20.10) in deep-chested dogs.
- Oval hyperkeratotic plaques become ulcerated (Figure 20.11), fistulated with exudation due to secondary infection. Lesions are painful.
- Foreign body granulomas can form due to embedded hair.

Differential diagnosis

- As callus as well as
  - vasculitis
  - chronic scabies

Diagnosis

- History and clinical signs.
- Cytology of exudate reveals keratin debris, pyogranulomatous inflammatory infiltrate, free hair shafts and bacteria are usually also present.
- Culture and sensitivity of exudate, collected by squeezing lesion.
- Skin biopsy reveals signs as callus above.
- In chronic cases that have been poorly responsive to antibiotic therapy; tissue culture may also be useful in case of anaerobic infection.

Treatment

- As callus plus.
- Systemic antibiotics based on culture and sensitivity for 6–12 weeks at least 10 days beyond clinical cure, lesions reassessed by cytology every 2 weeks.
- Topical antibiotics without glucocorticoids based on sensitivity, e.g. fusidic acid, may be useful.
- Antibacterial soaks with benzoyl peroxide gel (2.5%) or salicylic acid; urea-based gels can be useful to moisturise and clean the area.

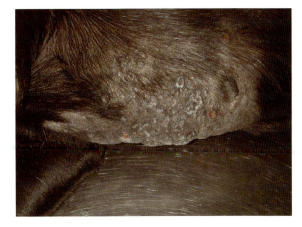

Figure 20.10 Callus dermatitis on sternum.

Pyotraumatic dermatitis

See Chapter 4.

Intertrigo

See Chapter 4.

Hygroma

Cause and pathogenesis

Hygroma is a cyst-like bursa that develops over a pressure point especially the hock. It is caused by repeated trauma to the site. Uncommon disease in dogs, not recorded in cats.

Clinical signs

- No sex predilection. Commonly seen in large and giant breeds.
- Lesions form as fluctuant areas of swelling over a bony prominence.
- Their distribution is the sane as for callus over the hocks, elbows and less commonly the sternum.
- Where the lesions are continually traumatised, they will become secondarily infected leading to the formation of granulation tissue within the 'cyst' of abscessation and fistulation.

Differential diagnosis

- Neoplasia
- Bacterial or fungal granuloma

These products should not be used without additional environmental measures else softening the lesions may aggravate the condition.
- Surgical excision is not recommended.

Diagnosis

- History and clinical signs.
- Cytology of uncomplicated lesions taken by fine needle aspirate reveals a haemorrhagic infiltrate with no evidence of inflammatory cells. Where lesions have become secondarily infected, bacteria and a pyogranulomatous inflammatory infiltrate are present.
- Skin biopsy reveals signs of cystic structures surrounded by areas of granulation tissue.

Treatment

- Padding either within the environment as a soft bed or on dog as, e.g., elbow pads, soft bandages for 2–3 weeks can prevent further trauma and can on occasions lead to resolution of the lesions.
- Systemic antibiotics based on culture and sensitivity are necessary for infected lesions; these can be required for 4–6 weeks.
- Surgical drainage and removal may be necessary in cases that do not respond to medical therapy and environmental modification. Risk of wound breakdown is high and this approach should only be employed when others fail.

Selected references and further reading

Dunstan, R.W. et al. (1998) The light and the skin. In: Kwochka, K.W. et al. (eds) *Advances in Veterinary Dermatology*. Vol. 3. pp. 3–36. Butterworth-Heinemann, Oxford

Medleau, L. and Hnilica, K. (2006) Miscellaneous cutaneous disorders of the Dog. In: *Small Animal Dermatology: A Color Atlas and Therapeutic Guide*. 2nd edn. pp. 327–342. WB Saunders, Philadelphia

Rosychuk, R.A. (2004) Environmental dermatoses. In: Campbell, K.L. (ed) *Small Animal Dermatology Secrets*. pp. 312–323. Hanley and Belfus, Philadelphia

Scott, D.W. et al. (2001) Environmental skin disease. *Muller and Kirk's Small Animal Dermatology.* 6th edn. pp. 1073–1111. WB Saunders, Philadelphia

Swaim, S.F. and Henderson, R.A. (1997) Specific types of wounds. In: Swaim, S.F. and Henderson, R.A. (eds) *Small Animal Wound Management.* 2nd edn. pp. 87–141. Williams and Wilkins, Baltimore

Walder, E.J. and Conroy, J.D. (1994) Contact dermatitis in dogs and cats: pathogenesis, histopathology, experimental induction and case reports. *Vet Dermatol*, 5, 149–162

21 Neoplastic and non-neoplastic tumours

This chapter is not designed to be a definitive guide to neoplasia in the dog and cat. Only commonly occurring skin tumours will be described.

The reader is referred to more specialised texts for further details.

Epithelial neoplasia

Epithelial tumour can be categorised according to their origin and can be subdivided into different subgroups; see Table 21.1 below. The most common tumours in each group are described in the dog in Tables 21.2–21.6 and in the cat in Tables 21.7–21.9.

Table 21.1 Epithelial tumours in the dog and cat.

1) Epidermal tumours	2) Hair follicle tumours
☐ Papilloma	☐ Fibroadnexal hamartoma
☐ Viral plaques	☐ Follicular cyst
☐ Actinic keratosis	☐ Infundibular keratinising acanthoma
☐ Bowenoid in situ carcinoma	☐ Tricholemmoma
☐ Basal cell carcinoma	☐ Trichoblastoma
☐ Basosquamous carcinoma	☐ Pilomatrixoma
☐ Squamous cell carcinoma	☐ Trichoepithelioma

(*continued*)

Table 21.1 (continued)

3) Tumours of adnexal glands

Sebaceous gland ducts
- ☐ Sebaceous duct cyst
- ☐ Sebaceous ductal adenoma
- ☐ Sebaceous ductal adenocarcinoma

Sebaceous gland
- ☐ Nodular sebaceous hyperplasia
- ☐ Sebaceous haematoma
- ☐ Sebaceous nevus
- ☐ Sebaceous adenoma
- ☐ Sebaceous epithelioma
- ☐ Sebaceous carcinoma

Hepatoid gland
- ☐ Hepatoid gland adenoma
- ☐ Hepatoid gland epithelioma
- ☐ Hepatoid gland carcinoma

Apocrine ducts
- ☐ Apocrine ductal adenoma
- ☐ Apocrine ductal adenocarcinoma

Apocrine glands
- ☐ Apocrine cyst
- ☐ Apocrine cystomitosis (canine)
- ☐ Apocrine adenoma
- ☐ Complex and mixed apocrine adenoma
- ☐ Apocrine carcinoma
- ☐ Complex and mixed apocrine adenocarcinoma

Table 21.2 Epidermal tumours in dogs.

Epidermal tumour	Age incidence	Breed predisposition	Site/appearance	Therapy
Papilloma	See chapter on viral skin disease			
Actinic keratosis Common, epithelial plaques, not neoplastic induced by solar radiation can progress to squamous cell carcinoma (SCC)	Older dogs	Sunbathing dogs, Dalmatians, pit bull terriers, harlequin Great Dane, beagles	Single or multiple plaques, papillate lesions, crust, scale >1 cm. Commonly ventrum and thighs	Topical anti-inflammatory drugs
Basal cell carcinoma Uncommon low grade malignancy; incidence of recurrence and metastasis low	7–10 years	Cocker spaniel, Kerry blue terrier, Shetland sheepdog, springer spaniel, miniature poodle, Siberian husky	Plaques and umbilicated nodules <1 cm in diameter ulcerated and alopecic. Often pigmented black or blue. Site – usually truncal (Figure 21.1)	Surgical excision Electrosurgery Cryosurgery
SCC Locally invasive, slow to metastasise; sun and chronically damaged skin, papilloma virus all been implicated; very common	>9 years	Scottish terrier, Pekinese, Boxer, standard poodle, schnauzer, Dalmatians Nail bed – large breeds, black coated esp. Labradors	Proliferative – papillomatous often ulcerated Ulcerative – crateriform crusted ulcers (Figure 21.2) Site – trunk, limbs, digits, scrotum, lips and nose	Surgical excision Cryosurgery Electrosurgery Hyperthermia Radiotherapy

Table 21.3 Hair follicle tumours in the dog.

Hair follicle tumours	Age incidence	Breed predisposition	Appearance/site	Therapy
Fibroadnexal hamartoma Scar tissue formed post-inflammation results in entrapment and distortion of folliculosebaceous units; common	Middle-aged to old dogs	Large breeds especially Labrador retrievers, basset hounds	Solitary, firm, circumscribed dome-shaped masses 1–4 cm in diameter Site – distal legs, pressure points and interdigital areas	Topical and systemic retinoids; wide surgical excision
Follicular cyst Simple benign sac like structure with epidermal lining; cell type determined by level of follicle affected	Middle-aged to old dogs	Boxer, Shih-Tzu, miniature schnauzers and Old English sheepdogs	Solitary, firm, intradermal nodule 0.2–2.0 cm; cyst contents semisolid, caseous, granular or doughy	Benign neglect; surgical removal
Infundibular keratinising acanthoma Uncommon benign follicular neoplasm; not invasive or metastatic	<5 years	Norwegian elkhounds, keeshond, German shepherd dog, Old English sheepdog	Circumscribed dermal/sc masses 0.5–4.0 cm; pore opens onto surface containing keratinised plaque; anywhere on body (Figure 21.3)	Surgical excision; retinoids – isotretinoin or etretinate 1.0 mg/kg sid may need long-term
Tricholemmoma Rare benign follicular neoplasm; rarely invasive or metastatic	5–13 years	Afghan hounds	Firm, oval 1–7 cm; head and neck	Surgical excision
Trichoblastoma Replace most of tumour called basal cell tumours; uncommon benign follicular neoplasm, rarely metastatic	6–9 years	Poodles, cocker spaniel, Kerry blue terrier, Bichon Frise, Shetland sheepdog, husky	Solitary firm, alopecic, pigmented nodules dome-shaped, polypoid 1–2 cm; head (base of ear), neck	Surgical excision
Pilomatrixoma Uncommon benign follicular neoplasm; rarely invasive or metastatic	>5 years	Kerry blue terrier, poodle, Old English sheepdog	Well-circumscribed solid/cystic tumour 1–10 cm in diameter Site – shoulder, lateral thorax and dorsum	Surgical excision
Trichoepithelioma Uncommon benign neoplasm; rarely invasive or metastatic	>5 years	Golden retriever, basset, German shepherd dog, cocker spaniel, Irish setter	Usually solitary, solid or cystic, circumscribed 0.5–15 cm in diameter; ulceration and alopecic common; site – dorsum, thorax, limbs	Surgical excision

Table 21.4 Adnexal gland tumours of the dog – sebaceous gland.

Adnexal gland tumours (1) Sebaceous gland	Age incidence	Breed predisposition	Site/appearance	Therapy
Nodular sebaceous hyperplasia Common benign hyperplastic lesions	>9 years	Cocker spaniel, poodle, wheaten terrier, beagle, dachshund, Manchester terrier, miniature schnauzer	Solitary well-circumscribed yellow/white alopecia, firm, dome-shaped, papillate, plaque 3 mm to 1 cm; can be melanotic; limb, trunk, face (eyelids, ears)	Surgical excision; laser ablation; cryosurgery; isotretinoin 1–2 mg/kg po sid until lesion regression; acitretin 0.5–1.0 mg/kg po sid until regression; monitor liver function
Sebaceous adenoma Common benign neoplasms; no metastatic potential	>9 years	Cocker spaniel, husky, miniature poodle, beagle Samoyed, dachshund	Solitary or multiple, dome-shaped, papillate, yellow or opalescent <1 cm Eyelids and limbs (Figure 21.4)	Surgical excision; other treatment as nodular sebaceous hyperplasia
Sebaceous epithelioma Fairly common, can be locally aggressive, metastasis rare	>9 years	Shih-Tzu, Lhasa apso, malamute plus as sebaceous adenoma	As sebaceous adenoma 2 mm–3 cm. Eyelid and head	Surgical excision
Sebaceous carcinoma Rare malignant neoplasms, locally aggressive, metastasis rare	>9 years	Cocker spaniel, cavalier King Charles spaniel, Scottish terrier, husky	Solitary nodules similar appearance to sebaceous adenoma but 2.5–7.5 cm ulceration common. Head and limbs (Figure 21.5)	Surgical excision; radiotherapy

Table 21.5 Adnexal gland tumours of the dog – hepatoid gland.

Adnexal gland tumours (2) Hepatoid gland	Age incidence	Breed predisposition	Site/appearance	Therapy
Hepatoid gland adenoma Benign growths derived from circumanal or hepatoid glands; may be secondary to androgen stimulation; common benign lesion	Older intact male dogs >8 years	Cocker spaniel, Samoyed, husky, English bulldog and beagles	Multiple or solitary slow growing firm round to lobular dermal nodules; vary from several mm to 10 cm; site – perianal skin	Castration and tumour removal in intact males, removal alone in others; cryosurgery; laser ablation
Hepatoid gland carcinoma Malignant neoplasm of hepatoid gland; metastasis common in poorly differentiated carcinoma, rare in well-differentiated lesions	Older male and female dogs regardless of neuter status	Artic circle breeds and German shepherd dogs	Similar to adenomas but larger at 2 cm + in diameter; can be aggressive poorly circumscribed and ulcerated; site – perianal skin, rare	Not hormonal influenced; no response to castration, wide surgical excision combined with radiation or chemotherapy if excision incomplete

Table 21.6 Adnexal gland tumours of the dog – apocrine gland.

Adnexal gland tumours (3) Apocrine glands	Age incidence	Breed predisposition	Site/appearance	Therapy
Apocrine cyst Common non-neoplastic lesion; do not metastasise	>6 years	Old English sheepdogs, Weimaraner	Solitary, well-defined tense or fluctuant bullous nodules several mm–cm in diameter; cyst content clear and watery; site – head, neck, legs and dorsal trunk	Benign neglect; surgical removal
Apocrine adenoma Uncommon benign neoplasm derived from apocrine glands; do not metastasise	Average 9 years	Golden retriever, German shepherd dog, malamutes, chow chows	Solitary raised alopecic well-circumscribed dermal or subcut tumours with bluish colour; may be ulcerated size 0.5–4.0 cm; site – head, neck, trunk and legs	Benign neglect; surgical removal
Apocrine carcinoma Uncommon malignant tumour; locally invasive and recur; 20% go to lymph node and have systemic spread	Average 10 years	Golden retriever, German shepherd dog, Norwegian elkhound	Solitary growth similar to adenoma; 0.5–10 cm diameter; site – head neck, trunk and legs	Wide surgical excision

Table 21.7 Epidermal tumours in the cat.

Epidermal tumour	Age incidence	Breed predisposition	Site/appearance	Therapy
Papilloma	See chapter on viral skin disease			
Actinic keratosis Common, epithelial plaques induced by solar radiation can progress to SCC	Older animals	White cats	Single or multiple plaques, papillate lesions, crust, scale >1 cm; commonly pinna, nose and eyelids (Figure 21.6)	Topical anti-inflammatory drugs
Basal cell carcinoma Uncommon low grade malignancy; incidence of recurrence and metastasis low	Average age 10 years	No breed predilection recognised	Plaques and umbilicated nodules <0.5 cm in diameter ulcerated and alopecic; often pigmented black or blue; site – nose, face and ears (Figure 21.7)	Surgical excision; electrosurgery; cryosurgery
SCC Locally invasive, slow to metastasise; sun and chronically damaged skin, papilloma virus all been implicated	5 years + average age 11 years	White cats – risk is 13× higher than other coloured cats	Proliferative – papillomatous often ulcerated, ulcerative crateriform crusted ulcers (Figure 21.8); site – eyelids (Figure 21.9), nasal planum and pinnae	Surgical excision; cryosurgery; electrosurgery; hyperthermia; radiotherapy

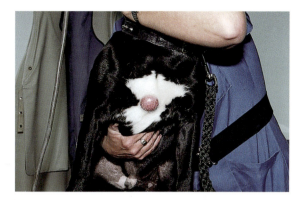

Figure 21.1 Solitary well-circumscribed basal cell carcinoma.

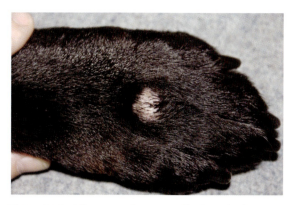

Figure 21.4 Sebaceous adenoma on the foot of a dog.

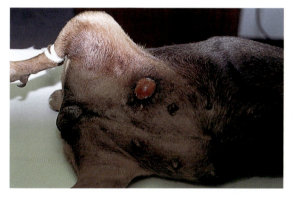

Figure 21.2 Ulcerative squamous cell carcinoma on the ventral abdomen of a Staffordshire bull terrier.

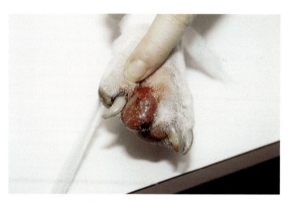

Figure 21.5 Sebaceous carcinoma of the interdigital space of an English bull terrier.

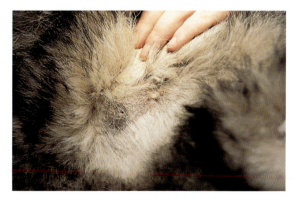

Figure 21.3 Intracutaneous cornifying epithelioma in a Norwegian elkhound.

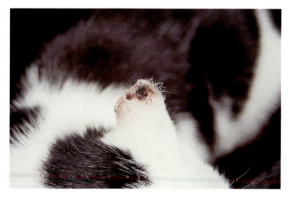

Figure 21.6 Actinic keratosis of ear tips.

Table 21.8 Adnexal gland tumours in the cat – sebaceous gland.

Adnexal gland tumours (1) Sebaceous gland	Age incidence	Breed predisposition	Site/appearance	Therapy
Sebaceous adenoma Common benign neoplasms; no metastatic potential	Average age 10 years	Persian cats	Solitary or multiple, dome-shaped, papillate, yellow or opalescent <1 cm; eyelids and limbs	Surgical excision; laser ablation; cryosurgery
Sebaceous epithelioma Fairly common, can be locally aggressive, metastasis rare	Average age 10 years	Persian cats	As sebaceous adenoma 2 mm–3 cm; eyelid and head	Surgical excision
Sebaceous carcinoma Rare malignant neoplasms, locally aggressive, metastasis rare	9–12 years	No breed predisposition recognised	Solitary nodules similar appearance to sebaceous adenoma but 2.5–7.5 cm ulceration common; head and limbs	Surgical excision; radiotherapy

Table 21.9 Adnexal gland tumours in the cat – apocrine glands.

Adnexal gland tumours (2) Apocrine glands	Age incidence	Breed predisposition	Site /appearance	Therapy
Apocrine cyst Common non-neoplastic lesion	>6 years	Persian cats, Himalayan	Solitary, well-defined tense or fluctuant bullous nodules several 2–10 mm in diameter; cyst content clear and watery; site – mostly head, especially eyelids (Figure 21.10)	Benign neglect; surgical removal
Apocrine adenoma Uncommon benign neoplasm derived from apocrine glands; do not metastasise	Average 11–12 years	None recognised	Solitary raised alopecic well-circumscribed dermal or subcut tumours with bluish colour; may be ulcerated size 0.5–4.0 cm; site – head	Benign neglect; surgical removal
Apocrine carcinoma	11–13 years	Siamese cats	Solitary growth similar to adenoma; 0.2–3 cm diameter; site – head especially lower lip and chin	Wide surgical excision

Neoplastic and non-neoplastic tumours

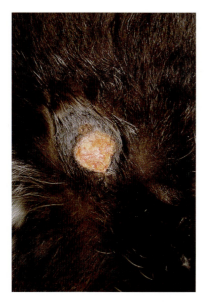

Figure 21.7 Well-demarcated basal cell carcinoma on thorax.

Mesenchymal and other tumours

Mast cell tumour

Cause and pathogenesis

Common malignant neoplasm derived from dermal tissue mast cells. It is most common cutaneous tumour of the dog and second most common of the cat. Metastasis is common.

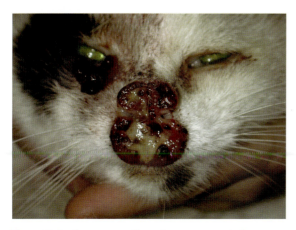

Figure 21.8 Squamous cell carcinoma on nasal planum.

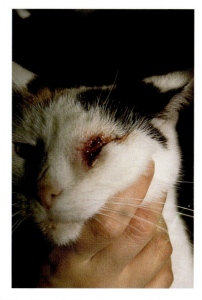

Figure 21.9 Crusted ulceration caused by squamous cell carcinoma of eyelid.

Clinical signs

- Age incidence approximately 8 years.
- Breed predisposition dogs include Boxer, Boston terrier, English bulldog, pug, golden retriever, Weimaraner (Figure 21.11). Cat predisposition includes the Siamese.
- Dogs:
  - Mast cell tumours are very variable in appearance and size:
    - Dermal or subcutaneous oedema, papules, nodules or pedunculated masses.

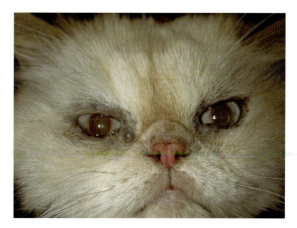

Figure 21.10 Apocrine cysts on the eyelid of a cat.

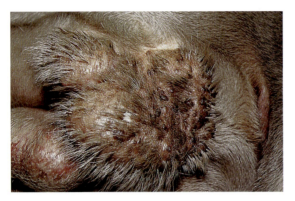

Figure 21.11 Mast cell tumour on the perineum of a Weimaraner.

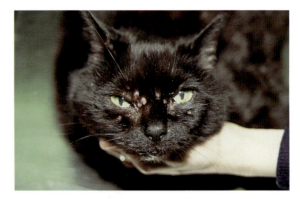

Figure 21.13 Multiple mast cell tumours on the head.

- Poorly or well circumscribed, soft or firm, alopecic or ulcerated (Figure 21.12).
- Size of lesions varies from a few millimetres to several centimetres.
  □ All tumours contain vasoactive substances that can produce localised oedema, inflammation and rarely anaphylactic shock if palpated.
  □ Tumours usually found on caudal half of body.
  □ Systemic signs gastro/duodenal ulceration, defective blood coagulation and thrombocytopaenia.
■ Cats:
  □ Mast cell tumours are very variable in appearance and size:
    - Solitary intradermal nodule that can be erythematous and alopecic or ulcerated; size varies from 0.2 to 3 cm.
    - Multiple clusters of subcutaneous nodules ranging in size from 0.5 to 1 cm can be seen in young cats (<4 years); these lesions may regress spontaneously (Figure 21.13).
  □ Tumours usually found on the head.
  □ Most tumours are well differentiated and benign.
  □ Systemic signs are rare.

Diagnosis

■ Cytology from an impression smear or fine needle aspirate taken with care reveals round cells with round nuclei that contain prominent basophilic granules. Granule staining depends on the degree of differentiation of the tumour (Figure 21.14).

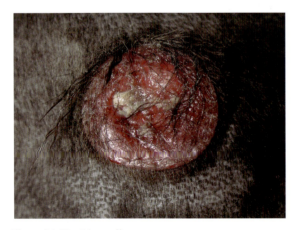

Figure 21.12 Mast cell tumour.

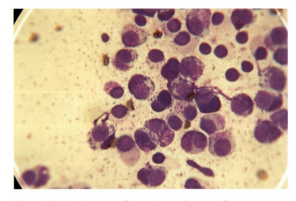

Figure 21.14 Fine needle aspirate of mast cell tumour.

Table 21.10 Mast cell tumour grading – some of the key points taken from Patnaik's grading system.

Histological grade	I	II	III
Extent of tumour	Dermis	Dermis and subcutis	Invades subcutis and deep tissues
Cellularity	Low to moderate cellularity	Moderate to high cellularity	Highly cellular
Cell morphology	Round monomorphic cells with distinct cell borders, medium sized granules	Moderately pleomorphic cells, distinct cell borders, fine granules	Pleomorphic cells, indistinct cell borders fine granules or none
Mitotic figures	Absent	0–2/HPF	3–6/HPF

- Skin biopsy reveals a non-encapsulated infiltrative sheet or densely packed cords of round cells with central nuclei, abundant cytoplasm and basophilic granules. Eosinophils are usually numerous in the section. Histology is essential to grade the tumour (see Table 21.10) and stage the disease to give indication for treatment and prognosis.

Treatment

- Dogs:
  - Single tumours (Grade I and II):
    - Surgical excision with a wide excision of 3 cm beyond palpable tumour. This can be curative for Grade I and II tumours. Post-operative follow up should be performed every 3 months.
    - Cryosurgery with premedication with antihistamines.
    - Electrosurgery with premedication with antihistamines.
    - Injection of deionised water or triamcinolone.
    - Radiotherapy.
  - Disseminated tumours:
    - Surgical excision even with a wide margin is rarely curative.
    - Chemotherapy:
      - Combination therapy with cyclophosphamide–vinblastine–prednisolone or cyclophosphamide–vincristine–prednisolone–hydroxyurea.
      - Lomustine may produce some response.
      - Cimetidine can be used for animals with gastrointestinal ulceration at a dose of 4 mg/kg po qid.
- Cats:
  - Surgical removal is curative in most cases.

Urticaria pigmentosa

Cause and pathogenesis

A benign proliferative mast cell disorder only seen in cats.

Clinical signs

- No sex predilection; urticaria pigmentosa is seen in young cats <1 year of age.
- Himalayan cats appear to be overrepresented.
- Lesions appear as areas of macular erythema and hyperpigmentation around the mouth, chin, neck and eyes.

Diagnosis

- History and clinical signs.
- Skin biopsy reveals signs of mast cell proliferation with areas of epidermal hypermelanosis.

Treatment

No treatment is necessary as spontaneous regression over a period of a few months.

Plasmacytoma

Cause and pathogenesis

Tumour of plasma cell origin. It is uncommon in dogs and rare in cats.

Clinical signs

- No sex predilection; most commonly seen in older animals.
- Cocker spaniel may be predisposed; no breed predisposition is recognised in the cat.
- Lesions are usually solitary well-circumscribed soft or firm, pedunculated or ulcerated dermal nodules.
- Size variable, from a few millimetres to a few centimetres in diameter.
- Most common sites are external ear canal (Figure 21.15), lip, trunks or digits.

Diagnosis

- History and clinical signs.
- Cytology of a fine needle aspirate reveals round cells with perinuclear halos or may have moderate amounts of dark basophilic cytoplasm and a 'clock-face' nucleus.
- Excisional biopsy is preferable. Histopathology reveals a well-circumscribed round cell tumour where cells are arranged in solid lobules. Cellular pleomorphism presents with a moderate mitotic rate.

Treatment

- Surgical excision is the treatment of choice; most lesions can be completely excised.
- In dogs plasmacytomas have a low metastatic potential and recurrence is rare so surgical removal offers a good prognosis for complete cure.
- In cats the risk of spread to lymph nodes and systemically is high so this tumour carries a much more prognosis in this species.

Transmissible venereal tumour (TVT)

Cause and pathogenesis

A TVT is a variably malignant tumour of unknown cell origin that may, due to its transmissibility, be virally induced. Transplantation of tumour cells is thought to occur during coitus but can also occur during normal grooming activity. Some tumours can spontaneously regress as dogs develop an antitumour immunological response. Disease found in tropical and subtropical climates. Only recorded in the dog.

Clinical signs

- Intact bitches appear to be predisposed; can affect dogs of any age or breed.
- Lesions found most commonly on external genitalia, but also on face and limbs.
- Single to multiple, firm to friable, erythematous, often haemorrhagic, dermal or subcutaneous nodules that may be papilliform.
- Size ranges from 1 to 20 cm in diameter.
- Ulceration and secondary infection is common.
- Metastasis is rare.

Diagnosis

- History and clinical signs.
- Cytology taken by fine needle aspirate reveals round cells with moderate amounts of mid-blue cytoplasm that contains characteristic vacuoles.

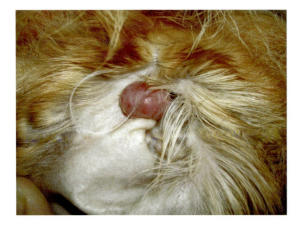

Figure 21.15 Plasmacytoma ear canal of dog.

Table 21.11 Benign mesenchymal tumours of the dog and cat.

Benign mesenchymal tumours	Age incidence	Breed predisposition	Appearance/site	Therapy
Fibroma Uncommon benign neoplasm arising from fibroblasts; non-invasive and non-metastatic	Middle-aged to older dogs and cats	Boxer, Boston terrier, Doberman, golden retriever, fox terrier Not recorded in the cat	Solitary, dome-shaped, pedunculated well-circumscribed nodules 1–5 cm may be melanotic; site: dog and cat – head and legs	Surgical excision; cryosurgery; electrosurgery; benign neglect
Nodular dermatofibrosis Rare condition where dermal fibrotic nodules are seen with renal cystic disease and in intact females uterine leiomyoma; poor prognosis usually fatal	Middle-aged to old dogs	German shepherd dog Not recorded in the cat	Multiple cutaneous nodules, firm well-circumscribed, dermal to subcut; size several mm – 4 cm; overlying skin thickened, ulcerated hyperpigmented; site limb head and ears	Ovariohysterectomy in females with uterine lesions; nephrectomy in dogs with renal lesions – renal disease often bilateral making surgery impossible
Fibropruritic nodule Uncommon benign nodular lesions associated with abnormal reaction to flea bites	Older dog	German shepherd dogs and their crosses Not seen in cats	Multiple firm alopecic nodules ranging from 0.5 to 2.0 cm may be erythematous and hyperpigmented; site – dorsal lumbosacral area	Treatment of flea bite allergy; surgical excision; anti-inflammatory therapy with glucocorticoids 1.0 mg/kg po sid for 2 weeks then every 48 hours tapering with a view to withdrawal
Feline sarcoid Uncommon papilloma-induced fibroblastic proliferation; lesion slow growing, infiltrative, recurrence after surgery common	Average age 12 months	Male cats predisposed Not recognised in dogs	Solitary or multiple nodules <2 cm diameter; firm often ulcerated; sites – philtrum, nares, upper lip, digits, tail tip and ears	Wide surgical excision including amputation if possible (ears, tail); cryosurgery; radiation therapy
Haemangioma Uncommon benign neoplasm from endothelial cells of blood vessels; solar damaged increased risk	9 years – dogs 9–11 years – cats	Boxer, golden retriever, German shepherd dog, English springer spaniel, Airedale – any light skinned sunbathing dogs; no breed predilection in cats	Solitary well-circumscribed, round blue/red black nodules 0.5–4.0 cm; site: dog – ventral abdomen, thorax; cat – head, legs and abdomen	Surgical excision; cryosurgery; electrosurgery; benign neglect; reduce subsequent sunlight exposure
Lipoma Common benign neoplasms from subcutaneous lipocytes	>8 years	Cocker spaniel, dachshund, Weimaraner, Doberman pinscher, miniature schnauzer, Labrador, Labrador retriever Cats – Siamese	Usually single well-circumscribed, soft fleshy dome-shaped tumours 1–30 cm; over thorax, abdomen and proximal limbs	Surgical excision, lesions will reduce in size with weight loss; intra-tumour injection of 10% calcium chloride; benign neglect

Table 21.12 Soft tissue sarcomas in the dog and cat.

Soft tissue sarcomas	Age incidence	Breed predisposition	Appearance/site	Therapy
Fibrosarcoma Uncommon neoplasm fibroblast origin; often rapid growth, frequent recurrence and metastases; in cats seen spontaneously or associated with feline sarcoma virus (FeSV) or vaccine induced	Older dogs Cats FeSV induced <5 years Others >5 years	Cocker spaniel, Doberman pinscher, golden retriever	Dog – solitary, poorly circumscribed irregular variably sized nodules 1–15 cm often ulcerated and alopecic; site – limbs and trunk (Figure 21.16) Cat – non-FeSV lesions solitary; FeSV-induced firm nodular to irregular, poorly circumscribed 0.5–15 cm; site – trunk, distal limb, pinna; (Figure 21.17) FeSV at injection sites	Poor prognosis; wide surgical excision; radiotherapy limited value; chemotherapy with doxorubicin, mitoxantrone may prolong survival
Haemangiosarcoma Malignant neoplasm from endothelium of blood vessels; solar damaged skin increased risk; local recurrence and metastasis common; dermal tumour better prognosis post-incision than subcut tumour	>10 years	GSD golden retriever BMD, Boxer – any light skinned sunbathing dogs White cats	Solitary/multiple poorly circumscribed red/dark blue plaques; haemorrhage, ulceration common; dermal form <2 cm; subcut form <10 cm; dogs – ventral thorax, abdomen, limbs (Figure 21.18); cats – head and ears (Figure 21.19)	Poor prognosis; radical surgical excision, often amputation; chemotherapy post-surgery with vincristine, doxorubicin, cyclophosphamide
Haemangiopericytoma Common neoplasms from vascular pericytes; locally invasive; local recurrence common despite surgery; metastasis rare	7–10 years	Boxer, GSD, cocker spaniel, springer spaniel, Irish setter No cat predilection	Solitary, firm multinodular well-circumscribed nodules <25 cm in diameter; alopecia, ulceration is common. limbs (Figure 21.20) (especially elbows and stifles)	Poor prognosis; radical surgical excision often amputation; radiation post-surgery may be beneficial
Liposarcoma Rare malignant neoplasms from subcutaneous lipoblasts; locally invasive, may metastasise	10 years	Dachshund, Shetland sheepdog, Brittany spaniel	Usually single, poorly circumscribed firm/fleshy nodules 1–10 cm; ventral abdomen, thorax, proximal limbs	Poor prognosis; radical surgical excision often amputation; chemotherapy with doxorubicin may be useful if excision is incomplete

- Skin biopsy reveals sheets of uniform round cells with a collagenous stroma interdispersed. Mitotic index is high.

Treatment

- Chemotherapy is the treatment of choice. Lesions usually respond well to vincristine given over 4–6 weeks. Doxorubicin may be used in cases that respond poorly to vincristine.
- Radiotherapy may be employed as these tumours are very radiosensitive.
- Surgical removal may be an option for small lesions but recurrence rates are high.
- Prognosis is good; most tumours will regress spontaneously or respond to chemotherapy.

Neoplastic and non-neoplastic tumours 339

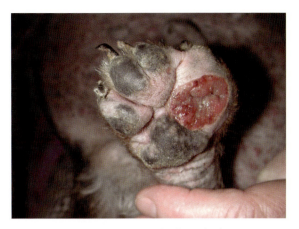

Figure 21.16   Fibrosarcoma on the foot of a dog.

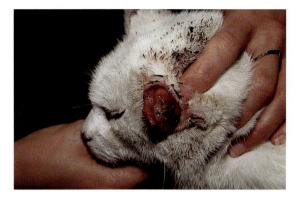

Figure 21.19   Dermal haemangiosarcoma on the ear of an elderly cat.

Benign mesenchymal tumours

These tumours all behave in a similar way. Therapy is not always necessary, provided they do not grow too large. The clinical presentation, age and breed predilection as well as most common sites are listed in Table 21.11.

Soft tissue sarcomas

Soft tissue sarcomas can affect the skin. They all behave in a similar way. The clinical presentation, age and breed predilection as well as most common sites are listed in Table 21.12. Diagnosis may be undertaken by fine needle aspirates of lesions and biopsy. These tumours respond poorly

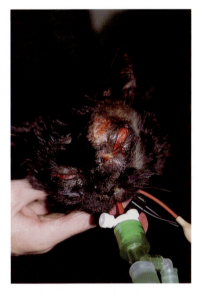

Figure 21.17   Fibrosarcoma on face showing typical poorly circumscribed alopecic ulcerated appearance.

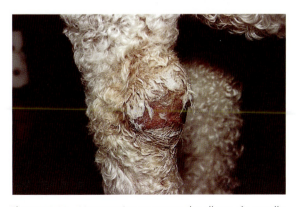

Figure 21.18   Haemangiosarcoma on the elbow of a poodle.

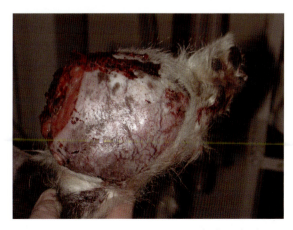

Figure 21.20   Haemangiopericytoma on the leg of a dog.

to chemotherapy or radiotherapy and need surgical removal. The results of tissue biopsy to establish aetiology plus such techniques as MRI allow the planning of adequate surgical margins for surgical removal, which needs to be extensive often resulting in amputation of a limb where it is found at this site.

Epitheliotropic lymphoma (mycosis fungoides)

Cause and pathogenesis

An uncommon neoplasm of T lymphocyte origin found in older dogs and cats.

Clinical signs

- Age incidence greater than 9 years of age in both dogs and cats.
- No sex or breed predisposition.
- Four clinical presentations:
  - Exfoliative erythroderma (erythema with pruritus and scale).
  - Mucocutaneous ulceration ± depigmentation (Figure 21.21).
  - Solitary or multiple plaques and nodules (Figure 21.22).
  - Infiltrative and ulcerative oral disease (usually misdiagnosed as chronic stomatitis) (Figure 21.23).
- Most cases occur as slowly progressive disease.

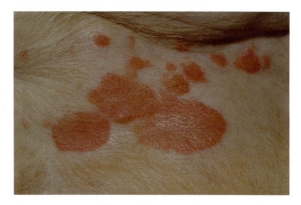

Figure 21.22 Nodules and plaques on the abdomen of a dog with epitheliotropic lymphoma.

Differential diagnosis

Due to the wide range of different clinical presentations, epitheliotropic lymphoma should be considered in all skin diseases of older dogs and cats.

Diagnosis

- History and clinical signs.
- Cytology as fine needle aspirate of nodules and plaques or impression smears of ulcers stained with Diff-Quik. Samples reveal abundant round neoplastic lymphoid cells with basophilic cytoplasm and an indented or lobular nuclei.

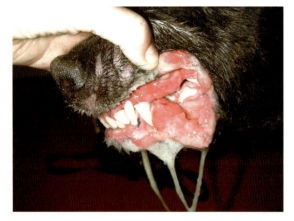

Figure 21.21 Mucocutaneous ulceration in a case of epitheliotropic lymphoma.

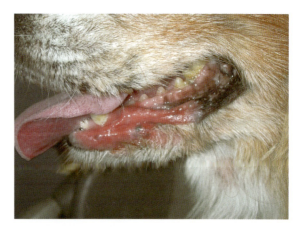

Figure 21.23 Ulcerative oral disease in a dog with epitheliotropic lymphoma.

Table 21.13 Histiocytic reactions in dogs.

Reactions (previous names)	Neoplastic	Subtype	Systemic involvement
Langerhans cell histiocytosis	Yes	Solitary cutaneous histiocytoma	No
	Yes	Multiple recurrent and persistent histiocytoma	No
	Yes	Persistent histiocytoma with lymph node involvement	No
	Yes	Langerhans cell histiocytosis	Yes, from skin metastasis to lymph nodes and internal organs
Histiocytic sarcoma (malignant histiocytosis)	Yes	Disseminated histiocytic sarcoma	Yes, metastatic spread from primary skin
	Yes	Localised histiocytic sarcoma	Can occur in subcutaneous tissue or other organs
Reactive histiocytosis (cutaneous and systemic histiocytosis)	No		Yes

- Skin biopsy reveals signs of a lichenoid infiltrate of neoplastic lymphocytes that infiltrate the superficial dermis and surface of follicular and sweat gland epithelium. Small intraepidermal clusters of cells called Pautrier's microabscesses are typical of epitheliotropic lymphoma.

Treatment

- Whatever treatment is used the disease carries a very poor prognosis; therapy may give short-term remission.
- Solitary lesions:
  - Surgical excision
- Multiple lesions:
  - Chemotherapy:
    - Combinations of prednisolone, cyclophosphamide, vincristine and methotrexate.
    - Lomustine (CCNU), peg – asparaginase or pegylated liposomal doxorubicin may be useful.
    - Retinoids, e.g. isotretinoin, for dogs 3–4 mg/kg po sid, and for cats 10 mg/cat po sid may improve clinical signs in some animals.
    - Interferon 1–1.5 million U/m² sq three times weekly produces some success.
  - Topical nitrogen mustard 10 mg of nitrogen mustard in 50 ml water or propylene glycol. Not for use in cats. Apply 2–3 times weekly until remission then every 2–4 weeks for maintenance. Operators should wear gloves when applying and dogs should wear collar to prevent ingestion of solution.

Tumours of histiocytic origin

Histiocytic lesions are relatively common in the dog, although rare in the cat. Lesions may be localised or generalised in the skin and may be confined to the skin or have concurrent systemic involvement. The different forms of reaction patterns in the dog are detailed in Table 21.13 and the signalment, breed and age predisposition as well as brief notes on therapy are detailed in Table 21.14.

Melanocytic neoplasms

Melanocytoma/melanoma

Cause and pathogenesis

- Benign or malignant proliferation of melanocytes in the skin. Eighty-five per cent

Table 21.14 Signalment for most common histiocytic disease in the dog and cat.

Histiocytic lesions	Age incidence	Breed predisposition	Appearance/site	Therapy
Langerhans cell histiocytosis Solitary cutaneous histiocytoma Common benign neoplasm derived from Langerhans cells	Dogs <2 years Rare disease in the cat	Many different dog breeds	Solitary, 'button-shaped' dermal tumour, often ulcerated. 0.5–4.0 cm in diameter (Figure 21.24); site – head, ear pinnae and legs	Surgical excision; cryosurgery; electrosurgery; benign neglect – most lesions undergo spontaneous remission in <3 months
Multiple recurrent and persistent histiocytoma Benign neoplasm derived from Langerhans cells	Any age, usually young dogs	Shar-pei and shar-pei cross dogs	Multifocal nodular lesions – seen at any site	As cutaneous histiocytoma immunosuppressive drugs contraindicated
Histiocytic sarcoma (malignant histiocytosis) Histiocytic sarcomas of dendritic cell origin Disseminated histiocytic sarcoma	Middle-aged to old dogs	Rare in the dog BMD, also Rottweilers, golden and Labrador retrievers Not recorded in cat	Most commonly causes malignancy of internal organs with wide-spread metastasis; skin can be involved with multiple firm dermal to subcut nodules that may be ulcerated	Treatment of no benefit; rapidly progressive fatal disease
Localised histiocytic sarcoma	Middle-aged to old dogs Cats 8–11 years	Common in dog, BMD Rottweilers, golden and Labrador retrievers Rare in cat	Lesions in subcut tissue, as well as spleen, tongue, lung, vertebral bone; firm nodules up to several cm; site – dogs when in skin – extremities (Figure 21.25)	Early wide excision of tumour often including amputation of extremity
Reactive histiocytosis (cutaneous and systemic histiocytosis) Reactive proliferation of dermal dendritic cells				
Cutaneous histiocytosis Rare benign proliferative disorder of histiocytes where lesions are confined to the skin	2–11 years	Canine breed predilection debatable; possible collies, Shetland sheepdogs, BMD Rottweilers, shar-pei, retrievers, Irish wolfhounds, Not seen in cats	Appearance – multiple dermal/subcut, plaques and nodules 1–5 cm; site – anywhere on body – head, neck, perineum, scrotum and extremities are commonly affected (Figures 21.26 and 21.27); nodules can be numerous up to 50	Chemotherapy – Prednisolone 1–2 mg/kg po sid until remission ~7–10 days then taper and stop; cyclosporine has been used in some cases with success; lifetime therapy often needed
Systemic histiocytosis Rare benign proliferative disorder of histiocytes where lesions are found in skin and internal organs	2–8 years	Many breeds especially BMD Not seen in cats	*Cutaneous signs* Plaques, nodules and ulcers over whole body especially muzzle (Figure 21.28), nasal planum, eyelids and scrotum *Systemic signs* weight loss, dyspnoea, lameness; disease waxes and wanes despite treatment	Treatment as cutaneous histiocytosis

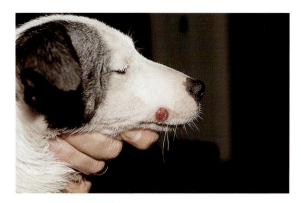

Figure 21.24 Histiocytoma in a young dog.

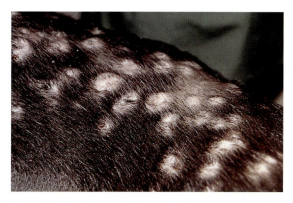

Figure 21.27 Close-up of Figure 21.26.

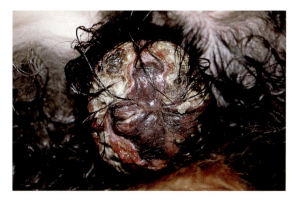

Figure 21.25 Histiocytic sarcoma in the scrotum of a Bernese mountain dog.

of cases are benign. Sunlight is not a causative agent. Genetic susceptibility may be a factor. Common tumour in old dogs, rare in cats.
- Tumour location is prognostic, most oral, and mucocutaneous lesions except (eyelid) are malignant. Fifty per cent of nail bed tumours are malignant.
- Breed is prognostic in that 75% of melanocytic neoplasms in the Doberman and miniature schnauzer are benign; 85% of those in miniature poodles are malignant.

Clinical signs
- Age incidence approximately 9 years.
- Breed predisposition in dogs includes Scottish terrier, Airedale, Boston terrier, cocker spaniel, springer spaniel, Boxer, golden retriever, Irish setter.

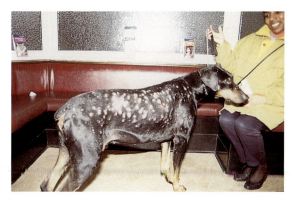

Figure 21.26 Cutaneous histiocytosis in a Doberman.

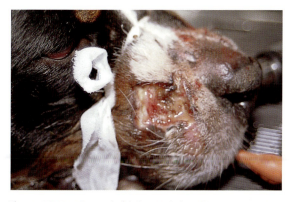

Figure 21.28 Systamic histiocytosis in a Bernese mountain dog.

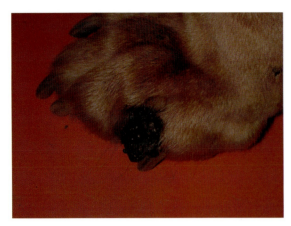

Figure 21.29 Melanoma on the toe of a dog.

- Breed predisposition in cats is not noticed.
- Melanocytoma:
  - Appearance – usually solitary, well-circumscribed, dome-shaped, alopecic brown/black pedunculated or wart-like growths 0.5–10.0 cm in diameter.
  - Site – head (especially eyelid and muzzle), trunk and paws.
- Melanoma:
  - Appearance – usually solitary, variable shape and colour (grey/brown/black or non-pigmented) 0.5–10 cm in diameter; often ulcerated and grow more quickly than melanocytoma (Figure 21.29).
- Dog lesions are found on the head, limbs, digits (including claw bed), scrotum, lip, trunk.
- Cat lesions most commonly seen on the head.

Diagnosis
- Fine needle aspirate of lesion reveals round, oval, stellate or spindle-shaped cells with moderate amounts of cytoplasm that contains brown to green/black pigment. Malignant melanomas may contain fewer pigment cells and show greater pleomorphism. Difference between benign and malignant very difficult on the basis of cytology.
- Skin biopsy will identify the mass as a melanocytic neoplasm but will not reliably differentiate melanocytoma from melanoma. Histopathology reveals accumulations of neoplastic spindle, epithelial or round cells with variable degrees of pigmentation.

Treatment
- Radical surgical excision.
- If excision is incomplete adjunctive therapy may include chemotherapy with intralesional cisplatin, radiation therapy, local hyperthermia and photodynamic therapy.
- Response to systemic chemotherapy with drugs such as mitoxantrone, doxorubicin, cisplatin often disappointing; may prolong survival but response otherwise poor.

Secondary skin neoplasms/paraneoplastic disease

Cause and pathogenesis

Secondary skin neoplasia results by metastatic spread of primary neoplasms in other organs to the skin, e.g. metastatic bronchial carcinoma. Paraneoplastic disease is where a distant tumour leads to evidence of cutaneous disease, which is non-neoplastic. Examples of this include thymoma or thoracic lymphoma and feline paraneoplastic alopecia.

Metastatic bronchial carcinoma/squamous cell carcinoma of the lungs

Cause and pathogenesis

Primary pulmonary lesions, which may be asymptomatic at the time of development of the secondary lesions produce metastatic disease to the nail beds. Seventy-five per cent of all pulmonary carcinomas in the cats metastasise to the nail beds.

Clinical signs
- No sex predilection; old cats and dogs are at increased risk, average age 12 years but can be seen in as young as 4 years.
- No evidence of a breed predilection.

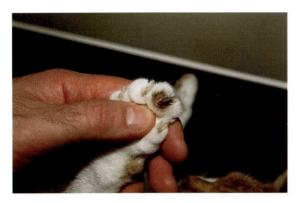

Figure 21.30 Metastatic bronchial carcinoma producing destructive paronychial lesions.

- Animals present with lameness and swelling of more than one digit.
- Lesions are seen on multiple digits but not all digits on one particularly paw need to be affected.
- Paronychial lesions are ulcerative and erosive (Figure 21.30) and may be pruritic; nails can be lost.
- Respiratory signs are not usually present.

Differential diagnosis

- Bacterial or fungal paronychial infection.
- Primary neoplasia, e.g. squamous cell carcinoma.

Diagnosis

- History and clinical signs.
- Skin biopsy of lesions on digits reveals signs of a poorly circumscribed neoplasm associated with bone lysis. The tumour morphology corresponds to the subtype of primary pulmonary tumour.
- Thoracic radiographs will identify the primary lesions in the cat's chest.
- Ultrasonography will identify pulmonary lesions.

Treatment

- The prognosis for this disease is grave. Mean survival time is 1–2 months.
- Treatment is unsuccessful.

Feline thymoma associated exfoliative dermatitis

Cause and pathogenesis

Rare paraneoplastic syndrome seen in the cat. Exfoliative skin disease precedes the development of systemic disease. It has only been reported in cats. As thymoma has not been recognised in all cases it is thought that in some circumstances this syndrome may represent an immunological reaction pattern.

Clinical signs

- No sex predilection or breed predisposition.
- Middle-aged to old cats are at an increased risk of developing disease.
- Lesions start on the head, pinnae and neck but rapidly generalise (Figure 21.31).
- Initially cats present with non-pruritic scaling lesions that lead to exfoliative erythroderma and alopecia (Figure 21.32) with oozing erosions and ulcers.
- Brown waxy keratosebaceous debris accumulates between the toes and claw beds.
- Malassezia may be seen as a secondary infection.
- Systemic signs include coughing and dyspnoea, lethargy and anorexia.

Differential diagnosis

- Dermatophytosis
- Cheyletiellosis

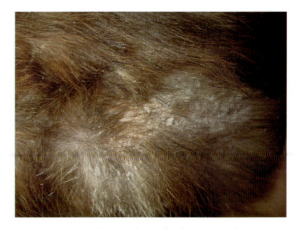

Figure 21.31 Scaling on the neck of a cat with thymoma.

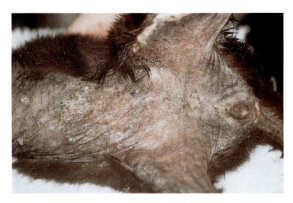

Figure 21.32 Typical exfoliative erythroderma seen secondary to thymoma. (Source: Picture courtesy of H O'Dair.)

- Primary keratinisation disorder
- Epitheliotropic lymphoma
- Pemphigus foliaceus

Diagnosis

- History and clinical signs.
- Skin biopsy of skin reveals signs that are very similar to erythema multiforme. There is mild apoptosis and an interface reaction.
- Thoracic radiographs to identify a thymic mass, which is found in most but not all cases.

Treatment

Thymomas are generally benign and thus successful surgical excision of the thoracic mass has been shown to lead to resolution of the skin disease.

Feline paraneoplastic alopecia

Cause and pathogenesis

Feline paraneoplastic alopecia is a rare but highly characteristic skin disease that is a marker for underlying visceral neoplasia. Most reported cases have had a pancreatic carcinoma of either the acinar cell or pancreatic duct origin. Metastasis to the liver appears to be common.

Clinical signs

- Old cats are affected: age 9–16 years.
- No breed or sex predilection.
- Cutaneous signs:

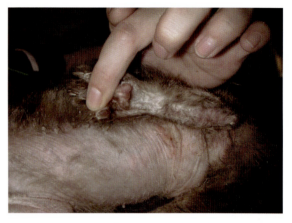

Figure 21.33 Ventral alopecia and 'shiny skin' in a cat with paraneoplastic alopecia.

- Lesions develop rapidly over 2–3 months.
- Acute onset; rapidly progressive alopecia involving the ventrum and legs initially but will generalise to involve the whole body (Figure 21.33).
- Hair is easily epilated in non-alopecic areas.
- Alopecic skin often smooth and 'glistening' (Figure 21.34).
- Pruritus usually minimal.
- Painful footpads, often thin, occasionally fissured; may have multiple concentric circular rings of scale that give a targetoid appearance.
- Secondary Malassezia infection is common.

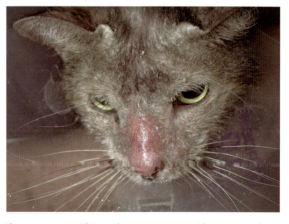

Figure 21.34 'Shiny skin' in a cat with paraneoplastic alopecia.

- Non-cutaneous signs:
  - Inappetence, lethargy
  - Weight loss

Differential diagnosis

- Hyperadrenocorticism
- Cutaneous fragility syndrome
- Telogen defluxion
- Traumatic alopecia (allergy, ectoparasites, psychogenic)
- Metabolic epidermal necrosis

Diagnosis

- History and clinical signs.
- Skin biopsy reveals signs of exfoliation of stratum corneum with laminated orthokeratosis alternating with focal parakeratosis. Follicular atrophy is a consistent finding.
- Diagnostic rule outs, i.e. haematology, biochemistry, ACTH usually unremarkable.
- Abdominal diagnostic imaging such as radiographs and ultrasonography to look for neoplasia.
- Exploratory laparotomy may be necessary in some to look for suspected neoplastic lesions.

Treatment

- None currently available.
- Grave prognosis; cats deteriorate rapidly and die.

Non-neoplastic tumours

Nevi

Cause and pathogenesis

Uncommon developmental defect characterised by hyperplasia of one or more skin components.

- Types of nevi:
  - Collagenous nevi – hyperplasia of collagen
  - Organoid nevi – hyperplasia of two or more skin components
  - Vascular nevi – cavernous dilatation of blood vessels
  - Sebaceous gland nevi
  - Apocrine sweat gland nevi
  - Epidermal nevi
  - Hair follicle nevi
  - Comedo nevi
  - Pacinian corpuscle nevi

Diagnosis

- History and clinical signs.
- Skin biopsy or excisional biopsy of the mass.

Treatment

- Small lesions can be monitored.
- Large, unsightly lesions may be removed surgically.
- Prognosis is good as tumours are not neoplastic.

Calcinosis cutis

Causes and pathogenesis

Uncommon disease manifested as calcification of the skin.

- Dystrophic calcification:
  - Calcinosis circumscripta – localised area of calcification due to
    - inflammatory lesions – foreign body granuloma, pyoderma, bite wounds
    - degenerative lesions – cysts
    - neoplastic lesions
  - Calcinosis universalis – generalised calcification due to
    - hyperadrenocorticism (Figure 21.35), especially dorsum, axilla and groin (naturally occurring or iatrogenic), diabetes mellitus
    - percutaneous absorption of calcium
- Metastatic calcification:
  - Chronic renal failure – lesions affect footpads
- Idiopathic calcification:
  - Calcinosis circumscripta of large breeds
  - Calcinosis universalis of young dogs:

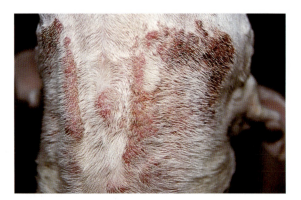

Figure 21.35 Calcinosis cutis on the dorsum of a dog with iatrogenic Cushing's disease.

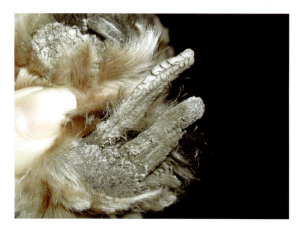

Figure 21.36 Cutaneous horn on the foot of a dog.

- Appearance – yellow/white firm plaques and nodules usually gritty.
- Often ulcerates can become secondarily infected.

Diagnosis

- History and clinical signs.
- Cytology is often not diagnostic but the gritty feel of calcium as the needle is inserted into the lesion is very characteristic. Cytological findings reveal amorphous white gritty material that becomes basophilic when it is stained.
- Skin biopsy reveals areas of finely or coarsely ground amorphous basophilic material in the deep dermal or subcutaneous tissue. It is often surrounded by granulation tissue.

Treatment

- Therapy of underlying causes where present will lead to spontaneous resolution of the lesions.
- In cases of idiopathic calcification surgical removal is curative.
- Prognosis is good.

Cutaneous horn

Cause and pathogenesis

Uncommon cutaneous lesion in the dog and cat. It may originate from papillomas, basal cell tumours, squamous cell carcinomas, or actinic keratoses.

Clinical signs

- No age or sex predilection.
- No breed predisposition.
- Lesions may be single or multiple. They appear as firm horn-like projections up to 5 cm in length (Figure 21.36).
- Solitary or multiple lesions on the footpads have been associated with FeLV infections.
- The lesions may occasionally be seen on the face.

Diagnosis

- History and clinical signs.
- Skin biopsy reveals signs of a well-demarcated area of papillomatous epidermal hyperplasia from which an extensive compact column of hyperkeratosis protrudes. Biopsies should always include the base of the horn.
- Cats with footpad lesions should be screened for FeLV.

Treatment

- Surgical excision is the treatment of choice where it is deemed necessary that these are removed.
- Prognosis is dependent on the underlying cause.

Selected references and further reading

Affolter, V. and Moore, P. (2000) Canine cutaneous histiocytic diseases. In: *Kirk's Current Veterinary Therapy XIII Small Animal Practice*. p. 588. WB Saunders, Philadelphia

Angus, J.C. and de Lorimier, L.P. (2004) Lymphohistiocytic neoplasms. In: Campbell, K.L. (ed) *Small Animal Dermatology Secrets*. pp. 425–442. Hanley and Belfus, Philadelphia

Beale, K.M. and Bolton, B. (1993) Canine cutaneous lymphosarcoma: epitheliotropic and non epitheliotropic, a retrospective study. In: Ihrke, P.J. et al. (eds) *Advances in Veterinary Dermatology*. Vol. 2. pp. 273–284. Pergamon, Oxford

Fan, T.M. (2004) Cutaneous mast cell neoplasia in the dog and cat. In: Campbell, K.L. (ed) *Small Animal Dermatology Secrets*. pp. 418–424. Hanley and Belfus, Philadelphia

Goldshmidt, M.H. and Shofer, F.S. (1998) *Skin Tumours of the Dog and Cat*. Butterworth-Heinemann, Oxford

Gross, T.L. et al. (2005) *Skin Diseases of the Dog and Cat: Clinical and Histopathologic Diagnosis*. 2nd edn. Blackwell Science, Oxford

London, C.A. and Seguin, B. (2003) Mast cell tumours in the dog. *Vet Clin N Am Small Anim Pract*, 33, 473–489

Medleau, L. and Hnilica, K. (2006) Neoplastic and nonneoplastic tumours In: *Small Animal Dermatology: A Color Atlas and Therapeutic Guide*. 2nd edn. pp. 393–447. WB Saunders, Philadelphia

Pulley, L.T. and Stannard, A.A. (1990) Tumours of the skin and soft tissue. In: Moulton, J.E. (ed) *Tumours in Domestic Animals*. 3rd edn. pp. 75–82. University of California Press, Berkeley

Scott, D.W. et al. (2001) Neoplastic and non-neoplastic tumours. In: *Muller and Kirk's Small Animal Dermatology*. 6th edn. pp. 1236–1414. WB Saunders, Philadelphia

Stokking, L.B. (2004) Epithelial neoplasms. In: Campbell, K.L. (ed) *Small Animal Dermatology Secrets*. pp. 393–401. Hanley and Belfus, Philadelphia

Index

A
abscesses 38
Acanthosis nigricans 249–250
acetate tape impression smear 14
acne 279–281
acquired aurotrichia in miniature schnauzers 250–251
acquired skin fragility 309
acquired symmetrical alopecia (feline) 225–226
acral lick granuloma 46, 268–271
acral mutilation syndrome 255
Acremonium spp. 70
acrodermatits 254–255
acromegaly 153–154
acromelanism 261
actinobacillosis 51
actinomycosis 50
acute moist dermatitis 26–28
adrenal gland tumours
    canine (table 21.1, 21.4, 21.5, 21.6) 327, 329, 330
    feline (table 21.8, 21.9) 332
adult onset impetigo 31
Aguirre syndrome 266–267
albinism 264
allergic miliary dermatitis 313–314
allergic skin disease 174–187
allergy testing 23–24
    intradermal 24
    serology 24
alopecia 214–230
alopecia areata 209
alopecia X 220–222
amyloidosis 208–209
anaerobic cellulitis 46
anal furunculosis 301–302
anal licking 274–275
anal sack disease 299–301
ancylostomiasis 133
angioedema 173–174
antibiotic therapy (table 4.2) 33
    (see also under individual diseases)
anti-inflammatory medication
    canine (table 10.1) 178
    feline (table 10.2) 184
aplasia cutis 244–246
argasid ticks 120
arrector pili muscle 4
aspergillosis 79–80
Aspergillus fumigatus 80
atopy
    canine 174–176
    feline 181–183
aurotrichia (acquired in miniature schnauzer) 250–251
autoimmune disease therapy
    canine (table 11.1) 190
    feline (table 11.2) 190

B

babesiosis 96–97
bacterial culture 21
bacterial folliculitis 34
bacterial pseudomycetoma 46–47
bacterial skin disease 26–56
    associated with primary immunodeficiency 54–55
    deep pyoderma 38–46
    superficial pyoderma 31–38
    surface pyoderma 26–31
    uncommon pyogranulomatous bacterial infection 46–54
basement membrane 2
biopsy 22
black/dark hair follicular dystrophy 218–219
Blastomyces dermatitidis 75
blastomycosis 75–76
blood vessels 4
Borrelia burgdorferi 54
borreliosis 54
botryomycosis 46
bullous pemphigoid 195–196
burns 318–320

C

C3 deficiency 55
calcinosis cutis 347–348
calici virus (feline) 91
callus 322
callus dermatitis 322–323
Candida albicans 66
candidiasis 66–67
canine
    atopy 174–177
    caryosporosis 94–95
    Chiari-like malformation 255–256
    distemper 82–83
    ehrlichoisis 94
    food hypersensitivity 179–281
    hyperadrenocorticism 143–148
    hypothyroidism 136–139
    leproid granuloma syndrome 50
    linear IgA dermatosis 208
    Rocky Mountain spotted fever 93–94
cattery management of dermatophytosis 62–65
cellulitis (anaerobic) 45
Chediak–Higashi syndrome 248–249
Cheyletiella (*blakei, parasitovorax, yasguri*) (table 7.2) 102
cheyletiellosis 102–104
Chiari-like malformation 255–256
chin pyoderma 42

coat brushing 13
Coccidiodes immitis 76
coccidiodomycosis 76–77
cold agglutinin disease (CAD) 201
collagenous fibres 3
colour dilution (mutant) alopecia 217–218
colour linked follicular dystrophy 217–219
congenital follicular dystrophy 215
congenital hypotrichosis 216
congenital skin disease 238–258
contact dermatitis (irritant) 230–231
contact hypersensitivity 177
contagious viral pustular dermatitis (Orf) 83
cryptococcosis 77–79
Cryptococcus neoformans 77
Ctenocephalides felis felis (table 7.10) 122–123
culture
    bacterial 21
    fungal 19–20, 61
Curvularia geniculata 70–71
cutaneous asthenia 251
cutaneous ecololgy 7
cutaneous horn 348
cutaneous mucinosis 256–257
Cuterebriasis 131–132
cyclic flank alopecia 223–224
cyclic haematopoiesis 55
cytology 18–19

D

deep pyoderma 38–41
demodex
    canis (table 7.3) 104–105
    cati (table 7.4) 110
    cornei (table 7.3) 104–105
    gatoi (table 7.4) 110
    injai (table 7.3) 104–105
demodicosis 104–112
    canine 104–109
    feline 109–112
Dermanyssus gallinae (table 7.8) 118
dermatological examination 12
dermatomyositis 246–247
dermatophilosis 37
dermatophyte test medium (DTM) 61–62
dermatophytosis 57–65
dermatosporaxis 251–252
dermis
    collagenous fibres 3
    elastin fibres 4
    epidermal appendages 4
    ground substance 4
dermoid sinus 244

diabetes mellitus 157–158
diagnostic tests 13–25
diascopy 14
dirofilariasis (heart worm) 135
discoid lupus erythematosus (DLE) 198–200
distemper (canine) 82–83
dracunculiasis 134
drug eruption 206–208
Dudley nose 263–264

E

ear cleaners (table 9.5) 169
ear margin dermatosis 289–290
ear wax – examination 20–21
ehlers–Danlos (cutaneous asthenia) 251–253
ehrlichiosis – canine 94
elastic fibres 4
endocrine skin disease 135–161
environmental skin disease 317–325
eosinophilic allergic syndrome 310–316
    investigation 315
    therapy 315–316
eosinophilic furunculosis of the face 185–186
eosinophilic granuloma
    canine 295–296
    feline 314–315
eosinophilic plaque 312–313
epidermal appendages 4
epidermal structure 2
epidermal tumours
    canine (table 21.2) 327
    feline (table 21.7) 330
epidermis
    keratinocytes 2
    Langerhans cells 2
    melanocytes 2
    Merkel cells 2
    structure 1–3
epithelial neoplasia 326–333
epitheliotropic lymphoma 340–341
erythema multiforme 202–204
eumycotic mycetoma 70–71
Eutrombicula spp. 116
examination of the animal 11

F

familial footpad hyperkeratosis 286
fatty acid deficiency 232–233
Felicola subrostratus (table 7.11) 126
feline
    acne 279–281
    acquired symmetrical alopecia 225–226
    acromelanism 261
    atopy 181–183
    calicivirus 91
    facial dermatitis in Persians 290–291
    food hypersensitivity 183–185
    herpes virus 90
    hyperadrenocorticism 148–151
    hyperthyroidism 140–143
    hypothyroidism 139–140
    immunodeficiency virus 88
    infectious peritonitis (FIP) 90
    leprosy syndrome 49–50
    leukaemia virus 86–87
    orofacial pain syndrome (FOP) 309–310
    paraneoplastic alopecia 346–347
    plasma cell pododermatitis 304–305
    pox virus 88
    preauricular and pinnal alopecia 226–227
    rhinotracheitis 90
    scabies 115–116
    thymoma associated exfoliative dermatitis 345–346
fibropruritic nodules 123–124
fine needle aspirate 19
flank suckers 273–274
fleas 121–126
flies 129–132
fly dermatitis 129
fly strike 130
focal metatarsal fistulation in the German shepherd dog 252–253
follicular dystrophy 215–219
folliculitis
    bacterial 34
    nasal 41
    pyotraumatic 41
food hypersensitivity
    canine 179–181
    feline 183–185
foot licking 273
footpad hyperkeratosis (familial) 286
frostbite 320
fungal culture 19, 61
fungal skin disease 57–81
furunculosis
    bacterial 39
    nasal 41

G

German shepherd dog pyoderma 44–45
giant cell dermatosis 87–88
granulocytopathy syndrome 55
ground substance 4

H

hair 5
- hair matrix 5
- hair papilla 5
- inner root sheath 5
- outer root sheath 6

hair cycle 6
hair cycle abnormalities 219–227
hair follicle tumours (table 21.3) 328
hard pad 82–83
heartworm 135
helminth parasites 132–135
hepatocutaneous disease 158–160
hereditary lupoid dermatosis of the German short-haired pointer 247–248
hereditary nasal parakeratosis of the labrador retriever 285–286
herpes virus (feline) 90–91
histiocytic tumours (table 21.13, 21.14) 341–342
Histoplasma capsulatum 79
histoplasmosis 79–80
history taking 9
hookworm dermatitis 132–134
hygroma 324
Hymenoptera 132
hyperadrenocorticism
- canine 143–148
- feline 148–151

hypereosinophilia syndrome 307
hyperoestrogenism 154
hyperthyroidism (feline) 140–143
hypervitaminosis A 234–235
hypothyroidism
- canine 136–139
- feline 139–140

I

ichthyosis (fish scale disease) 240–242
idiopathic bald thigh syndrome in the greyhound 225
idiopathic cyclic flank alopecia 223–224
idiopathic facial dermatitis in Persian cats 290–291
idiopathic periocular leukotrichia 266
idiopathic sterile granuloma and pyogranuloma
- canine 294
- feline 305–306

IgA deficiency 55
immune mediated disease 188–213
immunodeficiencies – bacterial skin disease 54
immunodeficiency virus (feline) 88
impetigo
- adult onset 31
- juvenile onset 31

impression smear 18–19
indolent ulcer 311–312
infectious peritonitis (feline) 90
inner root sheath 5
insects 121–132
interdigital cyst (pyoderma) 43
interstitial cell tumour 156–159
intertrigo complex 28
irritant contact dermatitis 320–322
ixodid ticks 120

J

juvenile cellulitis 296–297
juvenile impetigo 31

K

keratinisation defects 277–291
keratinocytes 2
kerion 59

L

lagenidiosis 74
Langerhans cells 2
leishmaniasis 97–99
lentigo 259–270
leproid granuloma syndrome 50
leprosy syndrome 49–50
leukaemia virus (feline) 86–87
L-form bacteria 54
lichenoid psoriasiform dermatosis of the English springer spaniel 242
linear IgA dermatosis 208
Linognathus setosus (table 7.11) 126
localised scleroderma 295
Lyme borreliosis 54
lymph oedema 253–254
lymph vessels 4
Lynxacarus radosky 119

M

Madurella spp. 70
malasseziasis 67–69
- *M. globosa* 67
- *M. pachydermatis* 67
- *M. sympodialis* 67

mast cell tumour 333–335
melanocytes 2
melanomas 341–344
melanotrichia 261
Merkel cells 2
mesenchymal tumours 333–340

metastatic bronchial carcinoma of the lungs 344–345
methicillin resistant *Staphylococcus aureus* (MRSA) 36–37
Microsporum spp. 57–59
    M. canis (table 5.1) 57–58
    M. gypseum (table 5.1) 57–58
    M. persicolor (table 5.1) 59
miliary dermatitis 313–314
morbillivirus 82
morphea (localised scleroderma) 295
mosquito bite hypersensitivity 129–130
mucinosis (cutaneous) 256–257
mucocutaneous pyoderma 32–33
mycobacterial infection 47
    opportunistic 48–49
Mycobacterium lepraemurium 49
mycoses
    subcutaneous 69–75
    superficial 57–69
    systemic 75–81
Myiasis (fly strike) 130–131

N

nasal depigmentation (Dudley nose) 263–264
nasal folliculitis 41
nasal parakeratosis of labrador retrievers 285–286
nasodigital hyperkeratosis 283–284
necrolytic migratory erythema 158–160
neoplastic and non-neoplastic tumours 326–349
neosporosis 95–96
Neotrombicula autumnalis (table 7.7) 116
nerves 4
neurodermatitis 275–276
nevi 347
nocardiosis 52
notoedric mange 115–116
nutritional skin disease 231–237

O

onychomycosis 59
opportunistic mycobacterial infections 48–49
Orf 83
orofacial pain syndrome (feline) 309–310
otitis externa 162–172
    diagnostic tests 168–169
    perpetuating factors (table 9.3) 162–163
    predisposing factors (table 9.2) 162–163
    primary causes (table 9.1) 162–163
    treatment 169–172
Otodectes cynotis (table 7.1) 100–102
outer root sheath 6

P

panepidermal pustular pemphigus 195
panniculitis (sterile nodular) 210–211
pansteatitis 233–234
papillomavirus 84–85
    cutaneous exophytic 84
    footpad 85
    genital 85
    inverted 85
    multiple pigmented epidermal plaques 85
    multiple viral 85
    oral 84, 85
    solitary cutaneous 86
paraneoplastic alopecia (feline) 346–347
parasitic skin disease 100–135
pattern baldness 222–223
pediculosis 126–128
pelodera dermatitis 133
pemphigus complex 188–195
    panepidermal pustular pemphigus 195
    paraneoplastic 195
    pemphigus erythematosus 193–195
    pemphigus foliaceus 189–193
    pemphigus vulgaris 188–189
perforating dermatitis 308–309
phaeohyphomycosis 71
pigment abnormalities 259–267
pili torti 216–217
pituitary dwarfism 151–152
plague 53
plasma cell pododermatitis (feline) 304–305
plasmacytoma 336
pododermatitis 43
post-clipping alopecia 220
post-inflammatory hyperpigmentation 260
pox virus (feline) 88–89
pre-auricular and pinnal alopecia 225–226
primary seborrhoea 238–240
proliferative arteritis of the nasal philtrum 211–213
protein deficiency 231–232
Prototheca wickerhamii 80
protothecosis 80–81
protozoal disease 94–99
pruritic alopecia 227–228
Pseudoallescheria boydii 70
pseudomycetoma
    bacterial 46–47
    fungal 59–60, 69–70
pseudorabies ('mad itch') 83–84
psychogenic alopecia 227–228
psychogenic dermatitis 275–276
psychogenic skin disease 268–276

pyoderma
    chin 42
    deep 38–46
    German shepherd dog 44–45
    superficial 31–38
    surface 26–31
pyogranulomatous bacterial infection 46–54
pyotraumatic folliculitis 41
pythiosis 72–73
Pythium insidiosum 72

R

relapsing polychondritis 210
reticular fibres 4
rhinotracheitis (feline) 90–91
Rickettsia rickettsii 93
rickettsial disease 93–94
Rocky Mountain spotted fever 93–94

S

sarcocystosis 96
Sarcoptes scabiei (table 7.5) 112
sarcoptic mange 112–114
scarring alopecia 229
schnauzer comedo syndrome 242–243
scleroderma (localised) 295
seasonal flank alopecia 223–224
sebaceous adenitis 287–288
sebaceous gland 6
seborrhoea 277–279
selective IgA deficiency 55
self-nursing 274
seminoma 156
Sertoli cell tumour 155–156
severe combined immunodeficiency 54–55
skin fold pyoderma 28
skin scraping 15
    deep 15–16
    superficial 15
soft tissue sarcomas (table 21.12) 338–339
solar dermatitis 317–318
Sporothrix schenckii 74
sporotrichosis 73–74
sterile eosinophilic pustulosis 293
sterile granuloma and pyogranulomas (idiopathic)
    canine 294
    feline 305–306
sterile nodular panniculitis 210
strangles (puppy) 296–297
stratum
    basale 2
    corneum 3
    granulosum 3
    lucidum 3
    spinosum 2
structure of skin 1
subcorneal pustular dermatosis 292–293
subcutaneous abscesses 38
subcutis 7
superficial pyoderma 31–38
surface pyoderma 36–41
sweat gland 6
    atrichial 6
    epitrichial 6
symmetrical lupoid onychodystrophy 297
syringomyelia 255
systemic lupus erythematosis (SLE) 196–198

T

tail biting 271–272
tail gland hyperplasia 281–282
tail sucking 272
telogen defluvium 224–225
testicular neoplasia 155–158
    interstitial cell tumour 156–158
    seminoma 156
    sertoli cell tumour 155–156
thymoma associated exfoliative dermatitis (feline) 345–346
ticks
    argasid ticks 120
    ixodid ticks 120
toxic epidermal necrolysis (TEN) 202–204
traction alopecia 228–229
transient hypogammaglobulinaemia 55
transmissible venereal tumour (TVT) 336–338
traumatic alopecia 227–229
trial therapy 24
Trichodectes canis (table 7.11) 126
trichography (hair plucks) 16–18
Trichophyton mentagrophytes (table 5.1) 47–48
trombiculiasis 116–117
tumour hypermelanosis 261

U

ulcerative dermatitis with linear sub-epidermal fibrosis 307–308
uncinariasis (hookworm) 132–133
urticaria 173
urticaria pigmentosa 335–336
uveodermatologic syndrome 264–265

V

vasculitis 204–206
vesicular cutaneous lupus 200–201

viral disease 82–93
vitamin A deficiency 234
vitamin A responsive dermatosis (table 13.1) 282–283
vitamin B deficiencies 235
vitiligo 262–263
Vogt–Koyanagi–Harada-like syndrome (VKH) 264

W

Waardenburg–Klein syndrome (WKS) 263
wet paper test 13

Wood's lamp examination 60

X

xanthoma 161

Y

Yersinia pestis 53

Z

zinc-responsive dermatosis 235–237
zygomycosis 73